D1292478

Transcatheter Aortic Valve Implantation

Transcatheter Aortic Valve Implantation

Tips and Tricks to Avoid Failure

Edited by

Patrick W. Serruys
Erasmus University Medical Center
Rotterdam, The Netherlands

Nicolo Piazza
Erasmus University Medical Center
Rotterdam, The Netherlands

Alain Cribier
Hôpital Charles Nicolle, University of Rouen
Rouen, France

John G. Webb
St. Paul's Hospital, University of British Columbia
Vancouver, Canada

Jean-Claude Laborde
Glenfield Hospital
Leicester, UK

Peter de Jaegere
Erasmus University Medical Center
Rotterdam, The Netherlands

informa
healthcare

New York London

First published in 2010 by Informa Healthcare, Telephone House, 69-77 Paul Street, London EC2A 4LQ, UK.

Simultaneously published in the USA by Informa Healthcare, 52 Vanderbilt Avenue, 7th Floor, New York, NY 10017, USA.

Informa Healthcare is a trading division of Informa UK Ltd. Registered Office: 37–41 Mortimer Street, London W1T 3JH, UK. Registered in England and Wales number 1072954.

©2010 Informa Healthcare, except as otherwise indicated

No claim to original U.S. Government works

Reprinted material is quoted with permission. Although every effort has been made to ensure that all owners of copyright material have been acknowledged in this publication, we would be glad to acknowledge in subsequent reprints or editions any omissions brought to our attention.

All rights reserved. No part of this publication may be reproduced, stored in a retrieval system, or transmitted, in any form or by any means, electronic, mechanical, photocopying, recording, or otherwise, unless with the prior written permission of the publisher or in accordance with the provisions of the Copyright, Designs and Patents Act 1988 or under the terms of any licence permitting limited copying issued by the Copyright Licensing Agency, 90 Tottenham Court Road, London W1P 0LP, UK, or the Copyright Clearance Center, Inc., 222 Rosewood Drive, Danvers, MA 01923, USA (http://www.copyright.com/ or telephone 978-750-8400).

Product or corporate names may be trademarks or registered trademarks, and are used only for identification and explanation without intent to infringe.

This book contains information from reputable sources and although reasonable efforts have been made to publish accurate information, the publisher makes no warranties (either express or implied) as to the accuracy or fitness for a particular purpose of the information or advice contained herein. The publisher wishes to make it clear that any views or opinions expressed in this book by individual authors or contributors are their personal views and opinions and do not necessarily reflect the views/opinions of the publisher. Any information or guidance contained in this book is intended for use solely by medical professionals strictly as a supplement to the medical professional's own judgement, knowledge of the patient's medical history, relevant manufacturer's instructions and the appropriate best practice guidelines. Because of the rapid advances in medical science, any information or advice on dosages, procedures, or diagnoses should be independently verified. This book does not indicate whether a particular treatment is appropriate or suitable for a particular individual. Ultimately it is the sole responsibility of the medical professional to make his or her own professional judgements, so as appropriately to advise and treat patients. Save for death or personal injury caused by the publisher's negligence and to the fullest extent otherwise permitted by law, neither the publisher nor any person engaged or employed by the publisher shall be responsible or liable for any loss, injury or damage caused to any person or property arising in any way from the use of this book.

A CIP record for this book is available from the British Library.

Library of Congress Cataloging-in-Publication Data available on application

ISBN-13: 9781841846897

Orders may be sent to: Informa Healthcare, Sheepen Place, Colchester, Essex CO3 3LP, UK
Telephone: +44 (0)20 7017 5540
Email: CSDhealthcarebooks@informa.com
Website: http://informahealthcarebooks.com/

For corporate sales please contact: CorporateBooksIHC@informa.com
For foreign rights please contact: RightsIHC@informa.com
For reprint permissions please contact: PermissionsIHC@informa.com

Printed and bound in the United Kingdom
Transferred to Digital Print 2011

Foreword

When you want to learn a new technique, the first option is to visit one of the centers with the largest experience and watch their procedures. The second option is to attend focused congresses or live courses. Both are expensive, time-consuming solutions and have the drawback to be highly influenced by the commercial interests of manufacturers, often sponsoring these events, with few chances to compare pro and cons of various devices. After some more time you may expect case reports, preliminary series, and review articles to appear in medical journals. Their focus is most often on science than on education. Books are the last place where you expect to find an update description of cutting edge techniques and to learn practical aspects of their application. This book has convinced me that if you find a motivated group of expert contributors you can timely produce a comprehensive in-depth analysis of the various aspects of a new technique—a theoretical introduction indispensable to assimilate and understand the procedural steps observed during live cases. This is the first book exclusively dedicated to transcatheter aortic valve implantation (TAVI) and mainly focuses on the two devices in current clinical use but with tips and tricks applicable to new iterations of the existing devices and to new systems in development.

As expected, you start with the anatomical features making degenerative aortic valve stenosis potentially treatable with a technique as crude as the displacement of the calcified cusps and the expansion of a new valve. Postmortem studies give us a clue on what can go wrong and why, an essential introduction to the following part, the definition of the parameters required to pose indications, and plan a successful TAVI procedure and handle its possible complications.

Many of the complications and failures of TAVI are not due to mistakes in their deployment but to poor handling of frail patients in the perioperative period. A chapter on anesthesia and two on postoperative care deal with these critical aspects. Elderly patients with degenerative aortic stenosis are often poor candidates to conventional general anesthesia. They often have coexistent pathology of the peripheral vessels, requiring pretreatment study of their size and pathology, and meticulous attention to vascular access and closure aspects are not always familiar to interventional cardiologists. Seven chapters deal with the practical steps of valve preparation, insertion, and deployment. The groups with the longest and largest world experience teach us how to cross the valve, how to perform an effective preparation of the valve with balloon dilatation, and how to advance the valve and deploy it exactly where required. The authors correctly focus on the most natural access site, transfemoral—already predominant now and due to become more frequent with further valve miniaturization. Transapical approach is still an important niche application of the technique and an important modality for cardiac surgeons to familiarize with these new devices. Imaging is ubiquitous in the book, from patient selection and device sizing to optimal positioning and assessment of results.

A quick look at the list of authors tells us a lot on the challenge these procedure represent for interventional cardiologists. Cardiac surgeons, anesthetists, radiologists, noninvasive cardiologist specialists in imaging and heart failure are key authors of this book and welcome newcomers in our catheterization laboratories. Coronary angioplasty is a lonely job: the cardiologist, surrounded by a handful of nurses and technicians around, is often responsible of the indications, treatment, and postoperative care. Interventionalists embarking in TAVI must change their mentality and accept to become members of a multidisciplinary team, sharing decisions and responsibilities.

Interventional cardiologists, however, have pioneered these procedures, overcoming skepticism and criticism when complications were high with the first crude devices, and have managed to demonstrate feasibility and efficacy of these procedures for selected indications in experienced hands. Education of the hundreds of interventional cardiologists needed to meet the expected demand for procedures required to treat a frequent pathology, often reserved to patients with no other options, is a daunting task. This book is an important step forward and an essential reading for interventional cardiologists and many others, from cardiac surgeons to noninvasive cardiologists, involved in the care of these difficult patients.

Carlo Di Mario, MD, PhD, FESC, FACC, FSCAI, FRCP
Consultant Cardiologist, Royal Brompton Hospital
Professor of Clinical Cardiology, Imperial College, London
President of the European Association of Percutaneous Cardiovascular Interventions (EAPCI)

Preface

It is human nature to develop and to evolve, to adapt and to adopt. These features are essential for the safeguarding of our future in an ever changing world. Transcatheter Aortic Valve Implantation (TAVI) is an example of such a development and evolution. Even in the absence of sound clinical data on its safety, efficacy, and durability, it is clear that we have to recognize its presence to which we must adapt and also assume our responsibility to improve TAVI from both a technological and clinical point of view.

This starts by a true understanding of all its components that ranges from an in-depth understanding of patient-related issues such as the anatomy of the aortic root, an in-depth understanding of the technology itself to the fine points of the procedure that not only include all facets of positioning and implantation but also the imaging techniques that are needed for guidance and evaluation, and last but not least, postoperative management of the patient.

The goal of this book is to help readers understand TAVI in its full spectrum and provide readers with the necessary information to perform a safe and successful transcatheter aortic valve implantation procedure. The "tips and tricks" captured in this first edition represent the learning experiences of the pioneers who contributed to the maturation and advancement of the technology. This textbook was written at the time when approximately 6000 transcatheter aortic valve implantation procedures were performed worldwide. Despite this, TAVI still is an experimental treatment since there is still much to learn, to understand, and to improve.

With the use of visual aids (over 200 color figures and 3 hours of DVD material), the authors attempt to explain, in detail, each step of the procedure. The textbook has been divided into three parts: (1) preprocedural, (2) intraprocedural, and (3) postprocedural "tips and tricks."

The initial chapters begin with a detailed description of the anatomy of the aortic valve that is essential to understand correct placement of the device and potential complications associated with the procedure. Also unique is a chapter on post-mortem examinations following transcatheter aortic valve implantation—such information will become crucial to unravel some of the mysteries of the procedure and causes of death in these individuals.

The second part of this book provides the intraprocedural tips and tricks that have been acquired through experience and mistakes and covers vascular access, advancement of the delivery catheter system, device placement and deployment, and acute procedural complications.

The third part of this book is dedicated to the postprocedural care of the patient and tries to address issues such as the length of stay in the intensive care unit, the indication and duration of temporary pacing, complications within the first 48 to 72 hours, antithrombotic/antiplatelet therapy post-implant.

The last section of the book provides a glimpse into the future for upcoming valve designs and ideas. Novel transcatheter aortic valve designs will soon enter the market. These devices will strive for lower profile catheters, durability of the valve prosthesis, and the ability to fully retrieve and/or reposition the device after assessing its function but before complete valve deployment.

There remain many unanswered questions with respect to patient selection (e.g., Should TAVI be restricted to high risk and inoperable patients?), to the selection of the appropriate valve size, and the etiology of complications that may occur (e.g., conduction abnormalities and paravalvular aortic regurgitation).

On behalf of all authors we hope that this book will enrich our understanding of TAVI in all its facets—from patient selection to its execution and postoperative management—and that it may inspire us to join forces in a multidisciplinary approach to thoroughly investigate TAVI from both a biomedical engineering and clinical perspective so that we continue the development with the ultimate goal of helping more patients in an appropriate way.

Special thanks go to Dr. Nicolo Piazza who was the mid-field in this endeavor. Thanks to his skills and detailed acquaintance with TAVI; he made sure that chapters of high quality were submitted in a timely fashion.

Patrick W. Serruys
Nicolo Piazza
Alain Cribier
John G. Webb
Jean-Claude Laborde
Peter de Jaegere

Contents

Contributors

Jodi Akin   Edwards Lifesciences, LLC, Irvine, California, U.S.A.

Jill Amstutz   Sadra Medical, Inc., Los Gatos, California, U.S.A.

Robert H. Anderson   Cardiac Unit, Institute of Child Health, University College, London, U.K.

Anita Asgar   Montreal Heart Institute, Université de Montréal, Montreal, Quebec, Canada

Vasilis Babaliaros   Emory University Hospital, Gruentzig Cardiovascular Center, Atlanta, Georgia, U.S.A.

Jeroen J. Bax   Department of Cardiology, Leiden University Medical Center, Leiden, The Netherlands

Anton Becker   Department of Pathology, University of Amsterdam, Academic Medical Center, Amsterdam, The Netherlands

Sabine Bleiziffer   Clinic for Cardiovascular Surgery, German Heart Center Munich, Munich, Germany

Peter C. Block   Emory University Hospital, Gruentzig Cardiovascular Center, Atlanta, Georgia, U.S.A.

Ad J. J. C. Bogers   Department of Cardiac Surgery, Erasmus University Medical Center, Thoraxcenter, Rotterdam, The Netherlands

Raoul Bonan   Montreal Heart Institute, Université de Montréal, Montreal, Quebec, Canada

Lutz Buellesfeld   Department of Cardiology and Angiology, HELIOS Heart Center Siegburg, Siegburg, Germany

Anson Cheung   St. Paul's Hospital, University of British Columbia, Vancouver, British Columbia, Canada

Alain Cribier   Department of Cardiology, Hôpital Charles Nicolle, University of Rouen, Rouen, France

P. de Feyter   Department of Interventional Cardiology, Erasmus University Medical Center, Thoraxcenter, Rotterdam, The Netherlands

Peter de Jaegere   Department of Interventional Cardiology, Erasmus University Medical Center, Thoraxcenter, Rotterdam, The Netherlands

Victoria Delgado   Department of Cardiology, Leiden University Medical Center, Leiden, The Netherlands

Todd Dewey   Heartcenter, Medical City, Dallas, Texas, U.S.A.

Itsik Ben Dor   Washington Hospital Center, Washington, D.C., U.S.A.

Gregory Ducrocq   Department of Cardiology, Bichat Claude Bernard Hospital, APHP, Paris, France

Hélène Eltchaninoff   Department of Cardiology, Hôpital Charles Nicolle, University of Rouen, Rouen, France

Hans Figulla   Division of Cardiology, University Hospital of Jena, Jena, Germany

John Gainor   Heart Leaflet Technologies, Inc., Maple Grove, Minnesota, U.S.A.

Ulrich Gerckens   Department of Cardiology and Angiology, HELIOS Heart Center Siegburg, Siegburg, Germany

Eberhard Grube   Department of Cardiology and Angiology, HELIOS Heart Center Siegburg, Siegburg, Germany

Joke M. Hendriks   Department of Vascular Surgery, Erasmus University Medical Center, Thoraxcenter, Rotterdam, The Netherlands

Dominique Himbert   Department of Cardiology, Bichat Claude Bernard Hospital, APHP, Paris, France

J. Hofland   Department of Cardiothoracic Anesthesia, Erasmus University Medical Center, Thoraxcenter, Rotterdam, The Netherlands

Zahid Junagadhwalla   Emory University Hospital, Gruentzig Cardiovascular Center, Atlanta, Georgia, U.S.A.

Samir R. Kapadia   Department of Cardiology, Heart and Vascular Institute, Cleveland Clinic, Cleveland, Ohio, U.S.A.

A. Pieter Kappetein   Department of Cardiac Surgery, Erasmus University Medical Center, Thoraxcenter, Rotterdam, The Netherlands

Jörg Kempfert   Universität Leipzig, Herzzentrum, Klinik für Herzchirurgie, Leipzig, Germany

Spencer H. Kubo   Heart Leaflet Technologies, Inc., Maple Grove, Minnesota, U.S.A.

Jean-Claude Laborde   Cardiology Department, Glenfield Hospital, Leicester, U.K.

Rüdiger Lange   Clinic for Cardiovascular Surgery, German Heart Center Munich, Munich, Germany

Georg Latsios   Department of Cardiology and Angiology, HELIOS Heart Center Siegburg, Siegburg, Germany

Leah Lepak   Sadra Medical, Inc., Los Gatos, California, U.S.A.

Samuel V. Lichtenstein   St. Paul's Hospital, University of British Columbia, Vancouver, British Columbia, Canada

Jurgen M. R. Ligthart   Department of Interventional Cardiology, Erasmus University Medical Center, Thoraxcenter, Rotterdam, The Netherlands

Axel Linke   Department of Cardiology, University of Leipzig—Heart Center, Leipzig, Germany

Reginald Low   University of California, Davis, Sacramento, California, U.S.A.

Ganesh Manoharan   Department of Interventional Cardiology, Heart Center, Belfast, U.K.

Ken Martin   Sadra Medical, Inc., Los Gatos, California, U.S.A.

Jean-Bernard Masson   St. Paul's Hospital, University of British Columbia, Vancouver, British Columbia, Canada

Rob Michiels   CONSILIUM Associates LLC and Consultant to Medtronic-CoreValve, Irvine, California, U.S.A.

William Mirsch   Heart Leaflet Technologies, Inc., Maple Grove, Minnesota, U.S.A.

Gaku Nakazawa   CVPath Institute, Inc., Gaithersburg, Maryland, U.S.A.

Fabian Nietlispach   St. Paul's Hospital, University of British Columbia, Vancouver, British Columbia, Canada

Stéphane Noble   Montreal Heart Institute, Université de Montréal, Montreal, Quebec, Canada

Yoshinobu Onuma   Department of Interventional Cardiology, Erasmus University Medical Center, Thoraxcenter, Rotterdam, The Netherlands

F. J. Orellana Ramos   Department of Cardiothoracic Anesthesia, Erasmus University Medical Center, Thoraxcenter, Rotterdam, The Netherlands

Peter M. T. Pattynama   Department of Radiology, Erasmus University Medical Center, Thoraxcenter, Rotterdam, The Netherlands

Nicolo Piazza   Department of Interventional Cardiology, Erasmus University Medical Center, Thoraxcenter, Rotterdam, The Netherlands

Augusto Pichard   Washington Hospital Center, Washington, D.C., U.S.A.

Jonas Runquist   Heart Leaflet Technologies, Inc., Maple Grove, Minnesota, U.S.A.

Amr Salaheih   Sadra Medical, Inc., Los Gatos, California, U.S.A.

Lowell Satler   Washington Hospital Center, Washington, D.C., U.S.A.

Martin J. Schalij   Department of Cardiology, Leiden University Medical Center, Leiden, The Netherlands

Richard Schroeder   Heart Leaflet Technologies, Inc., Maple Grove, Minnesota, U.S.A.

Joanne D. Schuijf   Department of Cardiology, Leiden University Medical Center, Leiden, The Netherlands

Gerhard Schuler   Department of Cardiology, University of Leipzig—Heart Center, Leipzig, Germany

Carl Schultz   Department of Interventional Cardiology, Erasmus University Medical Center, Thoraxcenter, Rotterdam, The Netherlands

Patrick W. Serruys   Department of Interventional Cardiology, Erasmus University Medical Center, Thoraxcenter, Rotterdam, The Netherlands

Pooja Sharma   Edwards Lifesciences, LLC, Irvine, California, U.S.A.

Laurens F. Tops   Department of Cardiology, Leiden University Medical Center, Leiden, The Netherlands

E. Murat Tuzcu   Department of Cardiology, Heart and Vascular Institute, Cleveland Clinic, Cleveland, Ohio, U.S.A.

A. Tzikas   Department of Interventional Cardiology, Erasmus University Medical Center, Thoraxcenter, Rotterdam, The Netherlands

Alec Vahanian   Department of Cardiology, Bichat Claude Bernard Hospital, APHP, Paris, France

Frank van der Kley   Department of Cardiology, Leiden University Medical Center, Leiden, The Netherlands

Lukas C. van Dijk   Department of Radiology, Erasmus University Medical Center, Thoraxcenter, Rotterdam, The Netherlands

Menno van Gameren   Department of Cardiac Surgery, Erasmus University Medical Center, Thoraxcenter, Rotterdam, The Netherlands

Robert Jan van Geuns   Department of Interventional Cardiology, Erasmus University Medical Center, Thoraxcenter, Rotterdam, The Netherlands

Renu Virmani   CVPath Institute, Inc., Gaithersburg, Maryland, U.S.A.

Marc Vorpahl   CVPath Institute, Inc., Gaithersburg, Maryland, U.S.A.

Ron Waksman   Washington Hospital Center, Washington, D.C., U.S.A.

Thomas Walther   Universität Leipzig, Herzzentrum, Klinik für Herzchirurgie, Leipzig, Germany

John G. Webb   St. Paul's Hospital, University of British Columbia, Vancouver, British Columbia, Canada

Robert F. Wilson   Heart Leaflet Technologies, Inc., Maple Grove, Minnesota, U.S.A.

Jian Ye   St. Paul's Hospital, University of British Columbia, Vancouver, British Columbia, Canada

1 | The Anatomy of the Aortic Valvar Complex

Robert H. Anderson
Cardiac Unit, Institute of Child Health, University College, London, U.K.

Anton Becker
Department of Pathology, University of Amsterdam, Academic Medical Center, Amsterdam, The Netherlands

Nicolo Piazza
Department of Interventional Cardiology, Erasmus University Medical Center, Thoraxcenter, Rotterdam, The Netherlands

INTRODUCTION

Interest in the anatomy of the aortic valvar complex had already arisen at the time of the Renaissance, as exemplified by the exquisite description and drawings provided by Leonardo (1). Since that time, investigations of the anatomy are numerous. Until now, however, little consideration has been given to understanding the anatomy with percutaneous valvar replacement in mind (2). The techniques for implantation of aortic valves by using a transcatheter approach are the topic of the larger part of this book. As will be described later, the chosen prosthesis is within the aortic root, and deployed so as to crush the diseased leaflets of the native valve against the supporting valvar sinuses. It is axiomatic, therefore, that detailed knowledge of the anatomy of the valve is required by those hoping to insert transcatheter valves in optimal fashion. We have often seen descriptions of the aortic valve concentrating exclusively on the leaflets. The leaflets, of course, are the working units of the valve. For those implanting valvar prostheses, however, the structure of the aortic sinuses of Valsalva that support the leaflets, along with the morphology of the surrounding cardiac structures, is just as, if not more, important. The overall valvar complex is best described, in our opinion, as the aortic root. As we will describe later, the root has significant length and is much more than a unidimensional ring, although all too frequently it is described in terms of an annulus. An appreciation of the overall anatomy of the root can help the operator position the prosthetic valve appropriately with respect to the coronary arteries, the mitral valve, and the conduction system. Such knowledge may also circumvent potential complications that can arise during implantation. Accurate knowledge of the structure of the valvar complex can also guide new designs and refinements of valvar prostheses. In this chapter, therefore, we describe the overall structure of the valvar complex.

THE AORTIC ROOT

The aortic root (3) is the direct continuation of the left ventricular outflow tract. Irrespective of the angle from which it is viewed, it forms the centerpiece of the heart (Fig. 1).

The valvar leaflets and their supporting sinuses, which together make up the root, are related to all four cardiac chambers. In its totality, the valvar mechanism guards the junction of the left ventricle with the aorta, with the root itself extending from the basal attachment of the leaflets within the left ventricle to their peripheral attachment at the level of the sinutubular junction. The latter junction marks the boundary between the expanded aortic valvar sinuses and the tubular part of the ascending aorta (Fig. 2).

When viewed relative to the frontal cardiac silhouette, the root is located to the right, and posterior, in respect to the subpulmonary infundibulum. As shown in Figure 2, an extensive tissue plane separates the freestanding infundibular sleeve of the right ventricle from the aortic root. Cuts in the short axis plane show that the posterior margin of the root is deeply wedged between the orifice of the mitral valve and the muscular ventricular septum (Fig. 3).

Approximately two-thirds of the circumference of the basal part of the aortic root is connected to the muscular ventricular septum, with the remaining one-third in fibrous

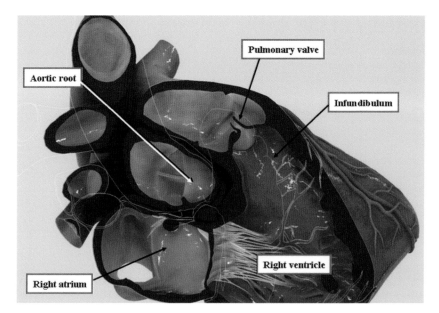

Figure 1 This illustration is obtained from virtual reconstruction of the heart. It shows the position of the aortic root as the cardiac centerpiece. *Source*: Photos courtesy of Dr Sue Wright and the team at Glassworks, who made it possible to produce the various virtual images used to illustrate this chapter.

continuity with the aortic (anterior) leaflet of the mitral valve. When viewed in short axis from the atrial aspect, the root is seen to be deeply wedged between the orifices of the mitral and tricuspid valves. This view shows well the origin of the coronary arteries, which arise from the sinuses adjacent to the pulmonary trunk, extending directly into the atrioventricular grooves (Fig. 4).

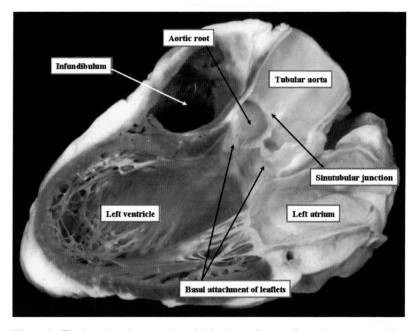

Figure 2 The heart has been sectioned in its long axis to replicate the parasternal long axis echocardiographic plane. The aortic root, extending from the basal attachment of the leaflets to the sinutubular junction, occupies the center of the heart. Note the freestanding muscular subpulmonary infundibular sleeve.

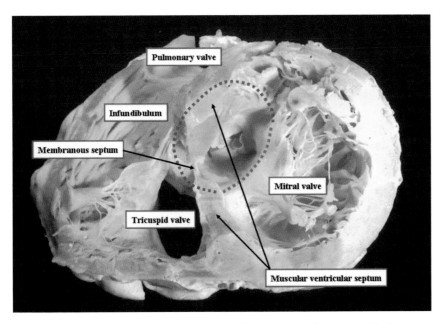

Figure 3 This section is taken across the short axis of the ventricular mass and is photographed from the cardiac apex. It confirms that the aortic root occupies the center of the heart when viewed in all three orthogonal planes and shows how two-thirds of the circumference of the root arise from the muscular ventricular septum (red dotted line), with the remaining one-third of the root supported by the aortic (anterior) leaflet of the mitral valve (green dotted line).

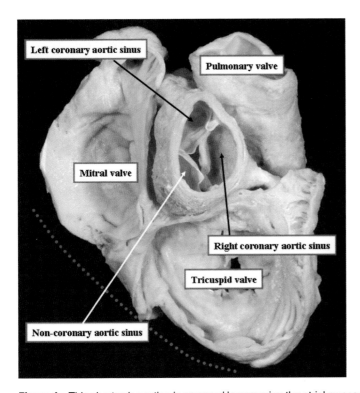

Figure 4 This short axis section is prepared by removing the atrial myocardium so that it is possible to visualize the mitral and tricuspid valvar orifices. The red dotted line shows the diaphragmatic surface of the heart. Note that the aortic root is the centerpiece of the cardiac short axis. Note also the extensive sleeve of freestanding infundibulum that lifts the pulmonary valve away from the base of the heart.

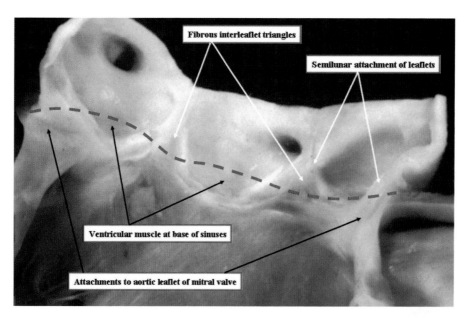

Figure 5 This specimen has been prepared by opening the aortic root through the area of aortic-to-mitral valvar fibrous continuity and removing the leaflets of the aortic valve. The anatomic ventriculo-aortic junction is shown by the red dashed line. As can be seen here, the semilunar attachments of the leaflets cross the junction, incorporating segments of muscle into the base of the two aortic sinuses giving rise to the coronary arteries.

The origin of the coronary arteries permits the aortic sinuses of Valsalva to be distinguished as the right and left coronary aortic sinuses, and the noncoronary aortic sinus. The walls of the sinuses are made of the same fibro-collagenous tissues as the aorta and support the valvar leaflets in semilunar fashion. As the expanded sinuses extend distally toward the sinutubular junction, they are separated by the triangles of much thinner fibrous tissue. This arrangement of the interleaflet fibrous triangles is best seen when the root is opened out, and the valvar leaflets are removed (Fig. 5).

The leaflets, the working components of the valvar complex, are themselves made up of a core of fibrous tissue, with endothelial linings on their arterial and ventricular aspects. They take a semilunar origin from the aortic sinuses, with the lines of attachment of each leaflet extending down from the sinutubular junction to a nadir within the left ventricular outflow tract, and then rising back to the sinutubular junction. The semilunar loci produced by the hinges of each leaflet together constitute the hemodynamic ventriculo-arterial junction, with all the cavities on the arterial aspect of the hemodynamic junction exposed to aortic pressure, but the cavities on the ventricular side exposed to left ventricular pressures. As these semilunar hinges course through the length of the aortic root, they cross the anatomic ventriculo-arterial junction. This latter junction is the circular locus over which the left ventricular structures support the fibroelastic walls of the aortic valvar sinuses and the intervening fibrous interleaflet triangles. Part of this locus is muscular and part fibrous, the latter being the area over which the leaflets of the aortic valve are in fibrous continuity with the aortic leaflet of the mitral valve (Fig. 6).

In the areas where the leaflets arise from the ventricular myocardium, their basal attachments are well below the level of the anatomic ventriculo-arterial junction (Fig. 5). It must have become clear by now that we are describing the working units of the valvar complex as the leaflets rather than cusps. This is, first, because using the term leaflet permits us to make direct comparison with the coapting components of the atrioventricular valves. It is also the case that leaflet is a more appropriate term of description, since the literal meaning of "cusp" is a point or elevation. Such elevations are seen only when the leaflets are viewed in closed position from the ventricular aspect. Cusp describes far more accurately the working surfaces of the molar or premolar teeth.

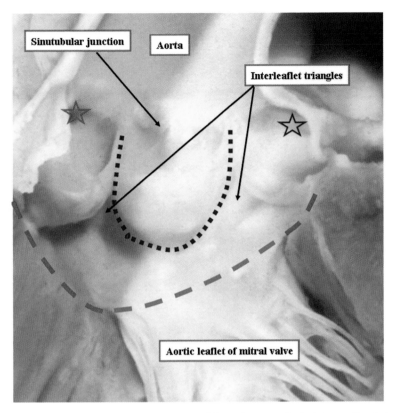

Figure 6 The aortic root has been opened through an anterior incision and is photographed from the front. Note the semilunar attachments of the leaflets, with the hinge of the leaflet supported by the noncoronary aortic sinus, highlighted as the blue dotted line. Note also that part of the leaflets arise from the muscular ventricular septum (red dashed line), but the remaining parts of the leaflets are in fibrous continuity with the aortic leaflet of the mitral valve (green dashed line). The orifice of the right coronary artery is shown by the red star, with the blue star marking the orifice of the left coronary artery.

THE RINGS WITHIN THE AORTIC ROOT

It is rare to find any description of the aortic root that does not use the term "annulus." When defined literally, an annulus is no more than a little ring. There are several such rings to be found within the aortic root, albeit not all correspond to discrete anatomic structures (3). Furthermore, the entity typically described by cardiac surgeons as the annulus does not correspond with any of these anatomic rings, be they real or virtual. It is the semilunar lines of attachment of the leaflets to the aortic valvar sinuses that the cardiac surgeons usually take to represent the annulus. When reconstructed in three dimensions, these semilunar attachments take the form of a three-pronged crown. Within the length of the aortic root supporting the leaflets, nonetheless, there are at least three potential or real circles, while the entire root could be cut from the heart and inserted on the finger in the form of a ring (Fig. 7).

Of these circles within the aortic root, it is the basal one, in other words the virtual ring formed by joining the points of the basal attachments of the leaflets, which echocardiographers usually define as the aortic annulus (Fig. 8).

In hemodynamic terms, this basal plane is the entrance from the left ventricular outflow tract into the aortic root. From the anatomic stance, it is a geometric construction rather than a true entity. It is also the case that measurements taken from the basal attachment of one leaflet to the basal attachment of an opposite leaflet represent a tangent of the outflow tract rather than its full diameter. The full diameter is represented by a section taken from the hinge of one leaflet to the triangle separating the opposite leaflets (Fig. 9).

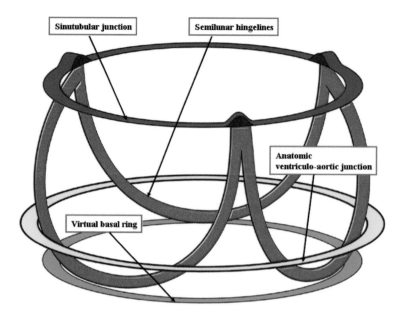

Figure 7   The cartoon shows how the attachments of the leaflets of the aortic valve, when reconstructed in three dimensions, take the form of a crown with three prongs (red construction). The attachments extend through the full extent of the aortic root. Within the root, there are then at least three structures that can be described as rings, namely the sinutubular junction (blue ring), the anatomic ventriculo-arterial junction (yellow ring), and the virtual basal ring constructed by joining together the basal attachments of the leaflets (green ring).

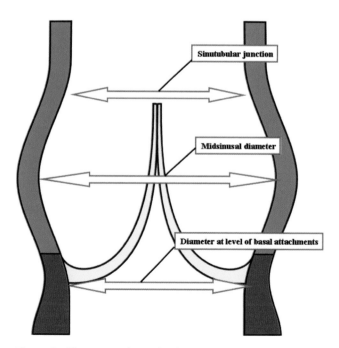

Figure 8   The cartoon shows that there are at least three significant diameters to be measured within the aortic root, namely, the sinutubular junction, the midsinusal diameter, and the diameter at the level of the basal attachment of the leaflets. It is this latter diameter that the echocardiographer usually defines as the valvar annulus, albeit it is no more than a virtual ring and does not correspond with the annulus defined by cardiac surgeons.

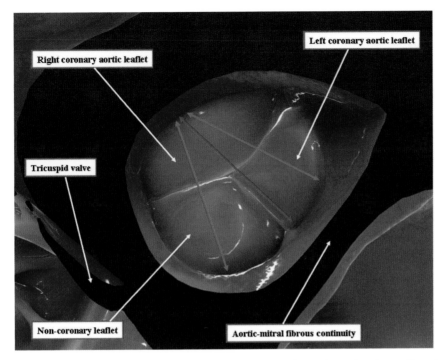

Figure 9 This image is created from the virtual heart (Fig. 1) and shows the view up the subaortic outflow tract as seen from the apex of the left ventricle. As can be seen, the orifice of the aortic valve is not truly circular. As a result, more than one diameter can be measured (e.g., maximum vs. minimum diameter). The diameter(s) of the ellipse should ideally be measured as the distance from the basal hinge of one leaflet to the space between the opposite leaflets (red double headed arrow). Measurements taken between the basal attachments of adjacent leaflets (green double headed arrows) typically cut tangents across the outflow tract.

The top of the crown, in contrast, is a true anatomical ring, namely the sinutubular junction. This ring is demarcated by the sinusal ridges. It is thickened at the sites of peripheral attachment of the zones of apposition between the valvar leaflets (Fig. 10).

This junction marks the outlet of the aortic root into the ascending aorta. The semilunar attachments of the leaflets cross another anatomic ring, this being the junction between the fibrous walls of the valvar sinuses and the supporting ventricular structures (specifically, the anatomic ventriculo-aortic junction). The overall arrangement is well seen when the aortic root is opened subsequent to removal of the valvar leaflets (Fig. 5). Examination of the opened root also confirms that the leaflets arise from ventricular muscle only over part of their circumference (Fig. 6). The larger part of the noncoronary leaflet of the valve, along with part of the left coronary leaflet, is in fibrous continuity with the aortic or anterior leaflet of the mitral valve. The ends of this area of fibrous continuity are thickened to form the so-called fibrous trigones that anchor the aortic–mitral valvar unit within the roof of the left ventricle. Thus, although it has become conventional wisdom to describe an annulus for the aortic valve, different specialists use the term in markedly varied fashion. Unless those using the term provide a definition of its meaning, its use can produce potential disagreement among those wishing to replace or repair the aortic valve. Rather than seeking to define an annulus, we prefer to describe the various components of the valve and account for the variable diameters of the root at its different parts (Fig. 8). The essence of the anatomic arrangement is that the leaflets are supported in crown-like fashion within the cylindrical root (Fig. 7).

In terms of its topology, the normal root has a consistent shape of varying size. Studies have demonstrated definable mathematical relationships between its diameter and clinically measurable dimensions of the leaflets (4,5). In general, the diameter at the level of the sinutubular junction exceeds that at the level of the virtual basal ring by up to one-fifth (6,7). The diameters of inlet and outlet, when expressed as a percentage of the largest diameter at the level of the

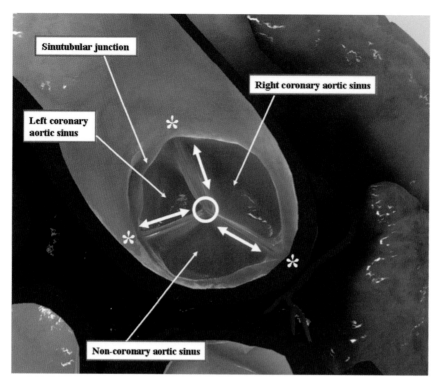

Figure 10   The image is again created from the virtual heart. It shows the closed aortic valve viewed from above, having cut away the parietal wall of the ascending aorta. It shows how the leaflets join together along trifoliate zones of apposition extending from peripheral attachments at the sinutubular junction (asterisks) to the centroid of the valvar orifice (circle). These zones of apposition (double headed arrows) are the true commissures, but usually only the peripheral attachments are defined in this fashion.

expanded aortic sinuses, have been calculated as 97% and 81%, respectively. Overall, therefore, the root can be considered in terms of a truncated cone (8) Moreover, the root is a dynamic structure, with its geometric parameters changing continuously both during the phases of the cardiac cycle and in relation to changes in pressure within the aortic root. (9) From diastole to systole, the diameter at the level of the outlet has been noted to increase by 12%, while the diameter at the base decreases by 16% (10,11).

In the setting of aortic stenosis, the aortic root is significantly larger, by at least 2 standard deviations, when compared to mean normal values (12), albeit no differences have been noted in the diameters of the virtual basal ring or at the midlevel of the sinuses of Valsalva. Bioengineers seeking to model prostheses should take cognizance of these changes in the geometry of the root, as should those inserting valves percutaneously. For instance, insertion of an oversized pros-thetic valve relative to the dimensions of the root can result in redundancy of the leaflets, with the creation of folds. Such folds can generate regions of compressive and tensile stresses, with corresponding changes in the function and durability of the valve (11). Insertion of prostheses too small for the patient will result in creation of a stenotic ventricular outflow tract. Accurate measurement of the various levels of the root, and selection of a prosthesis of appropriate size can prevent such potential problems. Those modeling the root should also note that it is not symmetrical. This can create problems should the asymmetric arrangement not be noted (13).

THE AORTIC VALVAR LEAFLETS

The normal aortic valve possesses three leaflets that close in a trifoliate fashion. Appropriate closure of the valve is dependent on the semilunar suspension of the leaflets within the root and on the integrity of the sinutubular junction (Figs. 10 and 11).

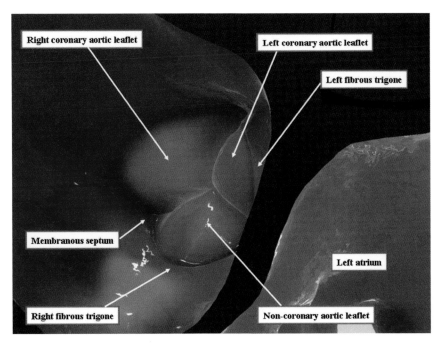

Figure 11 This image created from the virtual heart shows the aortic valve as seen from the cavity of the left ventricle. Note the semilunar attachment of the leaflets, and the attachment of the area of aortic-to-mitral fibrous continuity through the right and left fibrous trigones, these serving to anchor the aortic–mitral valvar unit within the base of the left ventricle.

It is paradoxical that, when the leaflets lose their semilunar hinge lines in the setting of diseases, achieving a more annular attachment, the valve becomes increasingly stenotic or regurgitant. It is often presumed that the leaflets are of comparable size in any given individual. This is far from the case. Variations exist not only between individuals in the dimensions of the root, but also in the same individual in terms of the dimensions of the different leaflets, including their height, width, surface area, and the volume of each of the supporting sinuses of Valsalva. A study of 200 normal hearts revealed that the average width, measured between the peripheral zones of attachment along the sinus ridge, for the right, the noncoronary, and the left coronary leaflets was 25.9, 25.5, and 25.0 mm, respectively (14). Important variations were found when the absolute width of each leaflet was expressed as a percentage of the width of adjacent leaflets. When the two leaflets from the coronary aortic sinuses were compared, these percentages varied between 75% and 159%. Comparisons of the leaflets guarding the noncoronary and right coronary aortic sinuses showed variations from 62% to 162%. For the comparison of the leaflets in the left coronary aortic sinus and the noncoronary sinus, the differences varied from 62% to 150%. Comparable variations were observed for the height. Out of the 200 hearts studied, leaflets of equal size were found in only five hearts. Evaluation of hearts removed from patients with aortic stenosis revealed similar findings with respect to the width, height, and surface area of the different leaflets (14). Such individual variations in geometry should be taken into account when measuring the aortic root prior to choosing a prosthesis for percutaneous insertion. The inequalities in the size of the leaflets can contribute to inaccurate measurements of the distance between opposing valvar hinge points as seen on a cross-sectional echocardiographic image. Variations in the height and width of the individual leaflets relative to the location of the coronary arteries also require special consideration.

LOCATION OF THE CORONARY ARTERIES

In the majority of individuals, the coronary arteries arise within the sinuses of Valsalva adjacent to the pulmonary trunk, with the arterial orifices usually positioned just below the level of the sinutubular junction. It is not unusual, however, for the arteries to be positioned superior relative to the sinutubular junction. A recent study that evaluated this feature by using computed tomography in 150 patients with normal hearts or only mild aortic stenosis, and in 19 patients with moderate or severe aortic stenosis, showed that the mean distance between the basal attachment of the leaflet and the orifice of the left coronary artery was 14.4 ± 2.9 mm, while the comparable distance for the orifice of the right coronary artery was 17.2 ± 3.3 mm (15). No significant differences were noted in the mean distances for subjects with or without severe aortic stenosis.

Knowledge of the location of the coronary arteries, of course, is essential for appropriate percutaneous replacement of the aortic valve. The valvar prostheses have been designed with a skirt of fabric sewn within the frame to help create a seal and prevent paravalvar leakage. Should the coronary arteries take a particularly low origin within the sinus of Valsalva, or should the prosthesis be placed too high, this skirt may obstruct their orifices, impeding the coronary arterial flow. Deployment of the valve, of course, necessitates crushing the leaflets of the native valve against the walls of the aortic sinuses. The combination of a relatively low-lying coronary arterial orifice and a large native valvar leaflet, therefore, can also obstruct the flow into the coronary arteries during valvar deployment (16). Furthermore, implantation of a transcatheter valve into a narrow (width) and/or short (height) sinus of Valsalva may contribute to compromising coronary arterial flow irrespective of the location of the coronary arterial orifice. All of these anatomic considerations mean that measurement of the height of the take-off of the coronary arteries relative to their supporting valvar sinuses and dimensions of the Sinus of Valsalva are crucial prior to valvar implantation.

THE INTERLEAFLET TRIANGLES AND THEIR RELATIONSHIP TO THE MITRAL VALVE AND MEMBRANOUS SEPTUM

As we have already explained, because of the semilunar attachment of the valvar leaflets, three triangular extensions of the left ventricular outflow tract reach to the level of the sinutubular junction (16). These triangles, however, are formed not of ventricular myocardium but of the thinned fibrous walls of the aorta between the expanded sinuses of Valsalva. The triangle between the right coronary aortic sinus and the noncoronary sinus incorporates, at its base, the membranous part of the cardiac septal structures. Its apical part, if removed, creates a communication with the rightward side of the transverse sinus of the pericardium (Fig. 12).

The triangle between the noncoronary and the left coronary aortic sinuses has its base in continuity with the aortic leaflet of the mitral valve. Removal of the apex of this triangle creates continuity with the mid-part of the transverse pericardial sinus (Fig. 13).

The triangle between the two coronary aortic sinuses is much smaller. Its base arises from the crest of the muscular septum, while its apex separates the aortic root from the freestanding sleeve of subpulmonary infundibular musculature (Fig. 14).

As we have emphasized frequently, the aortic valve itself is the cardiac centerpiece, and its leaflets are in continuity with some of the leaflets of both atrioventricular valves. The continuity with the aortic leaflet of the mitral valve is the most extensive. It is the ends of this area of fibrous continuity, which are thickened to form the left and right fibrous trigones; these fibrous structures anchor the conjoined aortic–mitral valvar unit in the base of the left ventricle (Fig. 11). As shown in Figure 13, the interleaflet triangle between the noncoronary and left coronary aortic sinuses is an integral part of this area of fibrous continuity, which in this area serves as the anterior annulus of the mitral valve. Inadvertent placement of the aortic valvar prosthesis too low within the left ventricular outflow tract, therefore, may impinge upon this leaflet of the mitral valve. The right fibrous trigone itself is confluent with the membranous septum, which as shown in Figure 12, is at the base of the interleaflet triangle located between the right coronary and noncoronary aortic sinuses. Together, the membranous septum and the right fibrous trigone form the central fibrous body of the heart. On the right side, the hinge of the septal leaflet of the tricuspid valve separates the membranous septum into its atrioventricular and interventricular components. This relationship is the key to the understanding of the relationship between the aortic valve and the conduction system.

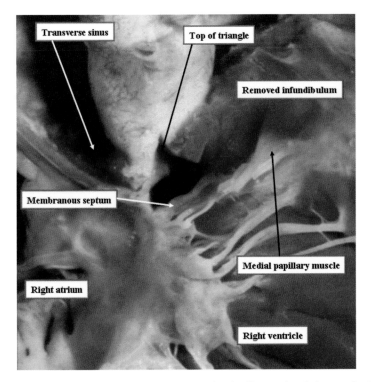

Figure 12 This image is created by removing the fibrous triangle interposing between the noncoronary and right coronary aortic valvar sinuses, and photographing the heart from the right side. Note that the apical part of the triangle opens to the transverse sinus of the pericardium.

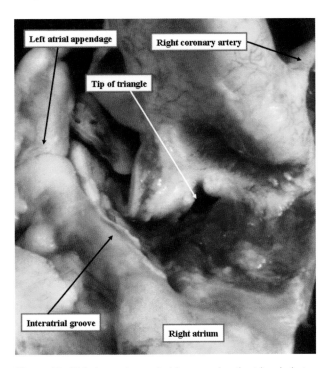

Figure 13 This image is created by removing the triangle between the non-coronary and left coronary aortic valvar sinuses, and photographing the heart from the back of the aorta. Note that the triangle opens into the transverse pericardial sinus.

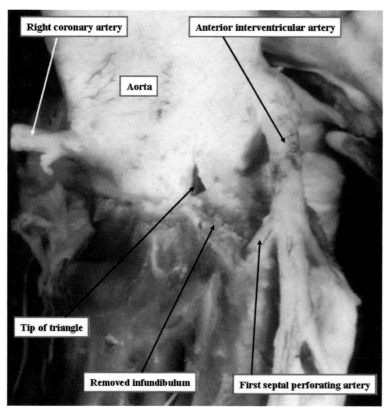

Figure 14 This image is created by removing the fibrous triangle interposed between the two aortic sinuses giving rise to the coronary arteries, and photographing the heart from the front, having also removed the subpulmonary infundibulum. The triangle opens into the tissue plane separating the aortic root from the freestanding infundibulum.

THE RELATIONSHIP BETWEEN THE AORTIC VALVE AND THE CONDUCTION SYSTEM

Within the right atrium, the atrioventricular node is located within the triangle of Koch. This important triangle is demarcated by the tendon of Todaro, the attachment of the septal leaflet of the tricuspid valve, and the orifice of the coronary sinus (Fig. 15).

The apex of this triangle is occupied by the atrioventricular component of the membranous septum. The atrioventricular node is located just inferior to the apex of the triangle adjacent to the membranous septum, and therefore, the atrioventricular node is in fact in close proximity to the subaortic region and membranous septum of the left ventricular outflow tract. It is this relationship that allows us to understand why pathologies involving the aortic valve can lead to complete heart block or intraventricular conduction abnormalities. The atrioventricular node continues as the bundle of His, piercing the membranous septum and penetrating into the left through the central fibrous body. On the left side, the conduction axis exits immediately beneath the membranous septum and runs superficially along the crest of the ventricular septum, giving rise to the fascicles of the left bundle branch. When viewed from the left, the bundle is intimately related to the base of the interleaflet triangle separating the noncoronary and right coronary leaflets of the aortic valve, with the superior part of the bundle intimately related to the right coronary aortic leaflet, as shown exquisitely in the reconstruction made by Tawara in his stellar monograph (Fig. 16) (6).

The illustration of Tawara shows how easily a prosthesis inserted too low within the outflow tract can impinge directly on the left bundle branch, with obvious implications for induction of abnormalities of conduction (7).

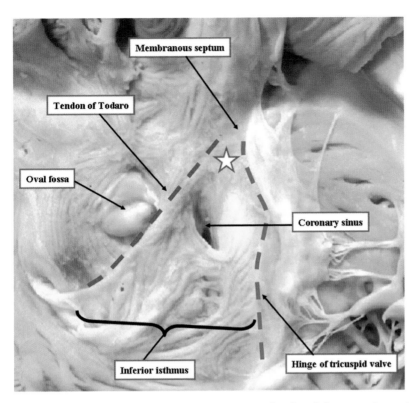

Figure 15 The dissection, made by Professor Damian Sanchez-Quintana, and reproduced with his permission, show the landmarks of the triangle of Koch. The tendon of Todaro is the continuation of the Eustachian valve, and is shown by the red dotted line. The star shows the location of the atrioventricular node.

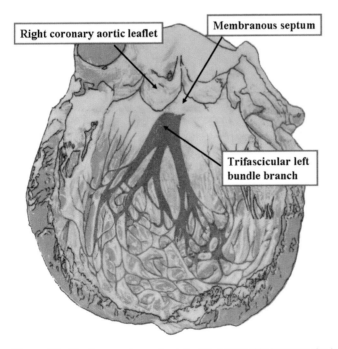

Figure 16 The image shows the intimate relationship between the leaflets of the aortic valve, particularly the right coronary aortic leaflet, and the atrioventricular conduction tissues. *Source*: Modified from Ref. 16.

CHANGES IN THE AORTIC ROOT WITH AGEING

The orientation of the aortic root relative to the surrounding cardiac structures is known to change with aging. This change in geometry was examined in a series of normal human hearts, comparing findings in individuals less than 20 years of age to those over 60 years of age (17). Several aspects are of note. First, examination of the angle between the outlet and apical trabecular parts of the ventricular septum showed significant differences. In hearts from individuals over 60 years of age, the angle varied between 90° and 120°. In those from individuals 20 years of age or less, the angle varied between 135° and 180°. In the younger patients, the left ventricular outflow tract represented a more direct and straight extension into the aortic root. In keeping with these findings, the majority of the circumference of the aortic inlet in all the hearts from the older subjects projected to the right of a line drawn through the outlet part of the muscular ventricular septum. In contrast, in the younger individuals, the majority of the circumference of the inlet projected either to the right or to the left. Thus, we can infer that, in elderly patients, the left ventricular outflow tract may not extend in straight fashion into the aortic root, but rather show a rightward dogleg.

The presence of a subaortic septal bulge, and an extension of this producing asymmetric septal hypertrophy, may create an obstacle to proper seating of the aortic prosthesis within the left ventricular outflow tract. Indeed, the presence of a significant subaortic bulge, or a hypertrophied septum, has been considered by some to be a relative contraindication to the transcatheter implantation of aortic prostheses.

THE DISEASED AORTIC VALVE

Aortic valvar disease can be congenital or acquired. When congenital, the valve most usually has only two leaflets and is usually termed a bicuspid valve, albeit that valves with one or three leaflets can also be malformed at birth. Acquired disease is most usually either rheumatic or degenerative and calcific. The most common indication for surgical replacement of the aortic valve in patients younger than 70 years is the bicuspid valve, whereas degenerative calcific disease is most frequent in the patients older than 70 years. In the following text, we provide insights into the pathogenesis of bicuspid, calcific, and rheumatic valves, and the implication it has for transcatheter implantation.

The prevalence of an aortic valve with two leaflets at birth is from 1% to 2%, affecting men three to four times more often than women. Although the abnormal valve is present at birth, patients typically present with symptoms in their sixth to seventh decade of life. In most instances, the two leaflets of the valve are unequal in size, with the larger leaflet having a midline raphe that represents incomplete separation, or congenital fusion, of two adjacent leaflets [Fig. 17(B)]. In three-quarters of patients, it is the leaflets arising from the sinuses giving rise to the coronary arteries that are fused, resulting in the more anterior leaflet being larger. In most other instances, the fused leaflet is made up of the right coronary and noncoronary leaflets. Turbulent flow across the diseased valve is thought to promote accelerated fibrosis and calcification at an earlier age. The most frequent primary complication is stenosis, seen in five-sixths, with insufficiency being the problem in the remainder of patients. Additional fusion along the zone of apposition between the leaflets is not typically observed. Severe calcification can make the diagnosis of the bicuspid valve a real diagnostic challenge.

Degenerative calcific stenosis of the aortic valve is present in approximately 2% of patients older than 65 years. Its precursor, thickening or calcification of the leaflets without obstruction to the left ventricular outflow tract, known as sclerosis, is observed in up to one-third of patients (18–21). Calcific aortic valvar disease results in symptoms in the eighth to ninth decade of life. The process of calcification begins at the base of the leaflets, where flexion is maximal, and extends into the sinuses of Valsalva. Ultimately, the process produces immobilization of the leaflets. The free edges of the leaflets are not involved, and typically there is minimal fusion along the zones of apposition between the leaflets [Fig. 17(C)]. In contrast to rheumatic disease of the aortic valve, the mitral valve is not involved.

Rheumatic aortic valvar disease is characteristically associated with adhesion and fusion along the zones of apposition between the leaflets, which are typically severely thickened. The free edges often retract and stiffen, resulting in the so-called "fish mouth" orifice [Fig. 17(D)].

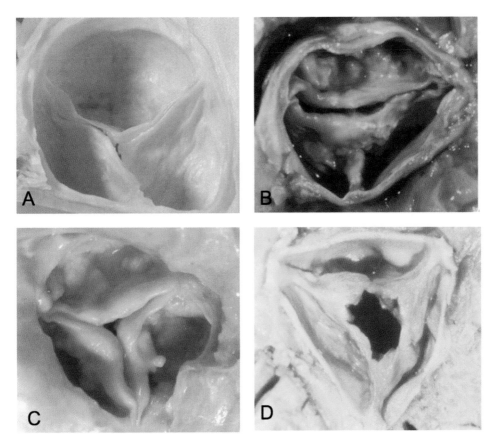

Figure 17 (**A**) Nondiseased tricuspid aortic valve viewed from the aortic aspect. (**B**) Stenotic bicuspid aortic valve with calcification and a midline raphe pointing at six-o'clock position. There is no fusion along the zone of apposition between the leaflets. (**C**) Calcific aortic valve disease with thickening of the leaflets and calcific deposits at their base. As in panel B, there is no fusion along the zones of apposition between the leaflets. (**D**) Rheumatic aortic valve disease with thickening of the leaflets and marked fusion along the zone of apposition between adjacent leaflets, producing the characteristic "fish mouth" orifice. (*Source*: From Ref. 23.)

Calcific nodules can be found on both sides of the leaflets. In rheumatic aortic valvar disease, stenosis and regurgitation can be of equal consequence.

Transcatheter implantation is currently reserved for high-risk elderly patients with calcific disease. Preimplantation balloon aortic valvoplasty is primarily performed to improve seating of the transcatheter prosthesis within the aortic root. Mechanisms of balloon dilation include splitting and/or cracking of the zones of apposition between the leaflets, cracking of calcific nodules, tears within the leaflets, and expansion of the walls of the valvar sinuses, known as "stretching," at sites where the leaflets themselves are not fused along their zones of apposition (22). The mechanism of action, therefore, is related to the etiology of the valvar disease. In the absence of fusion along the zones of apposition between the leaflets, as seen in congenital bicuspid and degenerative calcific disease, balloon dilation results in expansion of the walls of the root and fracture of the leaflets and calcific deposits. On the other hand, in the presence of fusion between the leaflets, as seen in rheumatic disease, balloon dilation results in splitting of the fused leaflets and cracking of the leaflets themselves. Balloon dilation is most effective in the setting of rheumatic disease, followed by calcific disease, and least effective for elderly patients with bicuspid valves.

Incomplete expansion of the balloon during preimplantation valvoplasty should serve as a clue that the leaflets that are severely noncompliant, with the subsequent possibility of incomplete expansion and malfunction of the prosthesis. Some believe this to be a contraindication to transcatheter implantation. Given the age and high-risk profile of patients, transcatheter aortic valves are implanted in the context of calcific aortic valvar disease. It is extremely rare for such valves to be implanted in patients with rheumatic aortic valvar disease. Although a bicuspid valve is currently considered a contraindication to transcatheter implantation, accumulating anecdotal experience suggests that it can be performed safely in selected individuals, but more evidence is needed before promoting such a practice.

CONCLUSION

Anatomical knowledge of the aortic valvar complex can be fundamental in understanding the key principles of percutaneous insertion of valvar prostheses. Appreciating the exact origin of the coronary arteries, and the location of left bundle branch, may help to minimize the risks of coronary ischemia and abnormalities of conduction that can occur during implantation. Knowledge of the limitations of measuring the so-called annulus by echocardiography, angiography or multislice computed tomography may decrease the possibility of creating a mismatch between the patient and the chosen prosthesis. Finally, an understanding of the variations in structure found not only between individuals, but also within the aortic valve of the same individual, can lead to refinements in the future designs of valvar prostheses.

ACKNOWLEDGMENTS

We are indebted to Dr Sue Wright and her colleagues at the National Heart Hospital, University College, London, and the team at Glassworks, for permitting us to reproduce images from the virtual heart they have created. Details of the virtual heart are available at www.heartworks. me.uk. We also thank Professor Damian Sanchez-Quintana, who prepared the exquisite dissection showing the landmarks of the triangle of Koch.

REFERENCES

1. Wells FC, Crowe T. Leonardo da Vinci as a paradigm for modern clinical research. J Thorac Cardiovasc Surg 2004; 127:929–944.
2. Piazza N, de Jaegere P, Schultz C, Becker AE, Serruys PW, Anderson RH. Anatomy of the aortic valvar complex and its implications for transcatheter implantation of the aortic valve. *Circ Cardiovasc Intervent* 2008; 1:74–81
3. Anderson RH. Clinical anatomy of the aortic root. Heart 2000;84: 670–673.
4. Rankin JS, Dalley AF, Crooke PS, et al. A 'hemispherical' model of aortic valvar geometry. J Heart Valve Dis 2008; 17:179–186.
5. Kunzelman KS, Grande KJ, David TE, et al. Aortic root and valve relationships. Impact on surgical repair. J Thorac Cardiovasc Surg 1994; 107:162–170.
6. Tawara S. Das Reizleitungssystem de Saugetierherzens. Eine Anatomich-hisologische Studie uber das Atrioventricularbundel und die Purkinjeschen Faden. Jena: Verlag von Gustav Fischer, 1906.
7. Piazza N, Onuma Y, Jesserun E, et al. Early and persistent intraventricular conduction abnormalities and requirements for pacemaking following percutaneous replacement of the aortic valve JACC Cardiovasc Interv 2008; 1:310–316.
8. Reid K. The anatomy of the sinus of Valsalva. Thorax 1970; 25:79–85.
9. Swanson M, Clark RE. Dimensions and geometric relationships of the human aortic valve as a function of pressure. Circ Res 1974; 35:871–882.
10. Brewer RJ, Deck JD, Capati B, et al. The dynamic aortic root. Its role in aortic valve function. J Thorac Cardiovasc Surg 1976; 72:413–417.
11. Thubrikar MJ, Piepgrass WC, Shaner TW, et al. The design of the normal aortic valve. Am J Physiol 1981; 10:H795–H801.
12. Crawford MH, Roldan CA. Prevalence of aortic root dilatation and small aortic roots in valvular aortic stenosis. Am J Cardiol 2001; 87:1311–1313.
13. Treasure T, Golesworthy T, Thornton W, et al. Unknown unknowns: The aortic root through the looking glass. Eur J Cardiothorac Surg 2009; 35(6):925–926.
14. Vollebergh FE, Becker AE. Minor congenital variations of cusp size in tricuspid aortic valves. Possible link with isolated aortic stenosis. Br Heart J 1977; 39:1006–1011.
15. Tops LF, Wood DA, Delgado V, et al. Nonivasive evaluation of the aortic root with multi-slice computed tomography: Implications for transcatheter aortic valve replacement. JACC Cardiovasc Imaging 2008; 1:321–330.
16. Sutton JP III, Ho SY, Anderson RH. The forgotten interleaflet triangles: A review of the surgical anatomy of the aortic valve. Ann Thorac Surg 1995; 59:419–427.

17. Becker AE. Middelhof CJFM Ventricular septal geometry: A spectrum with clinical relevance. In: Wenink ACG, et al., eds. The Ventricular Septum of the Heart. The Hague, The Netherlands: Matrinus Nijhoff Publishers, 1981.
18. Stritzke J, Linsel-Nitschke P, Markus MRP, et al. for the MONICA/KORA Investigators. Eur Heart J 2009; 30:2044–2053.
19. Otto CM, Lind BK, Kitzman DW, et al. Association of aortic valve sclerosis with cardiovascular mortality and morbidity in the elderly. NEJM 1999; 341:142–147.
20. Lindroos M, Kupari M, Heikkila J, Tilvis R. Prevalence of aortic valve abnormalities in the elderly: an echocardiographic study of a random population sample. JACC 1993; 21:1220–1225.
21. Stewart BF, Sisovick D, Lind BK, et al. Clinical risk factors associated with calcific aortic valve disease. Cardiovascular Health Study. JACC 1997; 29:630–634.
22. Waller F, McKay C, Vantassel JW, et al. Catheter balloon valvuloplasty of stenotic aortic valves. Part I. Anatomic basis and mechanisms of balloon dilation. Clin Cardiol 1991; 14:836–846.
23. Braunwald's Heart Disease: A Textbook of Cardiovascular Medicine, 7th Edition (Zipes DP, et al., eds.) 2004. W.B. Saunders Company.

2 | Accumulation of Worldwide Experience with Postmortem Studies of Transcatheter Aortic Valve Implantation—What Should We Be Avoiding?

Renu Virmani
CVPath Institute, Inc., Gaithersburg, Maryland, U.S.A.

Raoul Bonan
Montreal Heart Institute, Université de Montréal, Montreal, Quebec, Canada

Gaku Nakazawa
CVPath Institute, Inc., Gaithersburg, Maryland, U.S.A.

Stéphane Noble and Anita Asgar
Montreal Heart Institute, Université de Montréal, Montreal, Quebec, Canada

Marc Vorpahl
CVPath Institute, Inc., Gaithersburg, Maryland, U.S.A.

ANATOMY OF NATIVE VALVE

The underlying etiology of aortic valve stenosis is for the most part dependent on the age at which the patient presents. Since the need for percutaneous heart valve (PHV) replacement is mostly limited to high-risk patients presenting in their seventh and eighth decades, the most common indication for the procedure is senile calcific aortic stenosis and is more common in men than women. Calcification begins to accumulate in the base of the cusps on the aortic aspect and extends superiorly toward the mid-portion of the cusp with sparing of the free margin (closing edge). Calcification is typically more pronounced in the noncoronary cusp as compared to the coronary cusps. The mechanism of this finding may involve the relatively reduced diastolic pressure load imparted on the coronary cusps due to the presence of coronary ostia (1). Typically, the nodular calcific deposits are superimposed on a fibrotic cusp, whereas in the bicuspid aortic valve calcification occurs diffusely within the spongiosa (2). Commissural fusion classically is absent in senile aortic stenosis unless there has been an associated inflammatory or infectious disorder. The ventricular surface is mostly smooth with some degree of fibrosis. The pathogenesis of calcification of the tricuspid aortic valve is unknown. Mild asymmetry of valve cusps has been suggested as a potential precipitant of the calcification process (3,4). However, the high incidence of minor differences in cusp size (>50% in individuals) makes it unlikely to account for severe stenosis in most cases. Since calcification is commonly seen in atherosclerosis of coronary arteries, an association between coronary atherosclerosis including its epidemiologic risk factors has been suggested. In some studies, a significantly higher fasting cholesterol levels have been observed as compared to controls without aortic calcification (5,6).

Conflict of interest disclosures:
Raoul Bonan is clinical proctor and consultant to CoreValve. He has also received speaker honoraria from CoreValve Inc., Irvine, CA, United States. The other authors have nothing to disclose in relation to this article.
Renu Virmani, CVPath Institute Inc., received research grant for the evaluation of the animal and human explant hearts or valves from Edwards Lifesciences, Irvine, CA, United States, and prior to that from Percutaneous Valve Technologies, Ltd, Israel.
The other authors have no conflict of interest.

However, recent lipid-lowering trials failed to show a benefit of lipid lowering on calcific aortic stenosis. In a report from the Mayo Clinic, the average age of patients who underwent surgical aortic valve replacement for degenerative aortic stenosis was 74 years (range 49–92 years) and was performed more frequently in males (1.6:1) (7). The dominant lesion was stenosis (80%) with mild degrees of aortic regurgitation often present. In this study, aortic root dilatation was rarely observed (3%) (7).

Percutaneous aortic valve replacement has recently been proposed as a treatment for severe symptomatic aortic valve stenosis in patients refused or at high risk for conventional surgery. Since the first implantation by Cribier in 2002, more than 5000 patients have undergone transcatheter aortic valve implantation (TAVI). Two main technologies share the wealth of the experience to date: the Edwards SAPIEN valve® (Edwards Lifesciences, Irvine, CA) and the CoreValve ReValving system® (CoreValve Inc., Irvine, CA) (8).

The currently available transcatheter valves are bioprosthetic, that is, pericardial tissue valves. Bioprosthetic valves are prone to calcification and degeneration that can limit their long-term durability. The geometric relation or conformity of the device relative to the specific patient anatomy needs to be analyzed to better understand the seating of the prosthesis within the aortic root. Furthermore, the characterization of the histologic changes that occur over time in relation to valve frame, valve leaflets, and periaortic root structures needs to be better understood as well.

Retrieval analysis becomes an essential part of an accurate quality assessment protocol that requires a large involvement of doctors, patients, and manufacturers to be successful. Implant retrieval analysis might also have a substantial impact on design and clinical practice, improving the safety of artificial heart valves and curtailing implantation programs of unsafe valves.

In this chapter we provide gross and microscopic observations made in 15 explanted transcatheter heart valves (nine of Edwards and six of CoreValve). In all these patients, postmortem studies were performed after fatal complications related to patient comorbidities or procedural-related events—none were device-related events.

THE EDWARDS SAPIEN VALVE

Device Description

The first balloon-expandable Edward SAPIEN valve®, successor of the initially used Cribier–Edwards valve has a balloon-expandable stainless steel frame, fabric sealed cuff, and a bovine pericardial valve (Fig. 1). It is a trileaflet valve constructed with the bovine pericardium, which is sewn to the stent frame that is 14 mm in height. The first Cribier–Edwards valve prototype had the ventricular one-third of the stent frame covered with a fabric cuff designed to form a seal against the aortic annulus (9). However, the more recent prototype (Edward SAPIEN valve) has been modified using a similar stainless steel frame but the fabric skirt now covers two-thirds of the frame to improve sealing and reduce paravalvular regurgitation (Fig. 1) (8).

Animal Studies

To study the performance of the Cribier–Edward valve, transcatheter studies were initially performed in sheep models traditionally used for surgical valve implant studies. Currently, no animal model of aortic valve stenosis exists to adequately evaluate positioning, deployment, anchoring, and functioning of the transcatheter heart valves in the orthotopic position. The main limitations of these animal models include the short distance between the coronary artery ostia and aortic valve annulus, the small distance between the aortic valve annulus and mitral valve leaflets, and the relatively short length of the ascending aorta (10).

To overcome these anatomical limitations, Eltchaninoff et al. attempted to implant the prosthetic heart valve heterotopically in the descending aorta; however, the lack of a transprosthetic diastolic pressure gradient needed to close the valve led to the discontinuation of this model (11). Based on the Hufnagel concept (i.e., surgical correction of aortic regurgitation by implantation of a mechanical heart valve in the descending aorta), Cirbier et al. created a sheep model of aortic regurgitation by extracting small tissue fragments of the aortic valve by using bioptomes (12). The prosthetic heart valve was subsequently implanted percutaneously in the

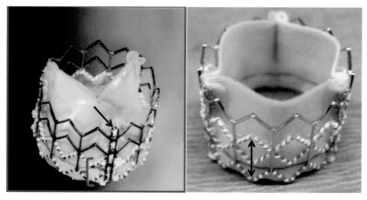

Cribier—Edward Valve   SAPIEN Valve (Edward Lifesciences)

Figure 1 Cribier–Edward percutaneous valve consists of three elements: the stainless steel balloon expandable frame, bovine pericardial valve tissue, and a PET skirt material. The leaflet tissue is secured within a fold in the PET skirt material, which is attached to the metal stent frame ({). The edges of the leaflets are attached to commissure bars (*arrow*). The fabric skirt in the Cribier–Edward valve covers the ventricular one-third of the frame, whereas in the SAPIEN valve, it covers the ventricular two-thirds of the frame to improve the sealing (*double arrow*). *Source*: From Ref. 18 (Cribier–Edward valve) and Ref. 17 (SAPIEN valve).

descending aorta just distal to the subclavian artery. Valve performance was followed for up to 21 weeks by angiography and echocardiography (10).

Four animals died of acute procedural complications, which included aortic perforation, mitral valve damage, hemothorax, and sheath dissection of the brachiocephalic artery. One animal had, via gross and radiographic inspection, a misaligned rotated PHV within the aorta, which lead to the valve assembly being perpendicular to aortic flow (10). The remaining nine implants appeared widely expanded in the aorta with the stent frames well apposed to the aortic wall. The entire assemblies were well aligned with aortic blood flow and correctly oriented for proper leaflet excursion. Radiographic examination of the implants showed all stent frames to be intact. No calcification was discernable from the X-rays within the device or leaflets. Grossly, all valve assembly stent frames, with the exception of the device in one animal (see earlier), all were well apposed to the aortic walls and completely incorporated with neointimal growth. Neointimal growth was also present along the basal attachment points of the leaflets, more so on the ventricular surface at 21 weeks. Neointimal growth was also present along the free edges of some of the leaflets. No fractures, tears, or fenestrations in the leaflets were grossly visible (Fig. 2).

In microscopic observation at 21 weeks, all devices, excluding the animal with the rotated PHV, showed widely patent lumens and good apposition of the stent frames to the aortic

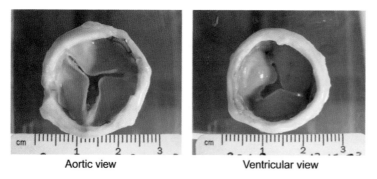

Aortic view   Ventricular view

Figure 2 Aortic and ventricular views of the valve assembly with surrounding ovine aortic root. The stent frame is expanded into a cylindrical shape and is well apposed to the native aortic surface. The valve leaflets are intact with no tears, calcification, or thrombosis. There is slight thickening of the leaflet free margins near the commissures and at the base along the PET skirt and suture lines (opaque white tissue).

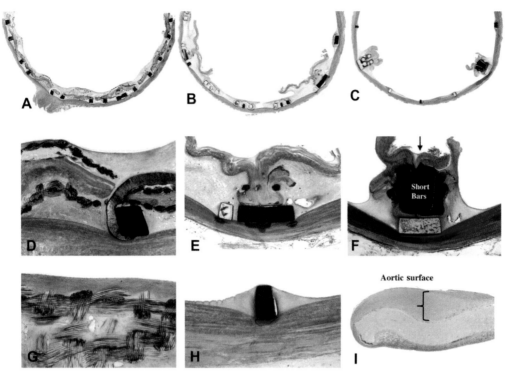

Figure 3 Histologic sections of the stent/valve assembly at three points: Photos (**A**) and (**D**) are low- and high-power views from the area of PET and valve tissue attachment to the stent frame. Photos (**B**) and (**E**) show basal commissure points with neointimal incorporated leaflet tissue. Photos (**C**) and (**F**) show distal commissure points and thin neointimal coverage of the stent frame struts (arrow). Photo (**G**) shows well-organized neointimal growth lining the luminal surface of the PET material. Photo (**H**) shows thin, well-organized neointimal growth over a distal stent frame strut. Photo (**I**) shows proteoglycan-rich neointimal growth incorporating the free edge of a prosthetic valve leaflet ({).

walls. The stent frames were completely incorporated with well-organized neointimal tissue composed of smooth muscle cells in a proteoglycan matrix (Fig. 3). Fabric skirt material and attachment sutures at the proximal end of the assemblies were also completely incorporated with neointima. There was essentially no inflammatory reaction to the stent frame or fabric skirt material. Support bar assemblies (i.e., longitudinal struts) at the commissure attachment points were intact with tight apposition of the leaflets at the commissures. Neointimal growth was greater around the commissures and generally showed less smooth muscle organization. The leaflet bases were also incorporated with neointima. Neointimal layers covering the stent frame struts were fully endothelialized (Fig. 3).

Analysis of the Retrieved Human Implants

To our knowledge, a total of nine postmortem studies have been performed in patients implanted with the Edwards PHV (Table 1). The majority of the prosthetic valves were explanted within 10 days of the procedure (range 1 to 55 days).

Gross and histologic observations involve prosthetic valve location, stent expansion, stent strut apposition to the aortic wall, integrity of the prosthetic valve leaflet, presence of thrombus, and bacterial endocarditis.

In our experience with seven explanted valves, the stent frame had been well deployed and anchored across the native valve annulus. The native valves were pushed and the stent frame was circular in all but one case where the frame was oval (Figs. 4 and 5). The mean external diameter of the frame was 26 ± 2 mm. The stent frame compressed the native valves into the aortic sinus such that no significant space could be visualized between the aortic and the left ventricular out flow tract. However, some leaks have been identified between the stent

Table 1   Retrieved Valves (Edwards)

Case #	Length of implantation (days)	Sex	Age (yr)	Valve generation	EuroSCORE (%)	Report from
1	1	Female	87	LC5649	18.81	REVIVE
2	3	Male	82	LA2022	50.74	Study
3	9	Male	85	9000TFX	28.83	REVIVAL
4	2	Female	89	9000TFX	16.56	Study
5	Unknown (Late, >2 months)	Unknown		PHV23	Unknown	
6	Unknown (acute)	Unknown		PHV23	Unknown	AFIP
7	Unknown (acute)	Unknown		PHV23	Unknown	
8	5	Male	87	PHV23 or 26	Unknown	Published (15)
9	2	Male	79	PHV26	14.15	Published (17)

Abbreviations: AFIP, Armed Forces Institute of Pathology; PHV, percutaneous heart valve. The REVIVAL trial, transcatheter endovascular implantation of valves; REVIVE, registry of endovascular implantation of valves.

frame and the native commissure. Generally, the lower edge of the valve prosthesis was located at the anatomic arterio-ventricular junction with tight apposition to the aortic root. The superior edge of the prosthetic valve was usually observed below the sinotubular junction. The coronary ostia are typically located at the rim of the sinotubular junction or just below it. In one of the autopsy cases, we observed definite obstruction of the left main coronary orifice by the prosthesis

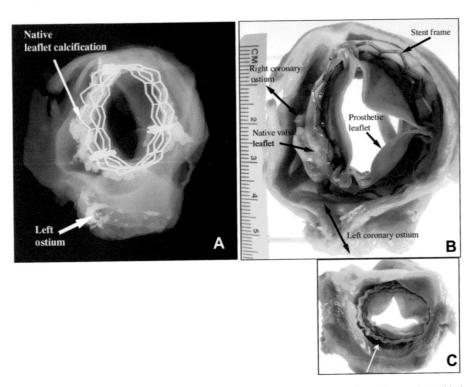

Figure 4   (Edwards Case #2 in Table 1.) Superior radiographic and gross view of the explant with the stent/valve assembly in situ. The native valve leaflets show marked calcification, especially the right coronary leaflet (*thin arrow*). The left and right coronary ostia are identified. The photo below of the inferior surface shows good apposition of the device to the aortic root adjacent to the left and noncoronary leaflets. A small gap is present adjacent to the right coronary leaflet (*arrow*) that resulted in a paravalvular leak secondary to poor expansion of the right coronary sinus due to heavy calcification.

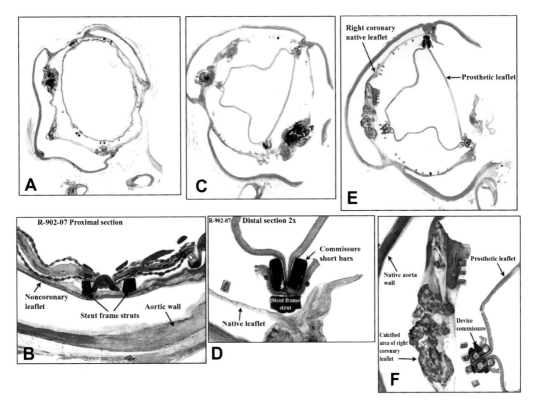

Figure 5 (Edwards Case #2 in Table 1.) (**A**) and (**B**) Low- and high-power cross-sectional views of the proximal end of the native aortic root and valve implant. The high-power image shows the skirt material on either side of the prosthetic valve tissue and stent frame struts apposed to the native noncoronary leaflet. Toluidine blue/basic fuchsin whole mount and 2×. (**C**) Low-power cross-sectional view of the mid-native aortic root and valve implant showing the prosthetic valve tissue secured within the three-stent frame commissures. Toluidine blue/basic fuchsin, whole mount. (**D**) Distal section showing another commissure point with securely fastened valve leaflet tissue. Toluidine blue/basic fuchsin 2×. (**E**) and (**F**) Low- and high-power cross-sectional views of the distal end of the native aortic root and valve implant. The high-power image shows a heavily calcified area of the right coronary leaflet. An adjacent prosthetic leaflet commissure is also pictured. Toluidine blue/basic fuchsin whole mount and 2×.

(Fig. 6). In one case, a cuspal tear was observed. In two valves, thrombus on the valve was seen as brownish-red material associated with white raised lesions (N.B. one of these cases involved an infective endocarditis). Inspection also revealed minor fibrin platelet thrombi on the valve leaflets mostly limited to the aortic surface but was not uncommonly seen on the ventricular surface as well (Fig. 7).

Considering the short-term implantation of the current series of valves, we observed up to two to three layers of acute inflammatory cells (i.e., mostly macrophages with or without giant cells and few neutrophils) covering the surface but not infiltrating into the valve leaflet itself. Neutrophils were prominent in the patient with bacterial endocarditis. In this case, the valve showed colonies of gram-positive cocci, mostly on the ventricular surface and infiltrating the leaflet collagen layers.

In longer term implants, portions of the stent frame, the mid-assembly sections taken at the level above the pericardial sleeve, and the area around the support bar (i.e., longitudinal strut) were slowly being incorporated with early fibrin deposition and smooth muscle cell infiltration and surface endothelialization. The basal portions of the valve leaflets were also infiltrated by neointimal tissue consisting of smooth muscle cells in a proteoglycan matrix. In the areas where the stent struts where in direct contact with the aortic wall, we observed fibrin deposition that was followed by mild neointimal growth and surface endothelialization (Figs. 8–10).

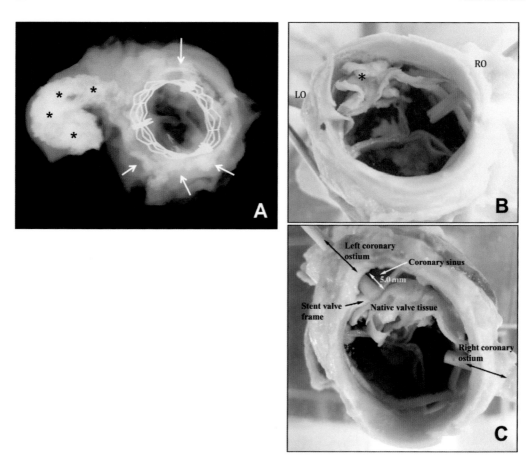

Figure 6 (Edwards Case #6 in Table 1.) Radiographic and gross views of aortic root with implanted prosthetic valve. Photo (**A**) shows a radiographic superior view of the explant with the stent/valve prosthesis in situ. There are areas of calcification in the adjacent mitral valve (*) and around the annulus (*arrows*). Photo (**B**) shows a gross superior view of the explant taken at the same angle as the X-ray. The right and left coronary ostia are identified. Evulsed native valve tissue is present in the upper left quadrant (*). Photo (**C**) shows an illustrated view of the aortic side of the implant. Left and right coronary ostia are tracked with probes. Evulsed native leaflet tissue is seen within the valve assembly adjacent to the left coronary cusp. *Abbreviations*: RO, right ostium, LO, left ostium.

THE COREVALVE REVALVING SYSTEM

Device Description
The CoreValve aortic bioprosthesis is the third generation of a trileaflet porcine pericardial tissue valve, mounted and sutured in a self-expanding nitinol frame, which is 53- or 55-mm long, depending on valve size (13). The frame is divided in three distinct zones of radial force or hoop strength. The lower portion has high radial force to expand and exclude the calcified leaflets and to avoid recoil. This portion extends to a small degree into the left ventricle. The middle portion features high hoop strength and carries the valve. The frame shape at this portion of the frame is designed to avoid the coronary arteries. The upper portion of the frame has low radial force and is flared outward to make contact with the ascending aorta, which serves to consistently align the valve to blood flow. Of note is that this device thus implants intra-annularly but functions supra-annularly.

Preclinical
The design was first tested on explanted human hearts (14). These hearts were explanted including the ascending aorta up to the root of the brachio-cephalic arterial trunk. After immobilizing the hearts, the distance between the arteriotomy and the aortic annulus was measured. The left

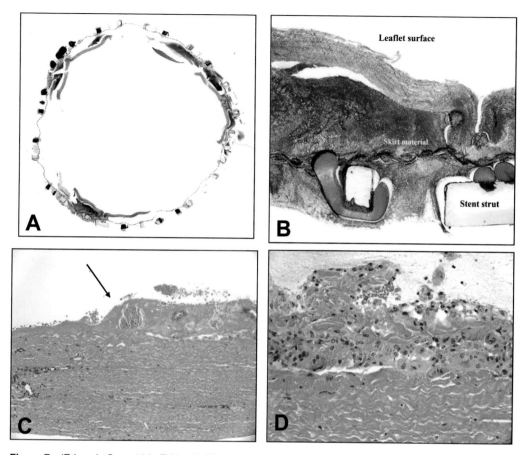

Figure 7 (Edwards Case #3 in Table 1.) (**A**) and (**B**) Low and high-power views of the middle valve assembly section showing early thrombus deposition between the leaflet material and the outer stent frame toluidine blue/basic fuchsin, whole mount and 4×. (**C**) Aortic side of same leaflet showing focal surface thrombus deposition with red blood cell extravasation (*arrow*). H&E 20×. (**D**) Macrophage infiltration of superficial collagen on the ventricular side of the leaflet. H&E 40×.

atrium was opened, the mitral valve was visualized, and its effective orifice area was measured. The prosthesis was loaded in the delivery catheter and the prosthesis was implanted. The following analysis was then carried out: (1) through the left atrium, verification of the mitral valve, appreciation of the mobility of the two mitral leaflets, and measurement of the mitral effective orifice area; (2) cut down of the aorta to the distal end of the prosthesis allowed verification of the patency of the left and right coronary arteries ostia by using a 1-mm coronary probe; (3) search for paravalvular leaks with a 1-mm metal tip inserted between the aortic wall and the external rim of the frame; (4) further dissecting the aorta to the annulus and verifying the adequate positioning of the prosthesis relative to the annulus and the subannular zone. In these studies, the prosthesis was never in contact with the mitral valve greater than 3 mm. (N.B.: The complete length of the anterior mitral valve leaflet is approximately 30 mm). No reduction of the effective orifice area was noted and there was no reduction in the mobility of the anterior mitral leaflet. The implantation of prostheses left a free passage to both coronary orifices. The prosthesis has a constraint mid-portion of the frame that allows for optimal valve prosthesis function and also does not allow the frame to interfere in any way with the coronary ostia.

In a few implantations, balloon expansions following the implantation of the prosthesis have shown further expansion of the frame inside the anatomic wall. Leaks of a lesser diameter were still observed but minimal, meaning that the 1-mm probe could be pushed in these leaks with repeated and strong applications. Definitive interpretation of these leaks has to be questioned at the time by the quality of the model, lacking the blood pressure that extends

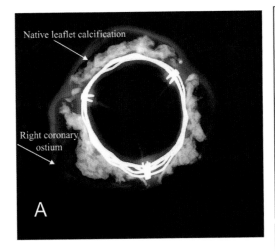

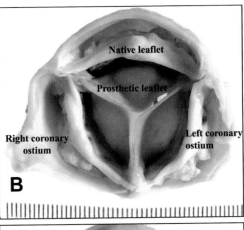

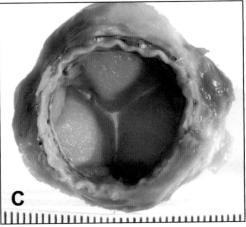

Figure 8 (Edwards Case #5 in Table 1.) Superior radiographic and gross view of the explant with prosthesis (stent valve) in situ (**A, B**). The X-ray shows marked calcification of the native valve leaflets. The left and right coronary ostia are identified in the gross view. The inferior view of the device shows good coaptation of the leaflet free edges (**C**).

the vessel and anatomy. Nevertheless, it may explain the paravalvular leak experience in clinic where a nontotal conformity between a self-expanded circular prosthesis in a noncircular native aortic annulus are mismatched.

Animal Model
The animal model chosen was the sheep, being the accepted model for valve testing in the orthotopic position (14). The anatomy above the valve annulus and especially the coronary sinuses are close to the human one. The CoreValve frame using one part located in the vicinity of these sinuses and bridging the coronary sinuses with an "ascending aorta segment" could therefore reproduce the advantage envisioned in humans.

However, one major difference to the human anatomy described in the literature and also encountered by other teams was confirmed. In the sheep model, there is no space between the aortic and mitral valve annulus (the so-called inter-aortico–mitral ridge) as it is well described in humans and noted by all surgeons performing heart valve replacements. Therefore, as the CoreValve frame is composed by an element that covers the subannular space and the inter-aortico–mitral ridge this causes various degrees of mitral interaction. Angiography of the ascending aorta and the left ventricle were carried out prior to and following the aortic ring measurement, for aortic valve or para-valvular leak evaluation with prosthesis implantation.

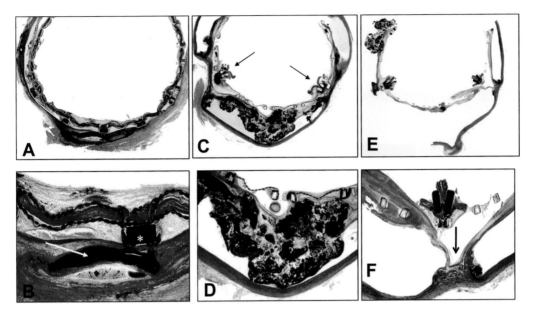

Figure 9 (Edwards Case #5 in Table 1.) (**A**) and (**B**) Low- and high-power cross-sectional views of the proximal end of the native aortic root and valve implant. The high-power image shows the skirt material on either side of the prosthetic valve tissue and stent frame struts apposed to the native leaflet (*). The underlying native valve shows focal calcification (*arrow*). Toluidine blue/basic fuchsin, whole mount and 2×. (**C**) and (**D**) Low- and high-power cross-sectional views of the mid-native aortic root and valve implant. The low-power image shows two intact frame commissures (*arrows*). The high-power image shows marked calcification of the native right coronary leaflet. Toluidine blue/basic fuchsin, whole mount and 1.25×. (**E**) and (**F**) Low- and high-power cross-sectional views of the distal end of the native aortic root and valve implant. The high-power image shows a native leaflet commissure (*arrow*) and prosthetic leaflet commissure above. Toluidine blue/basic fuchsin, whole mount and 1.25×.

The delivery of the device was precise, but in the first implantation, the absence of the retaining hooks lets prosthesis tend to jump out uncontrolled from the delivery system. Retaining hooks (connecting the frame to the inner catheter) have been applied to withhold the prosthesis until the external sheath is fully pulled back. This feature also permits, if necessary, to pull back the entire system to a more precise final position even when two-thirds of the sheath has been withdrawn.

The observed early migration of the device was corrected by (1) increasing the radial force of the lower portion of the device and oversizing the prosthesis relative to the native aortic valve annulus and (2) improving the quality of the tip of the delivery catheter thus preventing the encroachment in the distal frame during the retrieval.

Of the animals euthanized early, the evaluation showed: good adhesion, no impairment of coronary flow, no prosthesis migration and no valvular or paravalvular leak. Animals followed at 10 days and 6 weeks confirmed the intimate adhesion of the frame to the local tissue, absence of valve tear or calcification.

Analysis of the Retrieved Human Implants

A total of six implants have been retrieved and postimplantation time ranged from 3 to 425 days allowing for an appreciation of the early and mid-term gross and histologic changes that may occur after implantation (Table 2).

Postmortem studies have demonstrated the deposition of fibrin, platelets, and inflammatory cells (which eventually transform into pannus) around the valve frame. This pannus is well formed by three months and may even extend into the base of the valve leaflets.

In the five specimens from the Institut de Cardiologie de Montreal (ICM), the valve was divided into three distinct parts corresponding to the portions of the device described earlier. When implanted correctly, the lower part of the frame (i.e., Area 1) is in contact with the left ventricular outflow tract and native aortic valve leaflets; the mid part of the frame is constrained

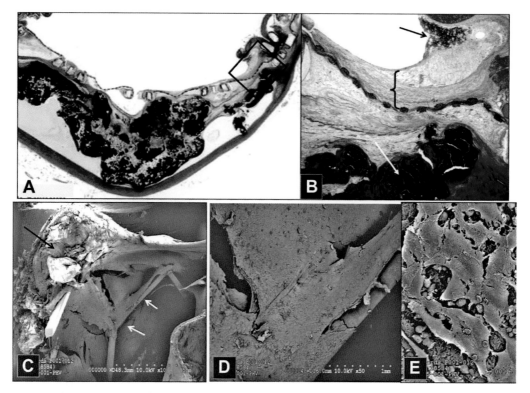

Figure 10 (Edwards Case #5 in Table 1.) (**A**) Mid-section of the valve assembly showing an intact valve frame (*boxed area*) with early neointimal covering of the fabric. Outside prosthetic valve assembly is the native heavily calcified valve. (**B**) The boxed area is magnified to show the area between the valve and the fabric is covered by neointimal tissue and is partially endothelialized the black arrow points to fibrin, and the white arrow shows the native heavily calcified valve adherent to the fabric. (**C**) Scanning electron microscopic images of the stent frame showing early coverage of the stent by neointima and focal adherent inflammatory cells. The black arrow points to the native calcified valve. The area between the white arrows is shown in (**D**) at higher magnification with adherent white cells and focal endothelialization better seen in (**E**) at higher magnification.

at the level of the coronary arteries and houses the prosthetic valve leaflets (i.e., Area 2); and the upper part of the frame sits in the ascending (i.e., Area 3) (Fig. 11). Sections were taken from the various regions including the valve leaflets and stained with H&E (hematoxylin and eosin) and Movat pentachrome stains. Two of the valves were processed in plastic including the nitinol frame with attached surrounding tissue and stained with toluidine blue and basic fuchsin.

ICM Case 1
An 85-year-old woman had a procedure-related death. Prosthetic valve placement was complicated 30 minutes following completion of the procedure by cardiac tamponade and arrest.

Table 2 Retrieved Valves (CoreValve)

Case #	Length of implantation (days)	Sex	Age (yr)	Valve generation	EuroSCORE (%)	Report from
1	3	Female	85	18 F	18.81	ICM
2	4	Male	85	21 F	69.00	
3	13	Male	77	18 F × 2	28.83	
4	104	Female	81	21 F	16.56	
5	350	Male	85	21 F	45.56	
6	425	Female	80	Unknown	7.08	Lepzig

Abbreviation: ICM, Institut de Cardiologie de Montreal.

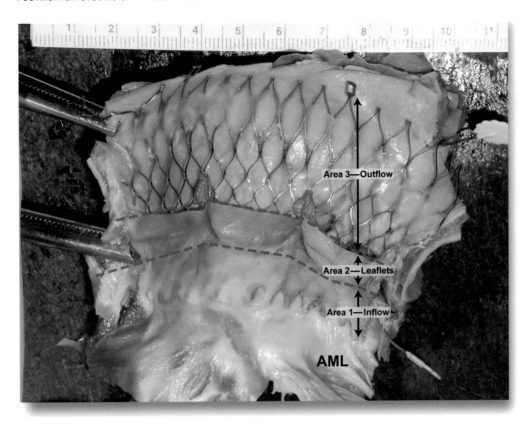

Figure 11 Heart opened along the left ventricular outflow showing CoreValve prosthesis in situ. The valve assembly is divided into three regions: Area 1—Inflow portion of the prosthesis that is typically in contact with the left ventricular outflow tract and native aortic valve leaflets; Area 2—Mid-portion of the prosthesis housing the porcine pericardial leaflets (*between red lines*); Area 3—Outflow portion of the prosthesis typically is seated in the ascending aorta. *Abbreviation*: AML, anterior mitral leaflet.

After emergency pericardiocentesis at bedside, the patient was rushed to the operating room where a perforation was identified in the aortic root close to the left main coronary takeoff. The patient died of multiorgan failure on the third day. On gross examination (Fig. 12), a thin layer of dull white endocardial tissue was seen on the interior surface of the device in Area 1 where the prosthesis was in close contact with the native valve. The prosthetic leaflets were fully functional. There was no tissue seen in the proximal portion of the prosthesis in Area 3. Small pieces of white dull tissue were visible on the inner surface, near the valve suture areas, on the frame. Microscopic examination revealed platelets, leucocytes, and fibrin (Fig. 12) with interspersed red cells surrounding Area 1 on the pericardial wrap of the valve frame.

ICM Case 2
An 85-year-old man underwent TAVI after consideration of comorbidities that included a recent myocardial infarction, left ventricular systolic dysfunction, type 2 diabetes, hypertension, hyperlipidemia, chronic obstructive pulmonary disease (COPD), and peripheral vascular disease. Furthermore, he had a 90% stenosis of the right internal carotid artery (15). Preoperative echocardiography revealed a calcified aortic valve with an Area of 0.4 cm^2 and a mean gradient of 41 mm Hg, consistent with severe aortic stenosis. The left ventricular ejection fraction was 35%. There was a Grade 2 mitral regurgitation and a Grade 3 tricuspid regurgitation. An angiogram of the descending aorta and iliac arteries revealed a calcified focal proximal left external iliac artery stenosis. To minimize difficulties with delivery catheter advancement, intervention first began with a left external iliac artery angioplasty. A 7 mm × 4 cm Powerflex balloon (Cordis Corp., Miami, FL) was inflated twice initially at 1 atm and then 2 atm.

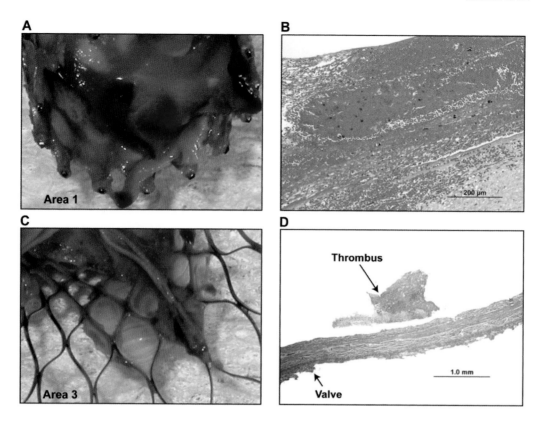

Figure 12 (CoreValve ICM Case #2.) (**A**) Area 1 shows a thin layer of white film, likely representing fibrin rich thrombus. (**C**) Area 3 shows the thin film covering focal areas of the frame. (**B**) and (**D**) are histologic sections taken from (**A**) and (**C**), respectively. (**B**) Focal presence of fibrin thrombus with interspersed red cells. (**D**) Prosthetic valve leaflet (*small arrow*) with a focal area of surface thrombus (*thin arrow*).

Following a reasonable increment in the diameter of this artery, the aortic valve intervention was performed under right femoro-femoral cardiopulmonary bypass (as it was recommended in early 2006) and angiographic guidance. A postimplantation angiogram was obtained, which demonstrated adequate positioning of the device. Transesophageal echocardiography (TEE) demonstrated a mean gradient of 8 mm Hg, and two areas of trace paravalvular leakage. The aortic valve area was 1.2 cm². The left ventricular ejection fraction was 30%. There was grade 1 mitral regurgitation. A 1.5 cm × 1.5 cm mobile mass was evident in the left ventricular out-flow tract and was retrieved using a bioptome. The mass appeared to be calcified vascular tissue originating from the left iliac artery. The patient remained unconscious and could not be weaned from ventilation. Clinical and computed tomographic assessments revealed signs of a major right hemispheric cerebral infarction. Postoperative echocardiography confirmed preserved bioprosthetic aortic valve function; however, he died on the fourth postoperative day. Autopsy examination revealed occlusive embolization of the left subclavian artery with material from the left external iliac artery "endarterectomy" site. There was evidence of right cerebral hemispheric infarction and severe aortic atherosclerosis (American Heart Association Grade VI). Cardiomegaly was evident (heart weight: 700 g) and was attributed to concentric left ventricular hypertrophy. The aortic valve prosthesis was well positioned within the axes of the left ventricular outflow tract and aortic root and the left and right coronary artery ostia were unobstructed. The self-expanding frame of the bioprosthesis had adapted itself cleanly to the geometry of the calcified annulus (Figs. 13 and 14).

ICM Case 3

A 77-year-old man had a first CoreValve prosthesis implanted too low, which resulted in an unacceptable aortic regurgitation (AR). To correct this AR, implantation of a second CoreValve

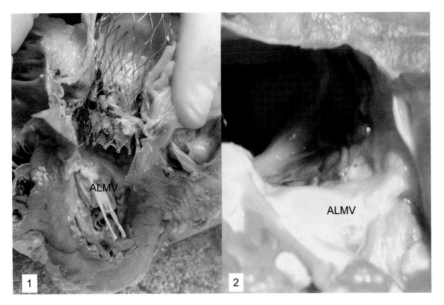

Figure 13 (CoreValve ICM Case #2.) Views of the CoreValve bioprosthesis in position. *Abbreviation*: ALMV, anterior leaflet of the mitral valve. (1) and (2) relation with the mitral valve.

prosthesis (prosthesis in prosthesis) was performed as a bail out. Transthoracic echocardiographic assessment at day 9 showed a reduction of mean gradient from 40 to 16 mm Hg and improvement of aortic valve area from 0.9 to 1.3 cm^2. Nevertheless, this patient who had previously been operated for coronary artery bypass grafts (CABG) died of cardiac failure in the context of a preexisting severe mitral regurgitation worsened by recent subendocardial anteroseptal myocardial infarction involving the anterior papillary muscle.

On gross evaluation (Figs. 15 and 16), two valves were present, one inside the other without local complication. In Area 1, white dull tissue was visible on the interior surface covering both prostheses. The first implant was placed too low in the outflow tract without any impedance of the anterior mitral leaflet; however, the valve was not well apposed to the outflow wall of the left ventricle. In Area 2, the second valve was functional with mild white dull tissue present in the aortic sinus. In Area 3, the interior surface of the frame was also covered by white dull tissue. Interestingly, both areas in close contact with the aortic and ventricular walls were covered by the same tissue, and no thrombus was observed in the area of blood flow toward the coronary ostia, whereas over the closed saphenous vein bypass graft a white dull tissue was observed on the frame of the valve (Fig. 16).

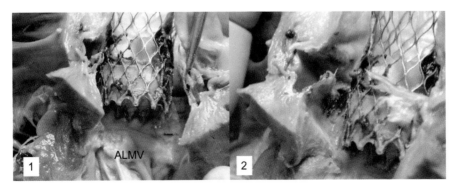

Figure 14 (CoreValve ICM Case #2.) Views of the CoreValve bioprosthesis in position. Relation with the native aortic leaflet: (1) The left anterior leaflet; (2) Magnification of the right anterior leaflet.

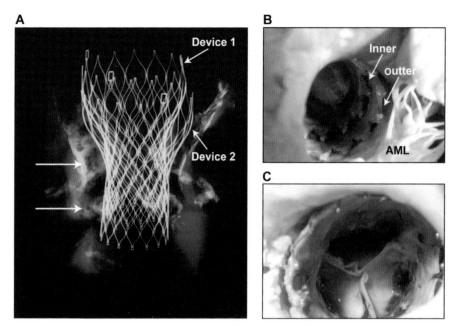

Figure 15 (CoreValve ICM Case #3.) (**A**). Radiograph of the aortic root with double valve implant in place for 13 days. The radiograph shows heavy calcification at the level of the native valves (*arrows*) and along the aortic wall (*arrows*). (**B**) and (**C**) Gross examination of the heart from the left ventricular outflow tract and ascending aorta, respectively. In (**B**), the double valve implantation can be appreciated with mild thrombus on the surface of the prosthetic valve. In (**C**), mild red thrombus can be appreciated near the leaflet attachment sites (*arrow*).

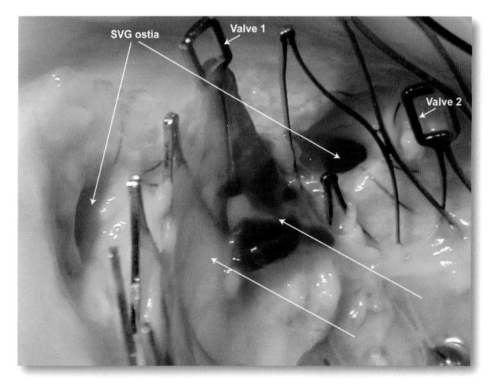

Figure 16 (CoreValve ICM Case #3.) Gross examination of the ascending aorta and Area 3 of the CoreValve prosthesis (labeled Valve 1 and Valve 2). Note that the ostia of the saphenous vein bypass grafts (SVG) are patent. The CoreValve frame in contact with the aortic wall is covered by fibrin and thrombus (*arrows*).

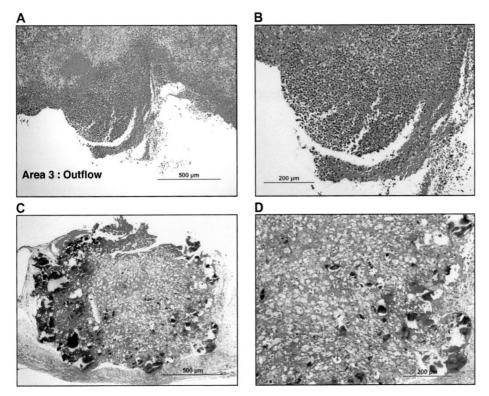

Figure 17 (CoreValve ICM Case #3.) (**A** and **B**) Histologic sections demonstrating thrombus formation (composed of red blood cells, fibrin, and inflammatory cells) over the struts in Area 3. (**C** and **D**) Calcified debris trapped between the device and the outflow tract in Area 3. In addition, there are surrounding foamy macrophages and occasional giant cells embedded in a fibrin and red cell rich matrix (Area 3) (**C** and **D**).

Microscopic assessment (Fig. 17) of the dull white intimal tissue revealed fibrin intermingled with acute inflammatory cells as well as red blood cells and platelets in Areas 1 and 3. In Area 1, underneath the device and in the outflow tract a focal area composed of fibrin and red cell rich matrix with calcification was identified. There were focal foamy macrophages and occasional giant cells noted.

ICM Case 4

An 81-year-old woman with moderate to severe mitral regurgitation prior to TAVI had been found dead in her bed 104 days postprocedure. On visual inspection (Fig. 18), struts in Area 1 were completely covered by a smooth glistening endocardial white tissue. The leaflets (Area 2) were fully functional. In Area 3, white intimal tissue was covering the distal spikes of the device only at areas, which were in contact with the aortic wall. Portions of Area 3 not in contact with the aortic wall were free of tissue coverage and allowed normal blood flow into the coronary ostia.

On microscopic examination of Area 1 (Fig. 19), the endocardial surface of the native aortic valve was covered by smooth muscle cells (SMCs) in a proteoglycan matrix that extended to cover the pericardial skirt of the prosthesis and spread to the basal portion of the valve leaflets in Area 2. A few inflammatory cells were identified including macrophages, lymphocytes, and giant cells (Fig. 19). Also, an area of foreign body giant cell reaction was seen where cotton fibers got deposited likely due to manipulation of the CoreValve device during manual loading. In Area 3, there was neointimal tissue growth surrounding the frame struts that were in contact with the underlying aortic wall.

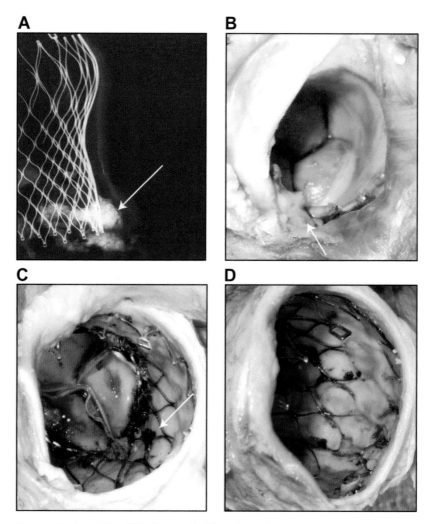

Figure 18 (CoreValve ICM Case #4.) (**A**) Radiograph and gross photographs of the CoreValve implant at 104 days. The radiograph of the aortic root with prosthetic valve assembly shows heavy calcification at the level of the native valves and along the aortic wall (*arrow*). (**B**). Gross photographs show struts in Area 1 completely covered by tissue and a calcified area inferior to the device is visible (*arrow*). Areas 2 (**C**) and 3 (**D**) show focal thrombus deposition on the inner surface of the frame (arrow in **C**).

ICM Case 5

An 85-year-old man with history of coronary artery bypass grafts to the left anterior descending (LAD) and posterior descending artery (PDA) performed eight years prior to presentation with progressive aortic valve stenosis died 350 days after CoreValve implantation in the context of renal failure and respiratory distress.

The autopsy revealed a well-functioning bioprosthetic valve and underlying massive cardiac amyloidosis of the heart. A transthoracic echocardiography assessment at 326 days showed a mean gradient of 15 mm Hg (43 mm Hg at baseline, 9 mm Hg at six months) and an aortic valvular area of 1.2 cm^2 (0.7 cm^2 at baseline, 1.6 cm^2 at six months).

By gross examination (Fig. 20), the frame struts and pericardial skirt of the valve from zone 1 were completely covered by a glistening white endocardial tissue. In Area 2, the endocardial white tissue was seen creeping over the valve sinus, both over the ventricular and aortic side. The left internal mammary artery (LIMA) to the LAD was patent and severe left proximal calcific coronary artery disease was also noted. In Area 3, the frame struts in contact with the aortic wall were totally covered by intimal glistening white tissue, but the upper and lower portion of the frame not in contact with the vessel wall remained totally bare (Fig. 20).

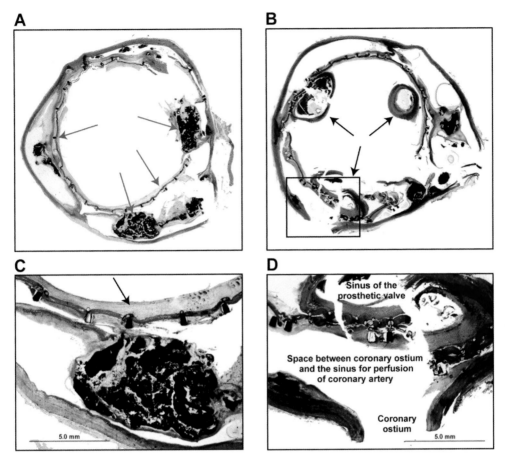

Figure 19 (CoreValve ICM Case #4.) Histologic transverse sections of the aorta with the prosthetic valve in situ. In (**A**) the native leaflets are heavily calcified (*green arrows*) and are excluded by the stent frame (*red arrows*). In (**C**) at higher magnification the calcified native leaflet is seen with neointima incorporating the stent frame (*arrow*). In (**D**) the boxed area of the coronary ostium from (**B**) is highlighting the space between the prosthesis and ostium through which coronary blood flow occurs.

Microscopic examination revealed the glistening white tissue to consist of SMCs within a proteoglycan collagenous matrix and covered by endothelium (Fig. 21). In Area 1, there were no signs of inflammation and the surrounding cardiac myocytes were focally separated and surrounded by amyloid deposits, consistent with senile amyloidosis (Fig. 21). In Area 2, on both sides of the prosthetic porcine pericardial leaflets there was presence of pannus, which consisted of SMCs in a proteoglycan-collagenous matrix (Fig. 22). Organizing granulation tissue was also observed focally around the struts of the frame (Fig. 22).

Lepzig Case (16)

An 80-year-old woman was admitted for shortness of breath (New York Heart Association Grade III) and stable angina pectoris (Canadian Cardiovascular Society [CCS] Grade II). Two years ago, the patient had a posterior wall infarction successfully treated by percutaneous coronary intervention and stent implantation. A low-gradient aortic stenosis with an aortic valve area of 1.1 cm^2 was also diagnosed but was considered to be clinically insignificant at the time. Because of the progression of symptoms within the last two years, a re-evaluation of coronary and aortic valve disease was performed. Coronary angiography revealed a one-vessel coronary disease with a patent stent in the right coronary artery without any evidence of restenosis. The left ventricular ejection fraction was only moderately impaired (55%). However, the aortic valve area, as determined invasively, had decreased to 0.5 cm^2. This was confirmed

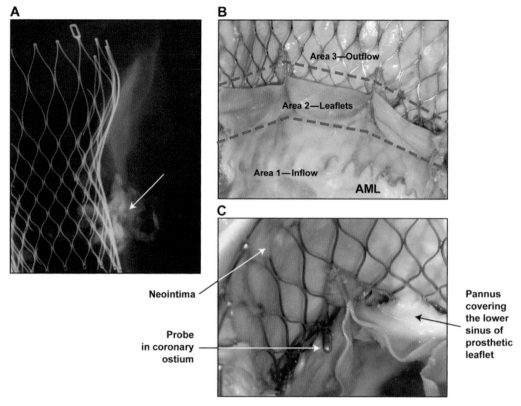

Figure 20 (CoreValve ICM Case #5.) Radiograph and gross photographs of the valve explanted at 350 days from the patient with senile amyloidosis. (**A**) The radiograph of aortic root with prosthetic valve assembly shows heavy calcification at the level of the native valves and along the aortic wall (*arrow*). (**B**) Gross photograph showing the three areas of the valve and pannus growth extending into the base of the prosthetic leaflets. (**C**) Higher magnification of the prosthetic valve and the metal frame. Patency of the coronary ostium is demonstrated using a probe (*arrow*). Pannus growth is seen in the prosthetic valve sinus near the ostium of the coronary artery (*arrow*). The CoreValve frame in Area 3 is covered by neointima (*arrow*). *Abbreviation*: AML, anterior mitral leaflet.

by echocardiography; the cusps of the aortic valve were calcified and their motion was impaired. Since the patient was anxious and refused conventional aortic valve replacement, percutaneous treatment of the aortic stenosis using the second generation of the CoreValve ReValving system) was proposed. As recommended at the time, under general anesthesia and extracorporeal circulatory support, a valvuloplasty was performed, followed by successful CoreValve implantation via a transfemoral access.

The patient was extubated the same day, recovered quickly after the procedure, and left the hospital 10 days later. At one-year follow-up, the mean gradient across the valve was 3 mm Hg, the aortic valve area was 1.7 cm^2, and there was no evidence of paravalvular leak. These changes in hemodynamics were accompanied by an improvement in symptoms in this patient. Unfortunately, the patient committed suicide 425 days after implantation.

The calcified native valve was pushed aside by the CoreValve frame, and neither the native cusps nor the implanted bioprosthesis had any interference with the coronaries. The bioprosthetic valve did not show any signs of morphological deterioration at autopsy. The lower part of the stent, which was covered by porcine pericardium and positioned in the left ventricular outflow tract, was completely enclosed by myofibroblasts. The ingrowths of the stent in the left ventricular outflow tract might explain why paravalvular leaks that are evident immediately after implantation disappear over time. Conversely, in the ascending aorta, only those struts of the frame that had close contact to the aortic wall were covered by endothelium. All other parts of the frame, in particular the struts at the top, which extended into the aorta, had a surface without discoloration. The Lepzig group postulate despite the high flow velocity

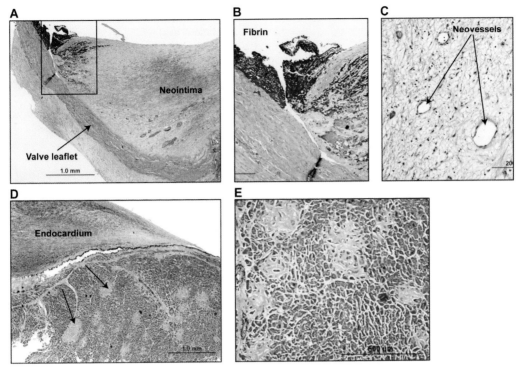

Figure 21 (CoreValve ICM Case #5.) (**A**). Prosthetic leaflets showing organized neointimal pannus growth covering both surfaces of the leaflet in the area of the commissures. (**B** and **C**) Higher magnifications of the boxed area from (**A**) and demonstrate organizing thrombus and neovascularization of the pannus, respectively. (**D** and **E**) Histologic sections of the myocardium taken from the left ventricular outflow tract showing endocardial thickening and focal infiltration of the myocardium by amyloid deposits (*arrows*).

in the aorta, these nonendothelialized and noncovered parts of the nitinol frame might be a place of origin for thrombi formation and thromboembolic events. Therefore, platelet inhibition for one year after CoreValve implantation might be considered.

Interpretation of Human Cases

The gross and microscopic examination of these explanted CoreValve prostheses at different time intervals provides insight into the pathological changes that may occur serially over time.

It appeared that the self-expanding frame of the CoreValve prosthesis, especially the inflow portion, conforms to noncircular local anatomies. The mid-portion of the frame being constrained was adequate distance from the coronary arteries to maintain their patency.

Gross examinations revealed neointimal tissue coverage in areas of the frame in contact with the aortic wall. Areas not in contact with the aortic wall or areas in the vicinity of high-velocity blood flow (i.e., patent SVG or native coronary ostia) did not show coverage by neointimal tissue. Neointimal growth was also visualized at the base of the prosthetic valve leaflets in the one patient with senile amyloidosis. It is possible that amyloidosis could have enhanced tissue proliferation in this patient. Nevertheless, in comparison with most surgical bioprosthesis, which are protected by a ring that mitigates tissue invasion, transcatheter heart valve leaflets simply sutured on a frame may be more vulnerable to neointimal growth invasion.

The histologic changes that may take place over time after implantation of the CoreValve prosthesis include the following: (*i*) the valve incorporation process starts with early fibrin deposition associated with an inflammatory response and some foreign body reaction. (*ii*) At approximately three months after implantation, fibrin deposition is replaced by smooth muscle cells (i.e., neointimal response). Focal areas of endothelialization and some residual inflammatory cells can be observed. (*iii*) After this time, neointimal tissue becomes less cellular but more fibrotic as proteoglycans and type III collagen get replaced with type I collagen.

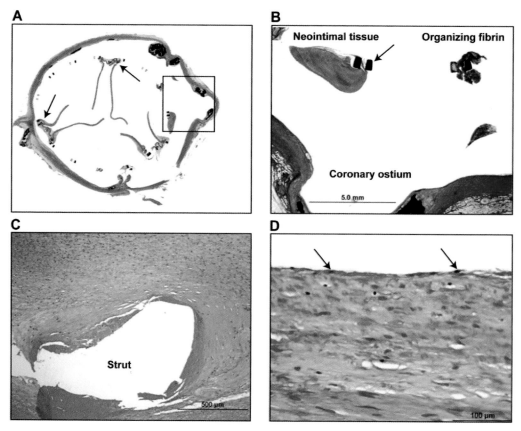

Figure 22 (CoreValve ICM Case #5.) (**A**) Transverse section of the aorta and valve assembly from the 350-day implant at the level of the prosthetic leaflet commissures (*arrows*). (**B**). High-power view of the boxed area showing patent coronary ostium and sinus space between stent frame (*arrow*) and ostium. Note the fibrin deposition and neointimal tissue growth around the stent frame focally. (**C**) From Area 3, a high-power view around the stent frame showing neointimal tissue consisting of smooth muscle cells in a proteoglycan collagen matrix. (**D**) High-power magnification of the neointima around the stent frame showing coverage of the neointima by endothelial cells (*arrows*).

In the majority of patients, in vivo examinations showed only trace to mild paravalvular regurgitation. In one patient (ICM case #3) in whom the valve was implanted too low, a second valve implantation (i.e., valve-in-valve) was required to mitigate the severe aortic regurgitation. Gross inspection confirmed the integrity of the anterior mitral valve leaflet even in the presence of an extremely low lying prosthesis. This observation further enforce the significant anatomic distance between the basal attachment points of the aortic valve leaflets and the hinge point of the anterior mitral valve leaflet.

In all these cases, and particularly in the two valves explanted at more than 350 days, the nitinol frame was intact with no fracture. Device fractures after percutaneous pulmonary valve replacement (Medtronic inc., Melody valve) have been reported to occur most commonly in the first 400 days after implantation (17% rate of platinum–iridium stent fracture) (17).

As a result of the information gleaned from these six postmortem studies of the CoreValve ReValving system, it appears that clopidogrel should be prescribed for *at least* three months after implantation during which time the prosthesis is "incorporated" within the aortic wall. Thereafter, when neointimal tissue growth and endothelialization have occurred, it should be theoretically safe to discontinue clopidogrel. Aspirin should be continued indefinitely.

CONCLUSION

At the time of this writing, structural failure of a transcatheter heart valve has not been reported—the question is not "if" it will occur but "when" and "how" will it occur. In this series of postmortem studies, observations such as cuspal tears, pannus invasion into the base of the prosthetic valve leaflets, and microthrombi visualized on the prosthetic valve leaflets are reminiscent of what has already been reported after postmortem studies of surgically implanted bioprosthetic valves. The cohort of patients currently undergoing TAVI (mean age ~82 years, high risk or inoperable) may not allow us to meaningfully understand the durability of these valves.

REFERENCES

1. Young ST, Lin SL. A possible relation between pressure loading and thickened leaflets of the aortic valve: A model simulation. Med Eng Phys 1994; 16(6):465–469.
2. Isner JM, Chokshi SK, DeFranco A, et al. Contrasting histoarchitecture of calcified leaflets from stenotic bicuspid versus stenotic tricuspid aortic valves. J Am Coll Cardiol 1990; 15(5):1104–1108.
3. Vollebergh FE, Becker AE. Minor congenital variations of cusp size in tricuspid aortic valves. Possible link with isolated aortic stenosis. Br Heart J 1977; 39(9):1006–1011.
4. Roberts WC. The structure of the aortic valve in clinically isolated aortic stenosis: An autopsy study of 162 patients over 15 years of age. Circulation 1970; 42(1):91–97.
5. Wilmshurst PT, Stevenson RN, Griffiths H, et al. A case-control investigation of the relation between hyperlipidaemia and calcific aortic valve stenosis. Heart 1997; 78(5):475–479.
6. Wierzbicki A, Shetty C. Aortic stenosis: An atherosclerotic disease? J Heart Valve Dis 1999; 8(4):416–423.
7. Dare AJ, Veinot JP, Edwards WD, et al. New observations on the etiology of aortic valve disease: A surgical pathologic study of 236 cases from 1990. Hum Pathol 1993; 24(12):1330–1338.
8. Webb JG, Lichtenstein S. Transcatheter percutaneous and transapical aortic valve replacement. Semin Thorac Cardiovasc Surg 2007; 19(4):304–310.
9. Cribier A, Eltchaninoff H, Bash A, et al. Percutaneous transcatheter implantation of an aortic valve prosthesis for calcific aortic stenosis: First human case description. Circulation 2002; 106(24):3006–3008.
10. Eltchaninoff H, Avadis-Nusimovici D, Baraliaros V, et al. Five month study of percutaneous heart valves in the systemic circulation of sheep using a novel model of aortic insufficiency. Eurointervention 2006; 1:438–444.
11. Boudjemline Y, Bonhoeffer P. Percutaneous implantation of a valve in the descending aorta in lambs. Eur Heart J 2002; 23(13):1045–1049.
12. Hufnagel CA. Surgical correction of aortic insufficiency. Mod Concepts Cardiovasc Dis 1955; 24(8):287–289.
13. Grube E, Schuler G, Buellesfeld L, et al. Percutaneous aortic valve replacement for severe aortic stenosis in high-risk patients using the second- and current third-generation self-expanding CoreValve prosthesis: Device success and 30-day clinical outcome. J Am Coll Cardiol 2007; 50(1):69–76.
14. Laborde JC, Grube E, Tixier D, et al. The CoreValve in the aortic position. In: Hijazi ZM, Bonhoeffer P, Feldman T, Ruiz CE, eds. Transcatheter Valve Repair. London: Taylor & Francis, 2006;175–186.
15. Berry C, Cartier R, Bonan R. Fatal ischemic stroke related to nonpermissive peripheral artery access for percutaneous aortic valve replacement. Catheter Cardiovasc Interv 2007; 69(1):56–63.
16. Linke A, Ilriegel R, Walther T, et al. Ingrowths of a percutaneously implanted aortic valve prosthesis (CoreValve) in a patient with severe aortic stenosis. Circ Cariovasc Interv 2008; 1:155–158.
17. Nordmeyer J, Khambadkone S, Coats L, et al. Risk stratification, systematic classification, and anticipatory management strategies for stent fracture after percutaneous pulmonary valve implantation. Circulation 2007; 115(11):1392–1397.
18. Webb JG, Chandavimol M, Thompson CR, et al. Circulation 2006; 113:842–850.

3 | Imaging—How Can It Help Before Transcatheter Aortic Valve Implantation?

Victoria Delgado, Laurens F. Tops, Frank van der Kley, Joanne D. Schuijf, Martin J. Schalij, and Jeroen J. Bax

Department of Cardiology, Leiden University Medical Center, Leiden, The Netherlands

INTRODUCTION

Transcatheter aortic valve implantation has been one of the main breakthroughs in the previous years for the treatment of patients with severe, symptomatic aortic stenosis at high risk or with contraindications for surgery. First experiences have demonstrated that, using either self-expandable or balloon-expandable valvular prostheses, transcatheter aortic valve implantation constitutes a feasible procedure and provides hemodynamic and clinical improvement with an acceptable procedure-related complication rate, given the high-risk characteristics of the patients (1–5). Future advances in devices profile will reduce the number of complications such as vascular injury, stroke or prosthesis malpositioning, or misdeployment with subsequent aortic regurgitation. Despite these technical issues, appropriate patient selection still constitutes the main determinant of procedural success. A multidisciplinary team comprising cardiologists, cardiovascular surgeons, imaging specialists, and anesthesiologists is recommended to select potential candidates for transcatheter aortic valve implantation. In the selection of candidates, confirmation of the aortic stenosis severity, evaluation of symptoms, life expectancy, and quality of life as well as risk of surgery together with the assessment of the feasibility of transcatheter aortic valve implantation should be considered.

Particularly, estimation of aortic stenosis severity, evaluation of the aorta, and surrounding structures and assessment of the ilio-femoral arterial system determine the inclusion/exclusion criteria for transcatheter aortic valve implantation and have important implications for pre-procedural planning of access approach (transfemoral or transapical) and valve sizing. In this regard, current imaging modalities, including echocardiography, multislice computed tomography (MSCT), and magnetic resonance imaging (MRI) enable the evaluation of the aortic valve morphology, severity of aortic stenosis, and anatomy of the aorta and ilio-femoral arterial system together with left ventricular dimensions and function.

This chapter provides a comprehensive overview on the role of current imaging techniques for evaluation of patients with severe aortic stenosis before transcatheter aortic valve implantation. Table 1 summarizes the key steps in the selection of patients and the role of echocardiography, MSCT, and MRI.

ECHOCARDIOGRAPHY

Qualitative diagnosis and assessment of aortic stenosis severity rely mostly on echocardiographic imaging techniques. Two-dimensional echocardiography enables the assessment of aortic valve anatomy (tricuspid/bicuspid) and function by direct visualization of the restrictive motion of one or more cusps. However, accurate estimation of aortic valve stenosis severity requires Doppler methodology. Assessment of aortic valve morphology and aortic stenosis severity is crucial before transcatheter aortic valve implantation. Only those patients with symptomatic severe aortic stenosis will be candidates for this procedure according to current recommendations (6). Furthermore, a bicuspid aortic valve may determine a prosthesis misdeployment, more elliptical rather than circular (7). In addition, echocardiography enables the assessment of left ventricular function and the evaluation of concomitant aortic regurgitation or mitral valve disease. Therefore, echocardiography and its different methodologies play a central role in the evaluation of patients before transcatheter aortic valve implantation.

Table 1 Selection of Patients for Transcatheter Aortic Valve Implantation: Role of Imaging

	TTE	TEE	MSCT	MRI
Aortic stenosis severity	+	+	+	+
Aortic valve morphology				
Tricuspid/bicuspid	+	+	+	+
Valvular calcifications	±	±	+	−
Aortic root and ascending aorta				
Aortic annulus diameter	+	+	+	+
Sinus of Valsalva and sinotubular junction diameters	+	+	+	+
Ascending aorta diameter	±	+	+	+
Ascending aorta angulation	−	−	+	+
Coronary ostia location	−	−	+	+
Coronary artery disease	−	−	+	+
Left ventricle				
Left ventricular dimensions and function	+	+	+	+
Intracavitary thrombus	+	+	+	+
Peripheral arteries and aorta				
Tortuosity	−	−	+	+
Atheromatosis	−	−	+	+
Bulky calcifications and porcelain aorta	−	−	+	−

Abbreviations: MRI, magnetic resonance imaging; MSCT, multislice computed tomography; TEE, transesophageal echocardiography; TTE, transthoracic echocardiography.

Aortic Valve Morphology

Prior to transcatheter aortic valve implantation, it is extremely important to determine the aortic valve anatomy and morphology, comprising the extent and location of calcifications. Transthoracic echocardiography can easily detect bicuspid aortic valve anatomy. In diastole, from the parasternal short-axis view, a normal tricuspid valve shows the typical "Y-closure" of the three cusps [Fig. 1(A)] whereas the bicuspid valve shows two cusps, with two sinuses and a single linear commissure [Fig. 1(B)]. Sometimes, a raphe may be present and, in heavily calcified aortic valves, commissural fusion is frequent, making the differentiation between bicuspid or tricuspid challenging. In systole, the presence of three different sinuses will help to define the aortic valve morphology. In those cases where the acoustic window does not permit adequate visualization of the aortic valve, transesophageal echocardiography will define aortic valve morphology [Fig. 1(C) and (D)]. The presence of a bicuspid valve has been proposed as contraindication for this procedure (6). However, few series have demonstrated that transcatheter aortic valve implantation may be feasible in this sort of valve morphology, although incomplete deployment may occur (7,8). Recently, Zegdi et al. (7) described a series of 16 severe aortic stenosis patients with bicuspid valves, undergoing transcatheter aortic valve implantation. In all patients a self-expandable prosthesis was used and in the majority of patients, a noncircular misdeployment of the stent was observed (7).

Strongly related to aging, calcification of aortic valve is a common finding in elderly patients with severe aortic stenosis deemed not suitable for surgical aortic valve replacement. The extent and location of calcifications may determine procedural success (7). Bulky calcifications located along the leaflets or at the commissures may hamper the anchorage and deployment of the device frame and eventually may lead to a life-threatening complication such as occlusion of coronary ostia (9). Nevertheless, the evaluation of extent and location of aortic valve calcifications will be covered more extensively in the MSCT section, the ideal imaging modality for this purpose.

Aortic Stenosis Severity

Current American College of Cardiology/American Heart Association guidelines consider several hemodynamic parameters to define aortic stenosis severity: maximum aortic velocity, mean transvalvular pressure gradient and continuity equation-derived valve area (10). These parameters can be obtained with Doppler echocardiography. An accurate estimation of aortic stenosis requires proper recording of the maximal jet velocity through the stenotic orifice, the

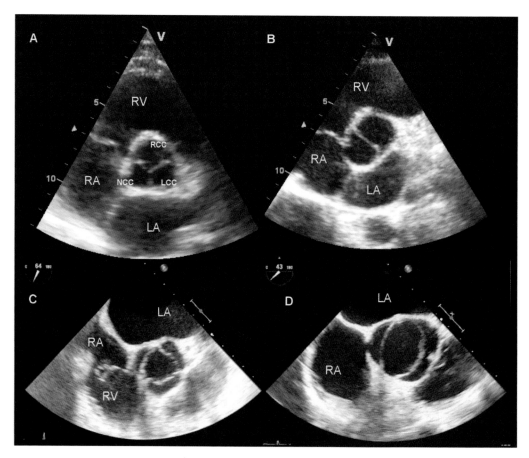

Figure 1 Echocardiography: evaluation of aortic valve morphology. Examples of tricuspid (**A**) and bicuspid (**B**) aortic valves imaged with transthoracic echocardiography. From the parasternal short-axis view, normal tricuspid aortic valve shows in diastole the typical "Y-closure" with the left, right and noncoronary cusps. In contrast, the bicuspid aortic valve shows only two cusps, two sinuses, and a single commissure. With transesophageal echocardiography, the aortic valve morphology can be clearly defined: in systole, normal tricuspid valve shows three different sinuses (**C**) whereas the bicuspid valve shows only two sinuses (**D**). *Abbreviations*: LA, left atrium; LCC, left coronary cusp; NCC, non-coronary cusp; RA, right atrium; RV, right ventricle.

most reproducible measurement and the strongest predictor of clinical outcome (11). From the transthoracic long-axis apical view, the Doppler ultrasound beam can be aligned with the direction of the blood flow through the stenotic orifice. Color Doppler imaging can be helpful to achieve an adequate alignment. From the continuous wave Doppler recording, maximal velocity can be measured (Fig. 2) and, based on the simplified Bernoulli equation, the maximum transaortic pressure gradient is calculated: $\Delta P_{max} = 4V_{max}^2$ (Fig. 2). The average of the instantaneous gradients over the ejection period results in mean pressure gradient and can be obtained by tracing of the Doppler envelope (Fig. 2).

Finally, to calculate the aortic valve area, the continuity equation is the most utilized method (11). This equation requires measurement of the cross-sectional area of the left ventricular outflow tract, velocity–time integral of the flow at the left ventricular outflow tract and at the stenotic orifice. In practice, velocity–time integrals are substituted by the maximal velocities and, subsequently, the simplified continuity equation results in: $AVA = CSA_{LVOT} \times V_{LVOT}/V_{AS}$ (where AVA is aortic valve area, CSA_{LVOT} is the cross-sectional area of the left ventricular outflow tract, V_{LVOT} is maximal velocity at the left ventricular outflow tract, and V_{AS} is maximal velocity at the aortic valve) (Fig. 2) (11). According to current guidelines, severe aortic stenosis is defined by a jet velocity >4 m/s, a mean pressure gradient >40 mm Hg, or and aortic valve area <1.0 cm^2 (10).

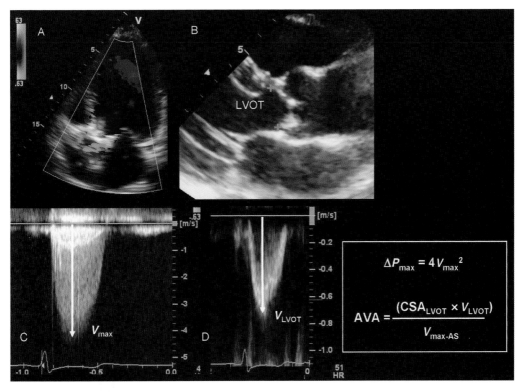

Figure 2 Estimation of aortic valve stenosis severity by Doppler echocardiography. Color Doppler echocardiography helps to align the ultrasound beam with the direction of the blood flow through the stenotic orifice (**A**). To calculate the aortic valve area, the cross-sectional area of the left ventricular outflow tract (**B**), the velocity through the stenotic orifice obtained at the continuous-wave Doppler recordings (**C**) and the velocity through the left ventricular outflow tract obtained at the pulsed-wave Doppler recordings (**D**) are required. In the continuity equation, velocity–time integrals or maximum velocities can be used. *Abbreviations*: ΔP_{max}, maximum transaortic pressure gradient; AS, aortic stenosis; AVA, aortic valve area; CSA, cross-sectional area; LVOT, left ventricular outflow tract; V_{max}, maximum velocity.

Aortic Valve Annulus Sizing

To avoid serious complications as prosthesis migration, and to minimize the risk of significant paravalvular leakage after prosthesis implantation, an accurate assessment of the dimensions of the aortic valve annulus is mandatory. However, there is no established gold standard method to measure the aortic valve annulus. Transthoracic echocardiography is the first approach to estimate the aortic valve annulus diameter. From the parasternal long-axis view, the aortic valve annulus diameter can be measured [Fig. 3(A)]. Similarly, transesophageal echocardiography, from a left ventricular long-axis view (135°) provides an excellent assessment of the left ventricular outflow tract, aortic valve annulus, and aortic root [Fig. 3(B)]. However, transesophageal echocardiography usually yields larger values than transthoracic echocardiography, as previously reported (12,13). Therefore, in controversial cases with borderline values, assessment with transesophageal echocardiography at the catheterization laboratory may help the decision making. Thus far, there are two different percutaneous aortic valves commercially available in two different sizes each: the balloon-expandable prosthesis (Edwards-SAPIEN valve; Edwards Lifesciences Inc., CA) in 23- and 26-mm sizes and the self-expandable prosthesis (CoreValve Revalving System; CoreValve Inc., Irvine, CA) in 26- and 29-mm sizes. Previous experience has shown that the 23-mm balloon-expandable valve is appropriate when the aortic valve annulus dimension ranges between 18 and 22 mm, whereas the 26-mm balloon-expandable valve is preferred in those cases with aortic valve annulus diameter between 21 and 26 mm (13). Concerning the self-expandable prosthesis, the 26-mm device is appropriate for aortic valve annulus size from 20 to 24 mm and the 29 mm prosthesis is more suitable for aortic valve

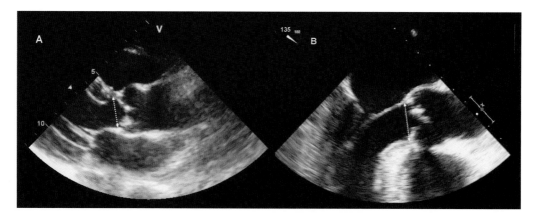

Figure 3 Aortic valve annulus sizing. Parasternal long-axis view on transthoracic echocardiography (**A**) or left ventricular long-axis view (135°) on transesophageal echocardiography (**B**) are the preferred views to assess the aortic annulus sizing (_arrow_), crucial to select the prosthesis size. _Abbreviations_: Ao, aorta; LA, left atrium; LVOT, left ventricular outflow tract.

annulus size from 24 to 27 mm (14). Finally, according to current recommendations (6), transcatheter aortic valve implantation should be contraindicated when the aortic valve annulus size is <18 mm or >25 mm, for balloon-expandable devices, and <20 mm or >27 mm, for self-expandable prosthesis (6).

Left Ventricular Dimensions and Function
In patients with severe aortic stenosis, left ventricular ejection fraction is one of the main determinants of the decision for surgical valve replacement (15). A depressed left ventricular ejection fraction (<30%) increases the operative risk but, in nonoperated patients, determines a poor prognosis (15). A less invasive procedure such as transcatheter aortic valve implantation may constitute a therapeutic option for those patients with severe left ventricular dysfunction. Transthoracic echocardiography is the most available method for left ventricular function evaluation. Left ventricular end-diastolic and end-systolic volumes can be measured by Simpson's rule and left ventricular ejection fraction can be derived (16). This two-dimensional echocardiographic method is the most accurate and reliable to measure left ventricular dimensions and ejection fraction in patients with abnormal left ventricular geometry, common finding in patients with severe aortic stenosis (17).

In addition, left ventricular hypertrophy is a common finding in these patients and a sigmoid septum is frequently observed [Fig. 4(A)] (17). In patients with a pronounced sigmoid septum, the transapical approach could be preferred instead of the transfemoral, because the positioning and anchorage of the prosthesis with the transapical approach may be more stable (6). Finally, one of the contraindications to perform transcatheter aortic valve implantation is the presence of left ventricular thrombus (6). Contrast-enhanced echocardiography constitutes a feasible imaging tool to rule out the presence of intracavitary mass [Fig. 4(B)].

All these evaluations can be noninvasively and easily performed with echocardiography. However, bearing in mind the three-dimensional nature of the aortic valve, measurement of the aortic valve annulus and left ventricular outflow tract size may be subjected to geometrical assumptions and consequent errors in the estimation of disease severity. Indeed, the aortic valve annulus is rather elliptical than circular and similarly, the left ventricular outflow tract may appear more elliptic-shaped, mostly when sigmoid septal hypertrophy exists. Therefore, three-dimensional imaging techniques may constitute more accurate methods to evaluate potential candidates for transcatheter aortic valve implantation. In this regard, initial experimental and clinical studies have demonstrated the higher accuracy of real-time three-dimensional echocardiography to assess aortic stenosis severity as compared to two-dimensional echocardiographic methods (17,18).

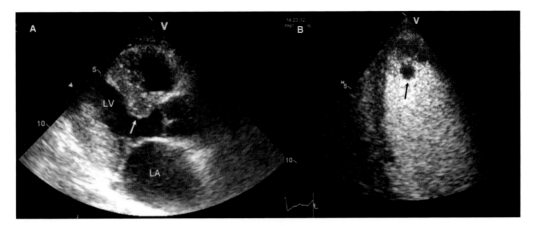

Figure 4 Evaluation of the left ventricle with echocardiography before transcatheter aortic valve implantation. The presence of severe left ventricular hypertrophy with a sigmoid basal septum (*white arrow*) may determine a transapical approach to achieve a more stable anchorage of the prosthesis (**A**). In addition, contrast echocardiography permits to rule out the presence of intracavitary thrombus (**B**, *black arrow*), that contraindicates the transcatheter aortic valve implantation. *Abbreviations*: LA, left atrium; LV, left ventricle.

MULTISLICE COMPUTED TOMOGRAPHY

Multislice computed tomography may be the most comprehensive noninvasive imaging modality to evaluate potential candidates for transcatheter aortic valve replacement. This three-dimensional imaging technique provides accurate information on anatomical aspects of the aortic valve, aortic root and surrounding structures (such as the coronary arteries), aorta, and peripheral arteries. First experiences have demonstrated the high accuracy of this technique to assess aortic valve area by planimetry of the stenotic orifice and furthermore, with the use of multiphase data sets obtained during ECG gating, motion of the cusps can be evaluated (19,20). Finally, left ventricular dimensions and function can be also assessed by using multiphase data sets reconstructed at each 10% of the R–R interval (21). According to current recommendations on patient selection for transcatheter aortic valve implantation (6), MSCT may be a valuable imaging tool for noninvasive confirmation of aortic stenosis severity, assessment of procedural feasibility, and device sizing.

Evaluation of the Peripheral Arteries and Aorta

The feasibility of transcatheter aortic valve implantation, particularly considering the transfemoral approach, depends strongly on the size, calcification, and tortuosity of the ilio-femoral arteries and aorta. Preprocedural angiography is still the imaging technique of reference. However, MSCT provides data on cross-sectional diameter, extent of calcification, and tortuosity along the course of the ilio-femoral arteries and abdominal and thoracic aorta (Fig. 5). Current devices require 18-, 22-, or 24-F introducer sheaths and, subsequently, cross-sectional diameters of the ilio-femoral arteries <6 to 9 mm would contraindicate a transfemoral approach (6). Bulky calcifications and pronounced angulations of the thoracic aorta may recommend a transapical rather than transfemoral approach. Particularly, in severe aortic stenosis patients with porcelain aorta, the transapical approach may constitute the only alternative to perform transcatheter aortic valve implantation, due to the high risk of vascular complications with the transfemoral approach (22). Finally, regardless of the vascular access, severe aortic dilatation at the level of the sinotubular junction (>45 mm) is considered a contraindication for self-expandable prosthesis (6).

Aortic Valve Anatomy, Morphology, and Stenosis Severity

The introduction of 64- and 320-slice MSCT systems has led to improved three-dimensional image quality with shorter scan times. Consequently, MSCT has become a valuable noninvasive imaging tool, enabling the exact depiction of the aortic valve anatomy and morphology. In

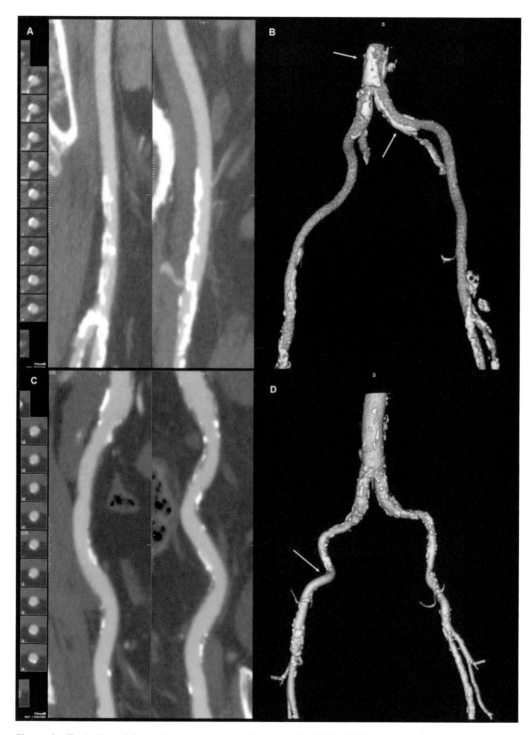

Figure 5 Evaluation of the peripheral arteries and aorta with MSCT. MSCT enables the assessment of the anatomy of the peripheral arteries and aorta. The extent of calcification and cross-sectional diameter can be quantified (**A**). The presence of bulky calcifications (*arrows*, **B**) or extremely tortuous peripheral arteries with sharp angulations (*arrow*, **C and D**) can be detected. These two characteristics may determine a transapical approach rather than transfemoral.

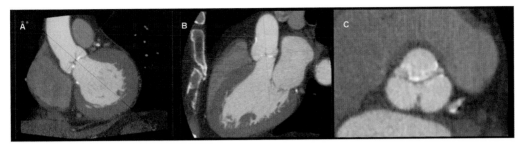

Figure 6 MSCT aortic valve assessment. The reconstruction of a coronal (**A**) and sagittal views (**B**) through the aortic valve and the correct orientation of both views yield the reconstructed double oblique transverse view of the aortic valve (**C**).

patients with a poor acoustic window and contraindications for transesophageal echocardiography (semi-invasive imaging modality), MSCT yields extensive data on aortic valve anatomy and the aortic root.

MSCT data acquisition is usually performed in a single breath-hold of about 5–10 seconds, synchronizing data acquisition with contrast enhancement. Intravenous nonionic contrast agent requirement is typically about 60 to 100 mL, depending on scanner type, patient size, and heart rate. When automated peak enhancement detection reaches +100 Hounsfield units in the descending aorta, data acquisition triggered to the ECG is initiated. Subsequently, retrospective multiphase data sets are reconstructed at each 10% of the R–R interval or at 30% to 35% and 75% after the R wave (systolic and diastolic phase, respectively) with a slice thickness of 0.5 mm and a reconstruction interval of 0.3 mm (23).

The postprocessing and image analysis start with the reconstruction of a coronal and a single oblique sagittal view through the aortic valve [Fig. 6(A) and (B)]. The correct orientation of both views yield the reconstructed double oblique transverse view at the level of the aortic valve [Fig. 6(C)] (23). From this latter view, the exact anatomy of the aortic valve (tricuspid/bicuspid) can be defined (Fig. 7) as well as the extent and location of calcifications: at the edge of the cusps, the commissures, or the joints of the cusps to the aortic wall (Fig. 8). From the coronal and sagittal views, the presence of bulky calcifications can be evaluated (Fig. 8). As mentioned before, these calcifications may pose resistance to the prosthesis deployment, resulting in a

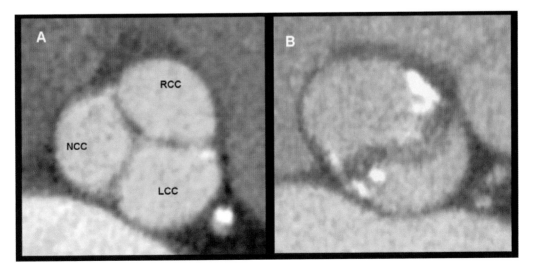

Figure 7 Assessment of aortic valve morphology by using MSCT. The normal tricuspid aortic valve (**A**) shows the three cusps (RCC, LCC,NCC) and the three different sinuses. A bicuspid aortic valve shows only two sinuses and a single commissure (**B**). *Abbreviations*: RCC, right coronary cusp; LCC, left coronary cusp; NCC, noncoronary cusp.

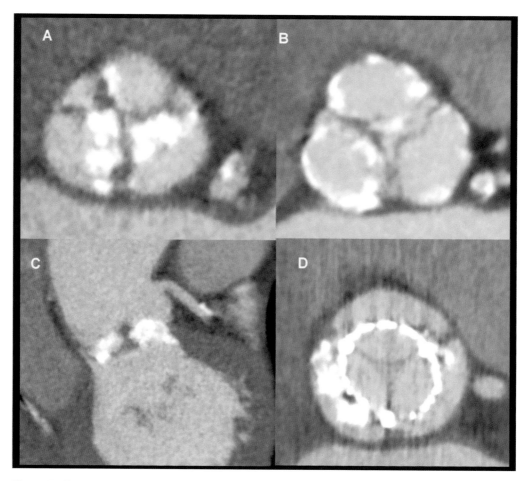

Figure 8 Evaluation of extent and location of aortic valve calcifications with MSCT. Aortic valve calcifications can be visualized at the free edge of the aortic cusps (**A**), at the joint of the cusps with the aortic annulus (**B**). The presence of bulky calcifications (**C**) may determine a noncircular deployment of the prosthesis (**D**).

noncircular deployment (Fig. 8), and may determine the occurrence of infrequent but life-threatening complications, such as occlusion of coronary ostia (9).

In addition, the area of the aortic valve can be estimated from the double oblique transverse view, through the tips of the cusps, reconstructed at the systolic phase. By delineating the edges of the cusps at the maximal systolic valve opening, aortic valve area can be accurately obtained, with high agreement, as compared to transesophageal echocardiography or MRI, and good reproducibility (19,20). In a previous series of 48 patients with aortic valve disease, Pouleur et al. (19) demonstrated that MSCT yielded planimetric aortic valve area measurements comparable to those obtained with transesophageal echocardiography or MRI, without significant bias (0.1 ± 0.3 cm^2 vs. transesophageal echocardiography, $p = 0.21$; 0.0 ± 0.3 cm^2 vs. MRI, $p = 0.99$) (19).

Aortic Annulus Sizing

One of the key points to achieve a successful transcatheter aortic valve implantation is accurate measurement of the aortic annulus. An undersized prosthesis may result in an unstable anchorage of the device, severe aortic regurgitation or device migration. In contrast, a prosthesis size too large may not be able to cross the aortic valve annulus. Three-dimensional imaging techniques such as MSCT enable an accurate evaluation of the shape and size of the aortic annulus. At the double oblique views, the aortic annulus appears as elliptic-shaped rather than circular-shaped, and the diameter obtained from the coronal view is usually larger than the diameter measured at the sagittal view (Fig. 9) (23). The sagittal view on MSCT would correspond to

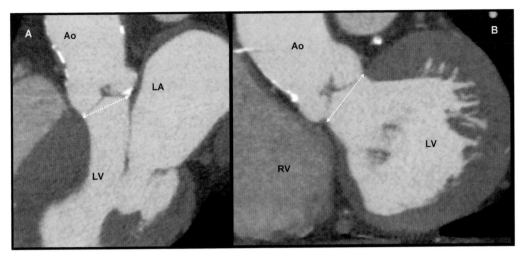

Figure 9 Aortic valve annulus sizing with MSCT. The sagittal view (**A**), that corresponds to the parasternal long-axis view of the echocardiography, usually yields smaller aortic valve annulus diameters than the coronal view (**B**), reflecting the ellipsoid shape of the aortic valve annulus. *Abbreviations*: Ao, aorta; LA, left atrium; LV, left ventricle; RV, right ventricle.

the parasternal long-axis on transthoracic echocardiography and, as previously demonstrated (23,24), both techniques yield comparable annulus sizes with a nonsignificant bias. However, the aortic valve annulus diameter measured at the MSCT coronal view cannot be assessed on two-dimensional echocardiography. Since the prosthesis size used should be the larger where possible, the decision should be based on the largest diameter of the aortic valve annulus and, in this regard, transthoracic echocardiography may be less accurate as compared to MSCT. However, thus far no prospective studies utilizing MSCT measurements to choose the prosthesis size have been performed.

Aortic Root Dimensions and Relation with Coronary Arteries
Similarly to aortic annulus sizing, aortic root dimensions can be measured with MSCT. The dimensions of the sinus of Valsalva may be assessed at the sagittal and coronal views and at the double oblique reconstruction. The particular trefoil shape of the aortic root at the level of the sinuses may have important implications for transcatheter aortic valve implantation (Fig. 10). In this view, three different sinus diameters may be assessed, from the root of the cusp to the contralateral commissure. However, the implication of these measurements in transcatheter aortic valve implantation needs to be elucidated in future studies.

In addition, the sinotubular junction diameter can be measured at the sagittal, coronal and double oblique views, showing often a circular shape. The accurate measurement of the sinotubular junction has serious implications for transcatheter aortic valve implantation. Particularly for self-expandable prosthesis, a diameter of the sinotubular junction >45 mm is considered a contraindication (6). Finally, the presence of transverse aorta may be evaluated. A pronounced angulation of the aortic root and ascending aorta relative to the left ventricle may indicate the transapical implantation of a balloon-expandable device (Fig. 11) (6).

Finally, the evaluation of the coronary arteries is mandatory before transcatheter aortic valve implantation. As previously reported, MSCT provides exact data on coronary anatomy and accurate quantification of coronary artery stenosis when present (25). Recent consensus reached by the European Association of Cardio-Thoracic Surgery, the European Society of Cardiology, and the European Association of Percutaneous Cardiovascular Interventions do not recommend transcatheter aortic valve implantation in those patients with severe proximal coronary artery stenosis not amenable for percutaneous coronary intervention (6). Last but not the least, the relative position of the coronary ostia to the aortic valve annulus and to the length of the aortic cusps should be assessed. Variable distance between the aortic valve annulus and the coronary ostia has been described previously, with a mean distance of 14.4 mm for the left

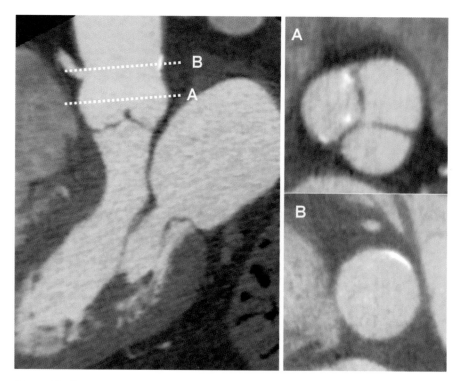

Figure 10 Assessment of aortic root dimensions with MSCT. The dimensions of the sinus of Valsalva (**A**) and sinotubular junction (**B**) can be measured either at the sagittal view or at the double-oblique view.

coronary ostium and 17.2 mm for the right coronary ostium (Fig. 12) (23). The height of the balloon-expandable prosthesis (Edwards-SAPIEN valve) is 14.5 mm and, despite the prosthesis struts that allow blood flow through, its positioning should be under the level of the coronary ostia. Self-expandable prosthesis (CoreValve Revalving System) has a height of 50 mm, but the characteristic design of this device with a waist in the middle part makes unlikely the occlusion

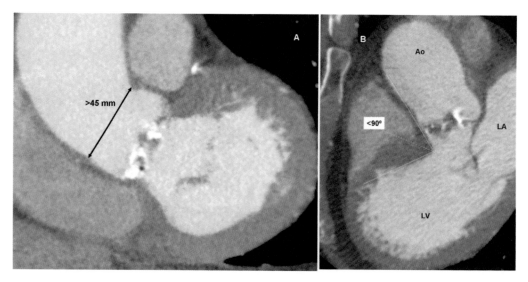

Figure 11 Evaluation of aortic root and ascending aorta by MSCT. The presence of dilated sinotubular junction (>45 mm) contraindicates the implantation of a self-expandable prosthesis (**A**). A transversal aorta, defined by an angle between the aorta and the left ventricle <90° (**B**), may recommend the transapical approach.

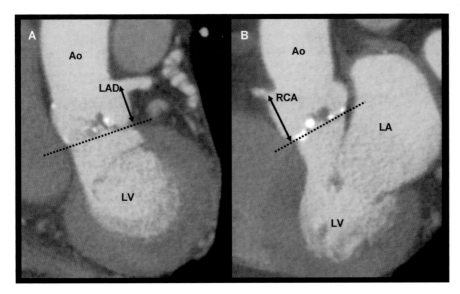

Figure 12 Assessment of relative position of coronary ostia to the aortic valve annulus. The height of the left coronary ostium (**A**) and the right coronary ostium (**B**) may be of importance to evaluate the risk of potential occlusion of one of these ostia during the prosthesis expansion by one of the native cusps. *Abbreviations*: Ao, aorta; LA, left ventricle; LAD, Left anterior descending artery; LV, left ventricle; RCA, right coronary artery.

of the coronary ostia. However, bearing in mind the sealing annular cuff located at the lower two-thirds of the device, there is still the possibility of this procedure-related complication if the distance between the coronary ostium and the aortic valve annulus is smaller.

Left Ventricular Dimensions and Function

From the same data set acquired for aortic valve evaluation, left ventricular function can be accurately evaluated with MSCT. Recently, automated algorithms to delineate the endocardial borders at the end-diastolic and end-systolic phases yield left ventricular volumes and ejection fraction measurements with good agreement with other imaging techniques (two-dimensional echocardiography and MRI) (21). In addition, other aspects that can determine or contraindicate the procedural approach, such as sigmoid interventricular septum or left ventricular thrombus, can be detected.

In summary, the main insights provided by MSCT are the exact depiction of the aortic valve, indicating the location and extent of the calcifications, the accurate aortic valve area estimation and aortic annulus sizing, and the aortic root dimensions together with its spatial relation with the coronary arteries. In addition, the study of the aorta and peripheral ilio-femoral arteries provides important information to decide on the procedural approach. Therefore, MSCT appears an excellent imaging technique to evaluate potential candidates for transcatheter aortic valve implantation. Nevertheless, the radiation exposure and the presence of high heart rates or cardiac arrhythmias may limit its feasibility.

MAGNETIC RESONANCE IMAGING

The technical advances and the increasing availability of the last years have increased the interest for cardiac MRI as a noninvasive imaging modality for cardiovascular diseases. Cardiac MRI is a three-dimensional imaging technique with high spatial resolution and does not use ionizing radiation. In the assessment of aortic valve disease, cardiac MRI yields accurate and highly reproducible estimates of various structural and functional variables. ECG-gated cine sequences acquired with the steady-state free-precession method or the true-fast imaging with steady-state precession method provide superior temporal and spatial resolution and optimized blood–myocardium contrast resulting in a more accurate delineation of the aortic cusps. These sequences allow the exact characterization of the aortic valve anatomy and dimensions, and provide quantitative data on aortic stenosis severity by assessing the peak flow velocity (26).

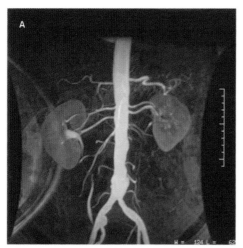
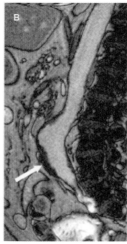
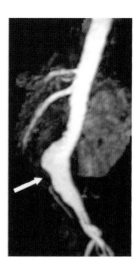

Figure 13   Evaluation of peripheral arteries and aorta by MR angiography. Gadolinium contrast-enhanced MR (**A**) allows for the evaluation of stenosis of the peripheral arteries. By using true-fast imaging with steady-state precession sequence acquisition (**B**), characterization of the vessel wall can be performed, detecting the presence of mural thrombus. *Source*: From Refs. 28 and 30.

In addition, MRI can provide valuable information on left ventricular dimensions, function, and accurate quantification of left ventricular mass (27). Finally, MR angiography enables the assessment of coronary artery disease and constitutes a robust imaging technique to evaluate the peripheral vascular system (28).

Therefore, MRI would be a valuable imaging technique to select potential candidates for transcatheter aortic valve implantation, giving information on the aortic stenosis severity, procedural feasibility, and device sizing. Nonetheless, MRI has several contraindications (patients with metallic implants, pacemakers, or claustrophobia) that limit a more widespread use of this technique.

Evaluation of Peripheral Arteries and Aorta

Although invasive angiography is the reference method to evaluate the size and tortuosity of the peripheral arteries, MR angiography may be an ideal noninvasive alternative imaging technique in patients with renal failure. Gadolinium contrast-enhanced MR angiography provides accurate assessment of the stenosis severity of iliac arteries [Fig. 13(A)] (28,29). In addition, true-fast imaging with steady-state precession sequence acquisition allows for vessel wall characterization with high image quality, and atherosclerosis and arterial wall thrombosis can be detected [Fig. 13(B)] (30). As already mentioned for MSCT, the cross-sectional diameter of the iliac arteries will determine the procedural approach, recommending the transapical approach when this diameter is <6 to 9 mm. In addition, the presence of thoracic or abdominal aortic aneurysms with mural thrombosis will contraindicate the transfemoral approach. In contrast to MSCT, extent and location of calcifications can not be evaluated with MRI.

Aortic Valve Anatomy and Valve Area Assessment

The aortic valve anatomy can be accurately evaluated at the double oblique axial cine images acquired using the steady-state free-precession or the true-fast imaging steady-state precession methods with ECG gating. In a series of 38 patients, Gleeson et al. (31) demonstrated a high accuracy (97%) of double oblique true-fast imaging steady-state precession MRI to distinguish tricuspid and bicuspid aortic valves (31). The assessment of aortic stenosis severity can be also performed with MRI. Either by direct planimetry of the stenotic orifice or by velocity-encoded techniques that quantify the peak flow velocity, aortic stenosis severity can be accurately evaluated (26,32). Several studies have demonstrated the accuracy of MRI to estimate the aortic valve area by planimetry, with excellent agreement as compared to transesophageal echocardiography or MSCT (32). However, this measurement does not reflect the workload of the left ventricle, more related to the effective orifice area, usually smaller than the anatomic aortic valve area. In this regard, velocity-encoded MRI enables the assessment of the effective orifice area providing comparable estimations as those obtained with Doppler echocardiography (26). Recently, in a series of 24 patients with mild to severe aortic stenosis, Caruthers et al. (26) demonstrated the accuracy of velocity-encoded MRI to estimate mean and peak transvalvular pressure gradient by means of the modified Bernoulli equation and the estimation of the aortic valve area by means of the continuity equation. The MRI-derived estimations showed a strong correlation with the parameters obtained by echocardiography (26). As a limitation, velocity-encoded cardiac MRI might underestimate the severity of the aortic stenosis when the velocity–time integral is >0.8 m (26).

Aortic Annulus Sizing

The exact size of the aortic annulus is one of the cornerstones of the procedural success. Similar to MSCT, MRI is a three-dimensional imaging technique that provides exact characterization of the geometry and size of the aortic annulus (33). Recently, Burman et al. (33) demonstrated in 120 studied individuals, the ellipsoid geometry of the aortic annulus that appears bounded by a combination of muscular and fibrous components without a clear ring structure (33). Consistently, the aortic annulus is significantly smaller in the sagittal plane (22.2 ± 2.4 mm for men and 19.9 ± 1.9 mm for women) than in the coronal plane (26.2 ± 2.3 mm for men and 23.0 ± 2.1 mm for women) (33). This finding highlights the great value of three-dimensional imaging techniques, such as MRI or MSCT, in the aortic annulus sizing with high impact on the accurate device size selection.

Aortic Root and Coronary Artery Evaluation

The largest series evaluating the aortic root dimensions with MRI has been published recently by Burman et al. (33). A total of 120 patients of different ages were evaluated providing a useful standardization of MRI measurements of the aortic root and yielding normal values (33). As previously indicated (see MSCT section above), the measurement of the sinotubular junction diameter has important implications for transcatheter aortic valve implantation, and in patients with a sinotubular junction diameter ≥45 mm the implantation of a self-expandable device may be contraindicated (6).

The assessment of the coronary anatomy is also crucial before transcatheter aortic valve implantation. Although the feasibility of MRI for non-invasive angiography has been demonstrated, the accuracy of MRI to detect coronary artery stenoses is lower as compared to MSCT (34).

Left Ventricular Dimensions and Function

MRI is considered the reference method for assessment of left ventricular dimensions, function and left ventricular mass (27). From sequential short-axis slices covering the entire left ventricle, the endocardial boundaries can be detected. Several automated algorithms for endocardial contour detection have demonstrated to provide accurate assessment of left ventricular dimensions and function, reducing significantly the postprocessing time. Cine sequences acquired with steady-state free-precession technologies have improved the image resolution resulting in reduced observer dependency of volumetric measurements (35). Finally, similar to MSCT, the left ventricular geometry and shape (hypertrophy) of the basal septum can be evaluated.

Magnetic resonance imaging constitutes a valuable noninvasive imaging technique for the selection of candidates for transcatheter aortic valve implantation. This imaging technique provides comprehensive evaluation of the aortic valve anatomy and function, aortic root dimensions, and characterization of the aorta and peripheral arteries together with the evaluation of left ventricular dimensions and function, without ionizing radiation. However, the several contraindications, such as metallic devices, pacemakers, or claustrophobia, and the long acquisition and postprocessing times needed, do currently not support widespread use of MRI.

CONCLUSIONS

Transcatheter aortic valve implantation is an emergent therapy that has become in the last few years a real expectancy for symptomatic patients with severe aortic stenosis deemed not suitable for surgical valve replacement. From the first-in-man experience in 2000 (1), outstanding technological advances have led to smaller profile delivery catheters and better prosthesis of different sizes. The initial antegrade approach with transeptal puncture has been abandoned in favor of the less invasive venous retrograde approach. Future technological advances and rigorous training in this promising field of interventional cardiology will result in higher success rates and reduce complication rates. However, the accurate selection of potential candidates for this therapy will remain one of the main determinants of procedural success. Cardiac imaging plays a central role in selection of patients. The wide availability and noninvasive character of transthoracic echocardiography make this imaging technique the first approach to characterize patients with severe aortic stenosis. However, in patients with poor acoustic window, assessment of several morphologic, and functional aortic parameters may be challenging. Furthermore, other important issues, such as the anatomy and status of the peripheral arteries cannot be evaluated with transthoracic echocardiography. MSCT and MRI are three-dimensional imaging techniques that provide extensive information on anatomy and function of the aortic valve, accurate sizing of the aortic annulus, exact characterization of the aortic root and its relations with surrounding structures, such as coronary arteries, and, finally, enable the assessment of the thoracic and abdominal aorta and peripheral arteries. Therefore, a cardiac multimodality imaging approach, combining echocardiography (transthoracic/transesophageal) with MSCT or MRI may constitute the best approach to evaluate symptomatic, severe aortic stenosis patients who are candidates for transcatheter aortic valve implantation.

REFERENCES

1. Cribier A, Eltchaninoff H, Tron C, et al. Early experience with percutaneous transcatheter implantation of heart valve prosthesis for the treatment of end-stage inoperable patients with calcific aortic stenosis. J Am Coll Cardiol 2004; 43:698–703.
2. Grube E, Laborde JC, Gerckens U, et al. Percutaneous implantation of the CoreValve self-expanding valve prosthesis in high-risk patients with aortic valve disease: The Siegburg first-in-man study. Circulation 2006; 114:1616–1624.
3. Grube E, Schuler G, Buellesfeld L, et al. Percutaneous aortic valve replacement for severe aortic stenosis in high-risk patients using the second- and current third-generation self-expanding CoreValve prosthesis: Device success and 30-day clinical outcome. J Am Coll Cardiol 2007; 50:69–76.
4. Lichtenstein SV, Cheung A, Ye J, et al. Transapical transcatheter aortic valve implantation in humans: Initial clinical experience. Circulation 2006; 114:591–596.
5. Webb JG, Pasupati S, Humphries K, et al. Percutaneous transarterial aortic valve replacement in selected high-risk patients with aortic stenosis. Circulation 2007; 116:755–763.
6. Vahanian A, Alfieri O, Al-Attar N, et al. Transcatheter valve implantation for patients with aortic stenosis: A position statement from the European Association of Cardio-Thoracic Surgery (EACTS) and the European Society of Cardiology (ESC), in collaboration with the European Association of Percutaneous Cardiovascular Interventions (EAPCI). Eur Heart J 2008; 29:1463–1470.
7. Zegdi R, Ciobotaru V, Noghin M, et al. Is it reasonable to treat all calcified stenotic aortic valves with a valved stent? Results from a human anatomic study in adults. J Am Coll Cardiol 2008; 51: 579–584.
8. Delgado V, Tops LF, Schuijf JD, et al. Successful deployment of a transcatheter aortic valve in bicuspid aortic stenosis: Role of imaging with multislice computed tomography. Circ Cardiovasc Imaging 2009; 2:e12–e13.
9. Webb JG, Chandavimol M, Thompson CR, et al. Percutaneous aortic valve implantation retrograde from the femoral artery. Circulation 2006; 113:842–850. DOI: 10.1161/CIRCIMAGING.108.809434.
10. Bonow RO, Carabello BA, Kanu C, et al. ACC/AHA 2006 guidelines for the management of patients with valvular heart disease: A report of the American College of Cardiology/American Heart Association Task Force on Practice Guidelines (writing committee to revise the 1998 Guidelines for the

Management of Patients With Valvular Heart Disease): Developed in collaboration with the Society of Cardiovascular Anesthesiologists: Endorsed by the Society for Cardiovascular Angiography and Interventions and the Society of Thoracic Surgeons. Circulation 2006; 114:e84–e231.

11. Otto CM. Valvular aortic stenosis: Disease severity and timing of intervention. J Am Coll Cardiol 2006; 47:2141–2151.

12. Babaliaros V, Liff D, Chen E, et al. Can Balloon Aortic Valvuloplasty Help Determine Appropriate Transcatheter Aortic Valve Size? JACC Cardiovasc Interv 2008; 1:580–586.

13. Moss R, Ivens E, Pasupati S, et al. Role of Echocardiography in Percutaneous Aortic Valve Implantation. JACC Cardiovasc Imaging 2008; 1:15–24.

14. Grube E, Buellesfeld L, Mueller R, et al. Progress and current status of percutaneous aortic valve replacement: Results of three device generations of the CoreValve Revalving system. Circ Cardiovasc Interv 2008; 1:167–175.

15. Iung B, Cachier A, Baron G, et al. Decision-making in elderly patients with severe aortic stenosis: Why are so many denied surgery? Eur Heart J 2005; 26:2714–2720.

16. Lang RM, Bierig M, Devereux RB, et al. Recommendations for chamber quantification: A report from the American Society of Echocardiography's Guidelines and Standards Committee and the Chamber Quantification Writing Group, developed in conjunction with the European Association of Echocardiography, a branch of the European Society of Cardiology. J Am Soc Echocardiogr 2005; 18:1440–1463.

17. Poh KK, Levine RA, Solis J, et al. Assessing aortic valve area in aortic stenosis by continuity equation: A novel approach using real-time three-dimensional echocardiography. Eur Heart J 2008; 29: 2526–2535.

18. Gutierrez-Chico JL, Zamorano JL, Prieto-Moriche E, et al. Real-time three-dimensional echocardiography in aortic stenosis: A novel, simple, and reliable method to improve accuracy in area calculation. Eur Heart J 2008; 29:1296–1306.

19. Pouleur AC, le Polain de Waroux JB, Pasquet A, et al. Aortic valve area assessment: Multidetector CT compared with cine MR imaging and transthoracic and transesophageal echocardiography. Radiology 2007; 244:745–754.

20. Reant P, Lederlin M, Lafitte S, et al. Absolute assessment of aortic valve stenosis by planimetry using cardiovascular magnetic resonance imaging: Comparison with transesophageal echocardiography, transthoracic echocardiography, and cardiac catheterisation. Eur J Radiol 2006; 59:276–283.

21. Henneman MM, Schuijf JD, Jukema JW, et al. Assessment of global and regional left ventricular function and volumes with 64-slice MSCT: A comparison with 2D echocardiography. J Nucl Cardiol 2006; 13:480–487.

22. Rodes-Cabau J, Dumont E, De LaRochelliere R, et al. Feasibility and initial results of percutaneous aortic valve implantation including selection of the transfemoral or transapical approach in patients with severe aortic stenosis. Am J Cardiol 2008; 102:1240–1246.

23. Tops L, Wood D, Delgado V, et al. Noninvasive Evaluation of the Aortic Root With Multislice Computed Tomography Implications for Transcatheter Aortic Valve Replacement. JACC Cardiovasc Imaging 2008; 1:321–330.

24. Doddamani S, Grushko MJ, Makaryus AN, et al. Demonstration of left ventricular outflow tract eccentricity by 64-slice multi-detector CT. Int J Cardiovasc Imaging 2009; 25:175–181.

25. Schuijf JD, Pundziute G, Jukema JW, et al. Diagnostic accuracy of 64-slice multislice computed tomography in the noninvasive evaluation of significant coronary artery disease. Am J Cardiol 2006; 98: 145–148.

26. Caruthers SD, Lin SJ, Brown P, et al. Practical value of cardiac magnetic resonance imaging for clinical quantification of aortic valve stenosis: Comparison with echocardiography. Circulation 2003; 108:2236–2243.

27. Constantine G, Shan K, Flamm SD, et al. Role of MRI in clinical cardiology. Lancet 2004; 363:2162–2171.

28. Auerbach EG, Martin ET. Magnetic resonance imaging of the peripheral vasculature. Am Heart J 2004; 148:755–763.

29. Swan JS, Kennell TW, Acher CW, et al. Magnetic resonance angiography of aorto-iliac disease. Am J Surg 2000; 180:6–12.

30. Iozzelli A, D'Orta G, Aliprandi A, et al. The value of true-FISP sequence added to conventional gadolinium-enhanced MRA of abdominal aorta and its major branches. Eur J Radiol 2008. DOI.org/10.1016/j.ejrad.2008.09.004.

31. Gleeson TG, Mwangi I, Horgan SJ, et al. Steady-state free-precession (SSFP) cine MRI in distinguishing normal and bicuspid aortic valves. J Magn Reson Imaging 2008; 28:873–878.

32. Pouleur AC, le Polain de Waroux JB, Pasquet A, et al. Planimetric and continuity equation assessment of aortic valve area: Head to head comparison between cardiac magnetic resonance and echocardiography. J Magn Reson Imaging 2007; 26:1436–1443.

33. Burman E, Keegan J, Kilner P. Aortic root measurement by cardiovascular magnetic resonance: Specification of planes and lines of measurement, and corresponding normal values. Circ Cardiovasc Imaging 2008; 1:104–113.

34. Schuijf JD, Bax JJ, Shaw LJ, et al. Meta-analysis of comparative diagnostic performance of magnetic resonance imaging and multislice computed tomography for noninvasive coronary angiography. Am Heart J 2006; 151:404–411.

35. Pujadas S, Reddy GP, Weber O, et al. MR imaging assessment of cardiac function. J Magn Reson Imaging 2004; 19:789–799.

4 | Risk Stratification for Transcatheter Aortic Valve Implantation

A. Pieter Kappetein, Menno van Gameren, Ad J. J. C. Bogers
Department of Cardiac Surgery, Erasmus University Medical Center, Thoraxcenter, Rotterdam, The Netherlands

Nicolo Piazza
Department of Interventional Cardiology, Erasmus University Medical Center, Thoraxcenter, Rotterdam, The Netherlands

INTRODUCTION

Transcatheter aortic valve implantation (TAVI) has led to a renewed interest in cardiac surgical risk modeling. This chapter focuses on the following questions: (1) What is the role of risk modeling in cardiac surgery? (2) What are the currently available cardiac surgery risk models? (3) What is the role of risk modeling in TAVI? (4) Which risk models should be used for TAVI? (5) How do risk models differ when applied to both low- and high-risk patients?

A brief discussion about the determinants of model quality can be found in the appendix of this chapter.

ROLE OF RISK MODELING IN CARDIAC SURGERY

Risk models can serve multiple purposes (Table 1).

Currently Available Cardiac Surgery Risk Models

Risk models for cardiac surgery can be divided into three broad categories: (*i*) general cardiac surgery models (1,2) (i.e., coronary artery bypass surgery, valve surgery, or other related cardiac surgery); (*ii*) general valve surgery models (3–9); and (*iii*) specific aortic valve surgery risk models (10,11).

Although a detailed description about each risk model is beyond the scope of this chapter, Table 2 provides a summary of currently available risk models with important determinants of model quality (see appendix for a discussion on the determinants of model quality).

Role of Risk Modeling in TAVI?

Risk models for TAVI can serve two distinct purposes, and therefore, two separate risk models may be required. First, a risk model is needed that can accurately identify high or prohibitive surgical risk patients for TAVI; this model should be constructed using a surgical cohort and can serve both clinical and research purposes. Second, a risk model is needed that can accurately estimate the risk of TAVI and therefore serve as a benchmark performance measure and improve the informed consent process; this model should be constructed using a TAVI cohort. Risk models for such purposes are not yet available.

Which Risk Model Should Be Used for TAVI?

Recently, attention has been directed towards the reliability of risk algorithms in predicting operative outcomes in high-risk patients undergoing aortic valve replacement (12–14). Patients who are currently evaluated for transcatheter or transapical AVR form a select population that is not representative of the populations that were used to develop existing risk models. It is axiomatic, therefore, that these models may not perform well when applied to this "outlier" population.

Justified or not, the logistic EuroSCORE and the STS (Society of Thoracic Surgeons) Predicted Risk of Mortality score are the most commonly used risk models to guide the recruitment of "high-risk" patients for TAVI trials. Furthermore, by comparing the "observed" versus "expected" mortality rates, these risk models are currently being used as TAVI performance

Table 1   Role of Risk Modeling in Cardiac Surgery

Performance measure or benchmark
Improve the informed consent process (individual risk)
Identify high-risk patients who may benefit from additional work-up or alternative treatment strategies
Identify high-risk patients who may experience longer lengths of stay
Inclusion/exclusion criteria for clinical trials
Appreciate the relative importance of risk factors of a model (beta-coefficients)

measures—a practice that can lead to complacency and acceptance of current results when there is definite room for improvement.

Osswald et al. have shown that although the logistic EuroSCORE can adequately stratify patients into low, intermediate, or high risk, it overestimates absolute 30-day mortality (13). The mortality risk may be overestimated by a factor of 2 to 3, especially in high-risk patients (12,14). Furthermore, the STS score was determined to be more accurate than the EuroSCORE or Ambler Risk Score in the prediction of operative and long-term mortality for high-risk patients undergoing surgical aortic valve replacement (12).

Currently, there is no validated risk model for the purposes of TAVI. Although some risk models may be more accurate than others, it does not necessarily mean they are appropriate for TAVI. Specific risk models to identify high-risk surgical valve patients should be the focus of future studies (15).

How Do Risk Models Differ When Applied to Both Low- and High-Risk Patients?

The predicted mortality rates for a particular patient can vary depending on the risk model used. These variations can be explained by the inclusion of different predictor variables as well as different relative weights assigned to similar variables included in the models.

Figure 1(A) and 1(B) shows the risk scores of a hypothetical low- and high-risk patient based on seven different risk models, respectively. Note that for a low-risk patient, the estimated mortalities are within similar range. For a high-risk patient, however, it can be seen that the estimated mortality varies considerably depending on the risk model. This must be kept in mind when clinically applying risk models for selecting high-risk patients for TAVI.

As was mentioned earlier, the EuroSCORE and STS score are commonly used for purposes of selecting high-risk patients for TAVI. TAVI trials have typically used a EuroSCORE $\geq$15% or STS score $\geq$10% as inclusion criteria. The calculated EuroSCORE and STS score of a hypothetical patient 80 years of age with a previous history of stroke is 16% and 2.9%, respectively. This patient would be included in a trial using a EuroSCORE $\geq$ 15% but this same patient would not be eligible for a trial using a STS score $\geq$ 10%. This example highlights the limitations of using current risk scores for clinical or research decision making.

THE WAY FORWARD

Ideally, a multicenter prospective database aiming to collect data on all valve interventions (i.e., surgical and transcatheter) would be optimal. This endeavor, however, would need endorsement by regulatory bodies and professional organizations. It is essential that the data collection be comprehensive and includes patient demographics as well as anatomic factors known to influence outcomes. Having said that, there needs to be a balance between being "comprehensive" and "parsimonious." Incorporating too many variables into the model calculations can result in "overfitting," that is, the model follows characteristics of the population it was derived from to the extent that it only "fits" that population. By using the Charlson comorbidity scale or Lee Score equivalent, one could attempt to stratify a patient on the basis of a limited number of risk factors only (e.g., age and sex). In a commentary to the Lee Score, De Craen states that the discriminative power of a model with age and sex as sole variables is almost comparable to that of the same model with 12 extra variables. Unfortunately, the effect of calibration was not discussed.

Table 2 Model Characteristics of Various Surgical Risk Algorithms

	Data set/reference	Region	Model design	Year of publication	Study period	Sample size	Sample size validation	Validation method	Discrimination results (ROC)	Calibration results (H–L)
1	– EuroSCORE (2)	European	CABG, valve surgery	1999	1995	13302	1479	Internal (time-split)	0.79	0.68
2	–STS (8)	USA + Canada	Ao/M without CABG	2000	1994–1997	49073	25460	Internal (time split)	0.77	0.23
			Ao/M with CABG		43463	25852			0.74	0.14
3	Single center (11)	Germany	Ao	2003	1996–2001	1400	1400	Internal	0.73	N/A
4	– NNE (4)	USA	Ao	2004	1991–2001	5793	Bootstrapped	Internal validation (bootstrapping)	0.75	0.16
			M	2004	1991–2001	3150	Bootstrapped	Internal validation (bootstrapping)	0.79	0.71
5	VA (7)	USA	Ao	2004	1991–2001	7450	Not validated	Not validated	N/A	N/A
			M	2004	1991–2001	1850	Not validated	Not validated	N/A	N/A
6	–PHS (5)	USA	Ao	2005	1997–2004	3324	Development population	Internal	0.79	0.94
			M	2005	1997–2004	1596	Development population	Internal	0.84	0.14
7	–SCTSGBI (9)	UK	Ao/M/ Combined Ao and M	2005	1995–2003	16679	16160	Internal, time split	0.77	0.78
8	STS score (3)	USA	Ao/M/T/P/ combined	2006	1994–2003	409100	Development population	Internal	0.74	N/A
9	New York State (6)	USA	Ao/M/T/P/ comb	2007	2001–2003	10702	Internal (time-split)	Internal (time-split)	0.79	0.52
			Ao/M/T/P/ comb + CABG	2007	2001–2003	8823		Internal (time-split)	0.75	0.04
10	Multicenter (10)	UK	Ao	2007	1997–2004	4550	816 + Boot-strapping	Split + bootstrap	0.78	0.73

Abbreviations: Ao, aortic valve; CABG, coronary artery bypass graft surgery; H–L, Hosmer–Lemeshow; ROC, receiver operator characteristics; M, mitral valve; NNE, Northern New England medical centers; PHS, Providence Health System Cardiovascular Study Group; P, pu.

Low-risk patient

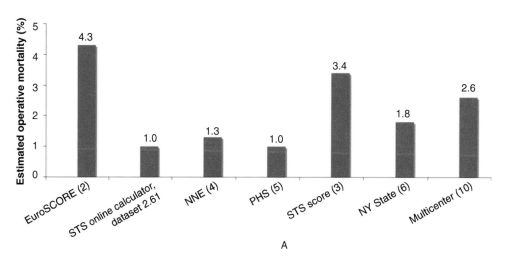

A

High-risk patient

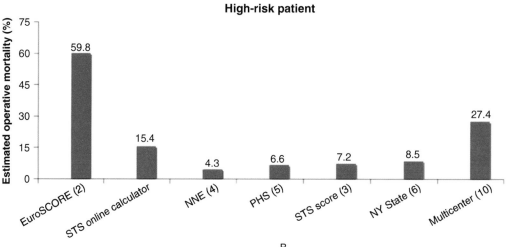

B

Figure 1 Estimated operative mortality based on seven different risk models of a hypothetical patient considered (**A**) low risk and (**B**) high risk. (**A**) Low-risk patient—75-year-old male with ejection fraction 55% and no other comorbidities. (**B**) High-risk patient—85-year-old female with ejection fraction 30%, renal dysfunction, and pulmonary hypertension.

CONCLUSION

Clinical judgment should play an integral role in the selection of patients for TAVI. Thus, risk scores should not dictate but guide clinical decision making

APPENDIX—MODEL BASICS AND MODEL ASSESSMENT
MODEL BASICS

Factors such as data quality, cohort characteristics, end-point definitions, and types of risk factor variables play an important role in the performance and general applicability of risk models.

Data Quality

The quality of the data set is crucial—a model is only as good as the data set it was derived from ("the garbage in–garbage out principle"). Data collection can be accomplished in a prospective or retrospective manner. Retrospective data collection carries relatively lower costs but can be limited by inaccurate or missing data that may lead to selection bias. Furthermore, the predictors and outcomes need to be accurately defined and then collected (16).

Prospective data collection is preferable—it is less vulnerable to missing data and allows for easier data auditing (source documentation, data source verification). Inclusion and exclusion criteria and predictor variables can be defined can be defined in advance. The clinical database used for score development can be derived from a single or several institutions and from one or several countries. Single center and voluntary databases (e.g., STS database) might be vulnerable to reporting bias, that is, centers with above-average clinical results might be more inclined to report their results.

Cohort Characteristics

To extrapolate a model correctly, it is crucial to appreciate the characteristics of the patient cohort (e.g., demographics, surgical, or TAVI patients) from which it was developed. Extrapolation of a model that was based on a single-centers' experience may be less desirable than a model based on multicenter experience.

The sample size of the original cohort has a direct influence on the number of independent variables that can be identified in the model. As a statistical rule of thumb, at least 5 to 10 events per predictor variable are required for model development (17). Although models derived from large cohorts may have the ability to identify a large number of independent variables, the clinical significance of variables always needs to be assessed.

End-Point Definition

Interpretation and comparison of model results should focus on the definition of the end-point variable. It is not uncommon that risk models intended for "similar" purposes use different definitions for short-term mortality; even for seemingly unambiguous end-point definitions like hospital mortality (e.g., in-hospital vs. 30-day mortality).

Variables

Most factors that contribute to risk are not independent of one another and correlation between two risk factors can lead to confounding. Univariate tests on the different risk factors would not reveal how these factors work together. In risk stratification models, however, we are less interested in confounding than we are with clinical trials. The goal is to identify important risk factors that work together to modify the risk of an outcome.

Some models have converted continuous variables (e.g., serum creatinine level) to binary or categorical variables using (arbitrary) cut-off points. Although this may improve the usability of the model, a degree of "predictability" may be lost. With multivariable regression analysis, the association between individual risk factors (also referred to as predictor variables or covariates) and outcomes can be determined, while holding constant the effect of others. Once the impact of each risk factor is established from a given population sample, it then becomes possible to estimate the probability of the outcome for patients having particular combinations of these risk factors.

MODEL ASSESSMENT

The fit of a risk stratification model is generally measured in terms of its discrimination and calibration. The process of measuring these terms is called validation.

Discrimination

Discrimination, which is measured using the *c*-index (area under the receiver operating characteristic curve) with 95% confidence limits (CI), captures the model's ability to distinguish between patients who will suffer from an event and those that will not—thereby measuring the trade-off between the specificity and sensitivity. It is defined as the proportion of the time that an event-free patient is assigned a higher probability of not suffering from an event than a patient who suffers from an event. A value of 1.0 is perfect, and a value of 0.5 denotes only random ability to distinguish between patients with and without events. In general, a value above 0.7 is considered good and above 0.8 excellent. In case of low discrimination, a risk model may accurately predict the percentage of patients that may experience a certain event but they might not be able to identify which patients experience the event.

Calibration

Calibration reflects the relationship between the observed number of events and the predicted probability of events and can be evaluated by the Hosmer–Lemeshow goodness-of-fit test (H–L). Models with Hosmer–Lemeshow p-values above 0.05 are generally considered to be well calibrated. Calibration plots can be used to give a graphical representation of model calibration.

Comparing mean event rates (predicted versus observed) to assess calibration is not sufficient. Calibration is less crucial than discrimination in the evaluation process because models can be recalibrated. Recalibration is done by adjusting the weights of the independent variables to the population one intends to use the model for, allowing for extrapolation and increased precision of the model when used in that population.

Validation Cohort

The predictive validity of a model is a measure of how well it performs on a data set other than the one from which it was developed.

Validation can be obtained by evaluating the model on new data with patients undergoing the same kind of treatment. The cohort used to validate a model greatly influences results. A model is "internally" validated when validation is performed using patients from the same population that the model was derived from.

Several approaches of internal validation are available: data splitting, cross-validation, or bootstrapping. Temporal validation is a form of data splitting and evaluates the performance of a model on subsequent patients within the same center(s).

Complementary to internal validation is external validation. This method uses a different population (e.g., from another center) to assess discrimination and calibration and lends the model to extrapolation. Having patient data across a wide variety of geographic areas increases the probability that the model will be suited for different populations, but the only way to determine the model's applicability is to verify the performance empirically in a representative sample.

Continuous evaluation of model performance is another aspect that is important to ascertain that classification performance does not degrade with time. Some models are redeveloped periodically to adjust for temporal trends.

REFERENCES

1. Parsonnet V, Dean D, Bernstein AD. A method of uniform stratification of risk for evaluating the results of surgery in acquired adult heart disease Circulation 1989; 79:I3–I12.
2. Nashef SA, Roques F, Michel P, et al. European system for cardiac operative risk evaluation (EuroSCORE). Eur J Cardiothorac Surg 1999; 16:9–13.
3. Rankin JS, Hammill BG, Ferguson TB Jr., et al. Determinants of operative mortality in valvular heart surgery. J Thorac Cardiovasc Surg 2006; 131:547–557.
4. Nowicki ER, Birkmeyer NJ, Weintraub RW, et al. Multivariable prediction of in-hospital mortality associated with aortic and mitral valve surgery in Northern New England. Ann Thorac Surg 2004; 77:1966–1977.
5. Jin R, Grunkemeier GL, Starr A. Validation and refinement of mortality risk models for heart valve surgery. Ann Thorac Surg 2005; 80:471–479.
6. Hannan EL, Wu C, Bennett EV, et al. Risk index for predicting in-hospital mortality for cardiac valve surgery. Ann Thorac Surg 2007; 83:921–929.
7. Gardner SC, Grunwald GK, Rumsfeld JS, et al. Comparison of short-term mortality risk factors for valve replacement versus coronary artery bypass graft surgery. Ann Thorac Surg 2004; 77:549–556.
8. Edwards FH, Peterson ED, Coombs LP, et al. Prediction of operative mortality after valve replacement surgery. J Am Coll Cardiol 2001; 37:885–892.
9. Ambler G, Omar RZ, Royston P, et al. Generic, simple risk stratification model for heart valve surgery Circulation 2005; 112:224–231.
10. Kuduvalli M, Grayson AD, Au J, et al. A multi-centre additive and logistic risk model for in-hospital mortality following aortic valve replacement. Eur J Cardiothorac Surg 2007; 31:607–613.

11. Florath I, Rosendahl UP, Mortasawi A, et al. Current determinants of operative mortality in 1400 patients requiring aortic valve replacement. Ann Thorac Surg 2003; 76:75–83.
12. Dewey TM, Brown D, Ryan WH, et al. Reliability of risk algorithms in predicting early and late operative outcomes in high-risk patients undergoing aortic valve replacement. J Thorac Cardiovasc Surg 2008; 135:180–187.
13. Osswald BR, Gegouskov V, Badowski-Zyla D, et al. Overestimation of aortic valve replacement risk by EuroSCORE: Implications for percutaneous valve replacement. Eur Heart J 2009; 30:74–80.
14. Brown ML, Schaff HV, Sarano ME, et al. Is the European System for Cardiac Operative Risk Evaluation model valid for estimating the operative risk of patients considered for percutaneous aortic valve replacement? J Thorac Cardiovasc Surg 2008; 136:566–571.
15. van Gameren M, Kappetein AP, Steyerberg EW, et al. Do we need separate risk stratification models for hospital mortality after heart valve surgery? Ann Thorac Surg 2008; 85:921–930.
16. Steyerberg EW. Clinical Prediction Models: A Practical Approach to Development, Validation, and Updating. Springer, 2009.
17. Vittinghoff E, McCulloch CE. Relaxing the rule of ten events per variable in logistic and cox regression. Am. J. Epidemiol 2006; DOI: 10.1093/aje/kwk052.

5 | Patient Selection—Risk Assessment and Anatomical Selection Criteria for Patients Undergoing Transfemoral Aortic Valve Implantation with the Edwards SAPIEN Prosthetic Heart Valve

Itsik Ben Dor, Lowell Satler, Ron Waksman, and Augusto Pichard
Washington Hospital Center, Washington, D.C., U.S.A.

INTRODUCTION

Preprocedural evaluation of patients for percutaneous aortic valve replacement (PAVR) is crucial to select the patients that will benefit the most and have the procedure done safely. This chapter focuses on risk assessment in the group of high operative risk or inoperable patients, currently considered potential candidates for PAVR. After determining appropriate operative risk one needs to determine the anatomical suitability. At our center, patients coming for evaluation for PAVR spend a full day at the hospital; they start with a complete echocardiogram, followed by cardiac catheterization and angiography of the coronaries, left ventricle (LV), and aorta.

PATIENTS SELECTION AND RISK ASSESSMENT

The percutaneous aortic valve is intended for use in symptomatic patients with severe calcific aortic stenosis requiring aortic valve replacement, who are at high risk for open chest surgery due to comorbid conditions, or patients who are inoperable. Defining high-risk surgical patients is not simple. An Society of Thoracic Sugeons (STS) risk score >10 and/or a logistic EuroSCORE >20 are most often used to define high risk (http://209.220.160.181/STSWebRiskCalc261/de.aspx,http://www.euroscore.org). The STS predicted risk of mortality most accurately predicts perioperative and long-term mortality for the highest risk patients having aortic valve replacement (1). The EuroSCORE overestimates the mortality risk of aortic valve replacement (2), and this overestimation is greatest in high-risk patients (3).

Patients can be at very high operative mortality risk but yet have low scores. There are numerous comorbidities not captured in either the EuroSCORE or the STS scoring systems such as porcelain aorta, chest wall radiation, chest wall deformity, highly compromised respiratory function, frailty, and others. There have been attempts to quantify frailty index (4), and correlate frailty index with outcome (5); however, the analysis of frailty is particularly difficult and is often not quantifiable. Clinical judgment of experienced cardiac surgeons has a key role in assessing operative mortality in these cases.

The currently available validated risk score systems have not captured the "nonoperable" patients. The definition of "inoperability" is difficult, and often requires the consensus of several surgeons. It is important to emphasize that those scoring systems are not intended to be used as substitutes for clinical decision making.

Many of these patients have decreased renal function. This is not a contraindication for the percutaneous valve procedure. We use contrast that is diluted 50% with normal saline, and we hydrate the patient before the percutaneous valve procedure. This has effectively prevented further deterioration of renal function post procedure.

ACCESS SITE PERIPHERAL ANATOMY

Adequate vascular access is one of the most important determinants of procedural success and/or complications. The 22- and 24-F sheath used for delivery of the 23- and 26-mm valves

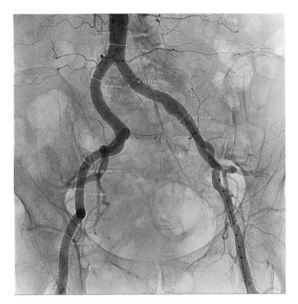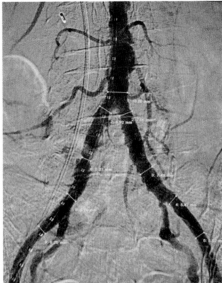

Figure 1 Abdominal aortography for measurement of vessel diameters with quantitative coronary angiography (QCA) and a reference marker pigtail (*left panel*). Digital subtraction for measurement of vessel diameters with QCA and a reference marker pigtail (*right panel*).

require a minimum vessel diameter of 7 and 8 mm, respectively. Three imaging modalities are available to evaluate the access vessels: angiography, contrast computed tomography (CT), and intravascular ultrasound (IVUS). Often there is discrepancy in the results obtained by these techniques. We find that high-quality CT is the most accurate and provides the most useful information to predict feasibility of transfemoral approach.

Angiography
Abdominal aortography gives excellent images. Digital subtraction allows for same or better images with smaller amount of contrast (10–15 cc). Vessel diameters are measured with QCA and a reference marker pigtail (Fig. 1).

Precise vessel measurements are performed in multiple sites in the common femoral, superficial femoral, external, and common iliac arteries. A minimal diameter of 7 mm for the 23-mm valve and 8 mm for 26-mm valve is required. Excess vessel tortuosity can prevent the large 22- or 24-F sheath from advancing to the abdominal aorta, like the left iliac in the Figure 2.

Tortuosity with a large lumen and no calcification is not a problem for use of the large sheaths (Figs. 3 and 4). Tortuosity without calcification that is straightened by a wire does not preclude the procedure (Figs. 5 and 6). Tortuosity with marked calcification does not allow the advancement of the large sheaths.

Calcification is often not well appreciated by angiography. We have seen many cases where the iliofemoral angio showed adequate vessels for percutaneous access, and the CT revealed severe calcification making us reject the patient for transfemoral access [Figs. 7(A) to (F) and 8].

Computerized Tomography
We routinely obtain the contrast CT by using 4-F pigtail placed in the abdominal aorta. This pigtail is left in place after catheterization. The injector is loaded with 20 cc contrast + 60 cc saline. The injection is performed at 4 cc/sec for 10 seconds (10 cc of contrast) (6). This technique gives better pictures than standard IV contrast and helps preserve renal function

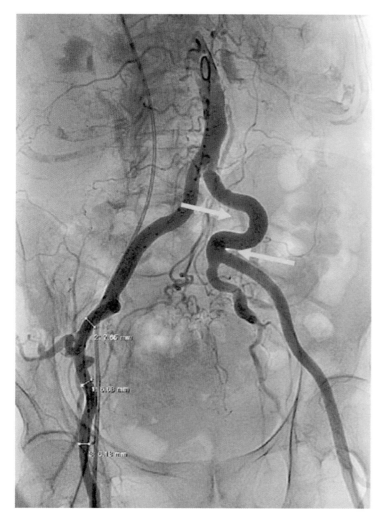

Figure 2 Abdominal aortography showing a very tortuous left iliac artery. This type of sharp angulation precludes the use of the 22 to 24-F sheath.

in this population of older patients with critical aortic stenosis [Fig. 9(A) and (B)]. A detailed CT analysis is very important and can predict possible access problems. The CT images are displayed in longitudinal, 3D, and axial views.

The *vessel diameter* is carefully assessed in longitudinal and axial views. We place the cursor in the abdominal aorta and bring it down millimeter by millimeter to get exact measurements in the entire length of the vessel considered for access. Examples of these measurements are given in Fig. 10(A) to (C). Occasionally the longitudinal images appear to have an adequate minimum diameter but the axial views do not: the real cross-sectional diameters are smaller than required for the large sheaths (Fig. 11).

Exact vessel diameter measurements require that the cursor be perpendicular to the longitudinal axis of the vessel, and this has to be adjusted for each segment of the iliofemoral arteries (Fig. 12).

Noncontrast CT is very important for quantifying the amount of calcification in both longitudinal and axial views. Again the cursor is moved millimeter by millimeter, looking for areas of significant calcification (Fig. 13). Significant calcification, especially in long segments, does not allow straightening.

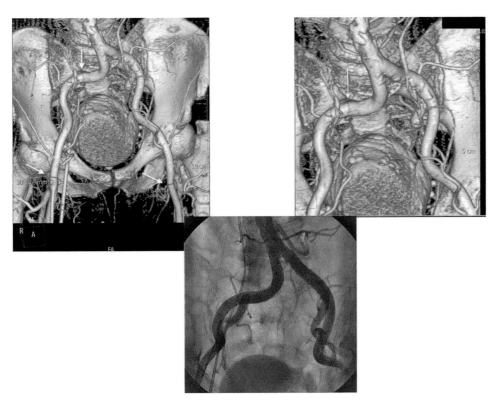

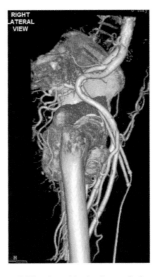

Figure 3 CT demonstrating severe tortuosity with large lumen diameter. Tortuosity with large lumen is no problem for the 22 to 24-F sheaths.

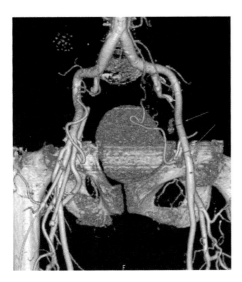

Figure 4 3D CT demonstrating tortuous vessel without calcification. Marked angulation as the iliacs go into the pelvic floor. As long as there is no calcification, these vessels straighten with a wire and usually allow for advancement of the large sheath.

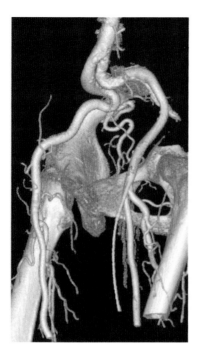
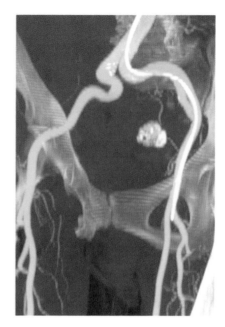

Figure 5   The left iliac is straightened by a wire.

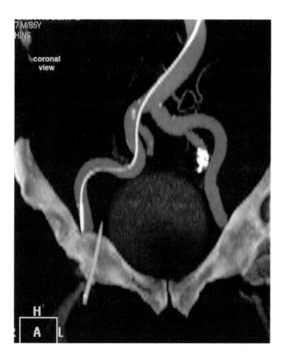

Figure 6   Tortuous vessels straighten with a wire and usually allow for advancement of the large sheath.

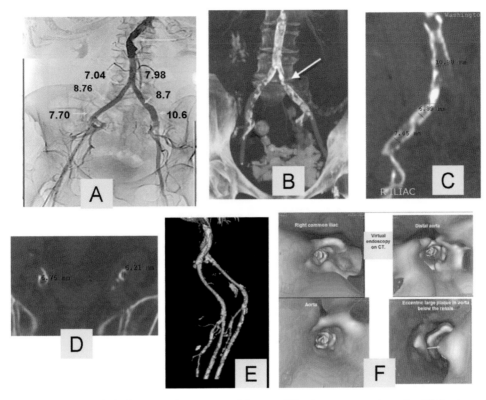

Figure 7 Iliac analysis demonstrating severe calcium on CT not seen on angiography. (**A**) Angiography with vessel-size measurement, (**B** and **C**) noncontrast CT demonstrating severe calcification, (**D**) axial view, (**E**) 3D longitudinal view, and (**F**) virtual endoscopy.

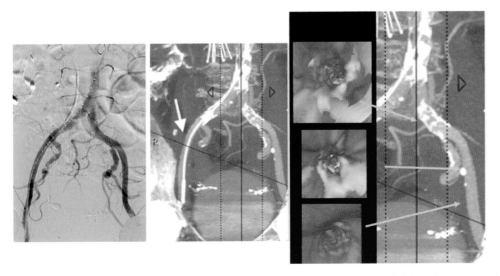

Figure 8 Excellent vessels on angiography, but CT shows calcification that precluded the advancement of 22-F sheath.

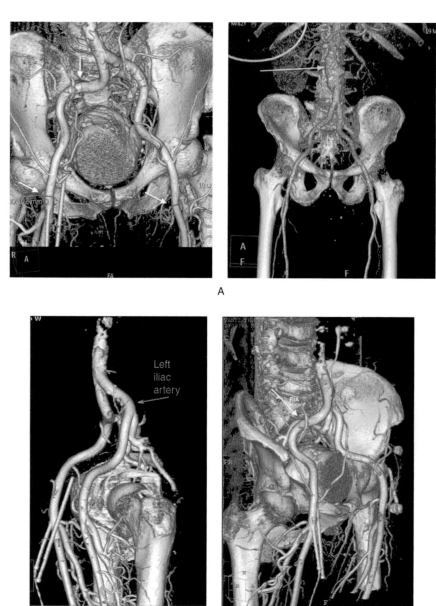

Figure 9 (**A**) Iliac analysis by CT using 4-F pigtail and 10 to 12 cc of contrast (*left panel*), iliac analysis by CT using 100 cc of IV contrast (*right panel*). (**B**) Iliac analysis by CT with 10 cc of contrast injected in the abdominal aorta with a 4-F pigtail.

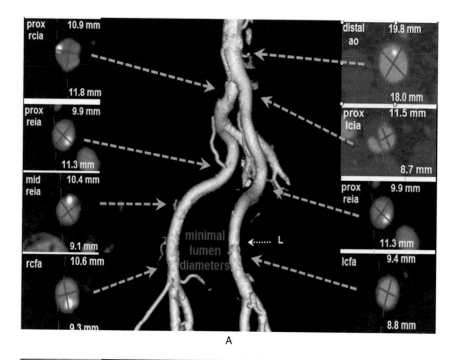

A

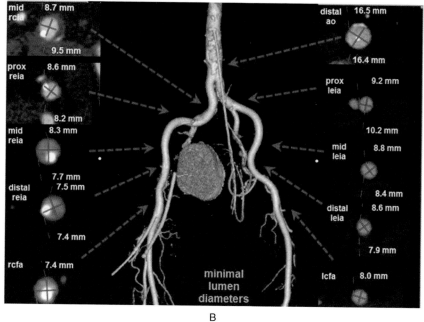

B

Figure 10 (A –C): Axial cuts for precise diameter measurement. (Continued on pg. 72).

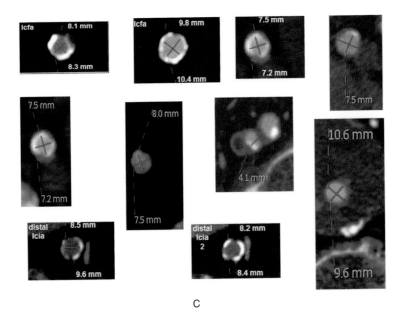

C

Figure 10 *(Continued) Lumen measurement have to exclude calcium.*

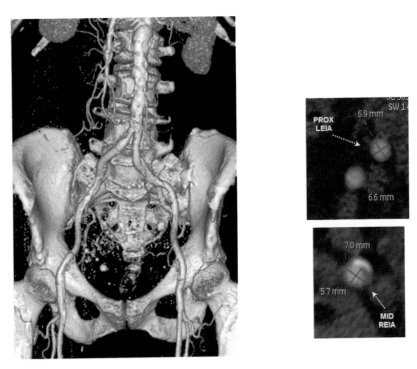

Figure 11 Adequate vessel dimensions on longitudinal view. Too small on axial views.

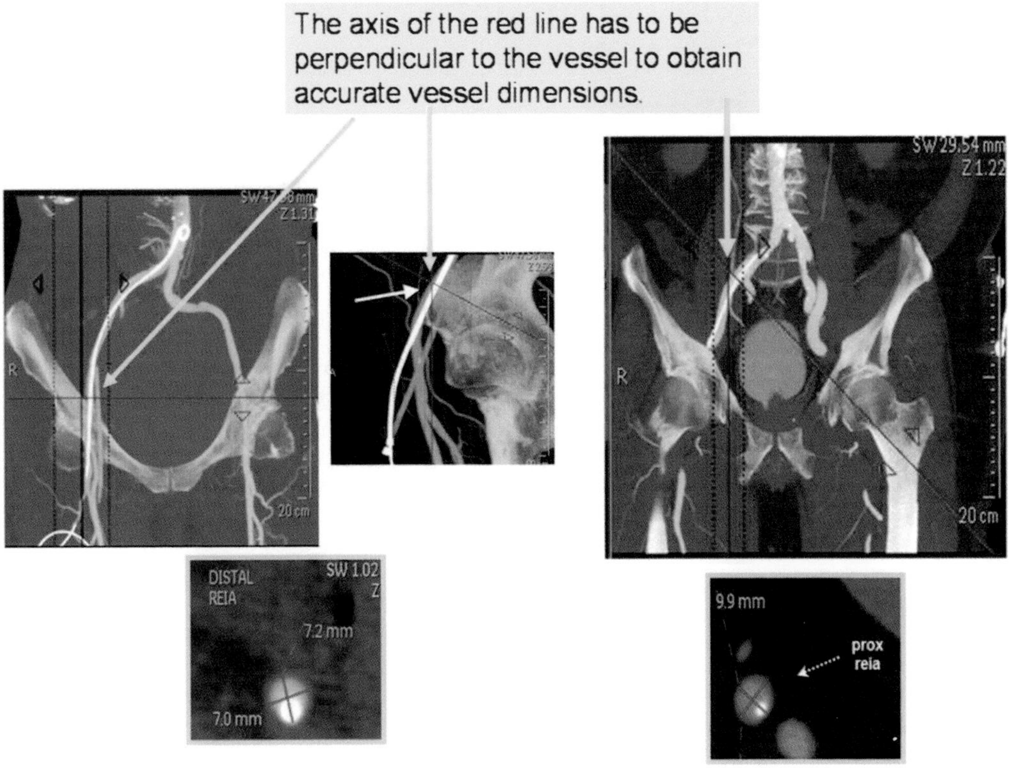

The axis of the red line has to be perpendicular to the vessel to obtain accurate vessel dimensions.

Figure 12 The axis of the red line has to be perpendicular to the vessel to obtain accurate vessel dimensions.

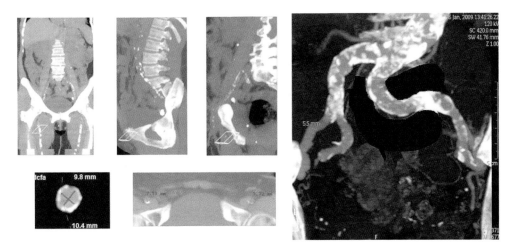

Figure 13 Noncontrast CT for measurements the amount of calcium.

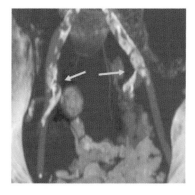

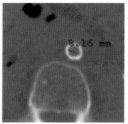

Figure 14   Severe calcification at the internal/external iliac bifurcation.

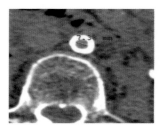

Figure 15   High-level blooming (*left panel*) dis-
tort vessel diameter measurement and evaluation of calcium severity. Low-level blooming (*right
panel*) allows for precise measurements.

Severe calcification at the bifurcation of internal and external iliac is of special concern as this area has no yield for expansion or movement: the internal iliac anchors the bifurcation down into the pelvis (Fig. 14).

Blooming artifact: Blooming has to be brought to a low level to perform adequate measurements of the vessels and to quantify the extent of calcification. The dimensions can change significantly after correction (Fig. 15; Video 1).

Tortuosity is best analyzed with contrast CT: 3D displays are rotated to best define tortuosity [Fig. 16(A) and 16(B)].

Virtual endoscopy with CT: This is at times useful to estimate the distribution of calcium within the lumen along the vessel being considered for access. See three examples with low amount of calcium (Video 2), mild spotty calcification (Video 3), and high amount of calcium with concentric arcs of calcium (Video 4). Concentric calcification can cause significant problem advancing or retrieving the delivery sheath.

Intravascular Ultrasound
We have used IVUS of the iliofemoral vessels when there is discrepancy in the results of angiography and CT. IVUS is excellent to measure vessel diameter but does not allow for good

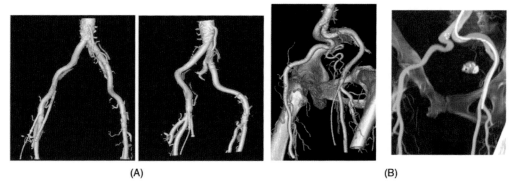

(A)   (B)

Figure 16   (**A**) and (**B**):3D contrast CT allows for analysis of tortuosity. (**A**) Mild tortuosity and (**B**) severe tortuosity.

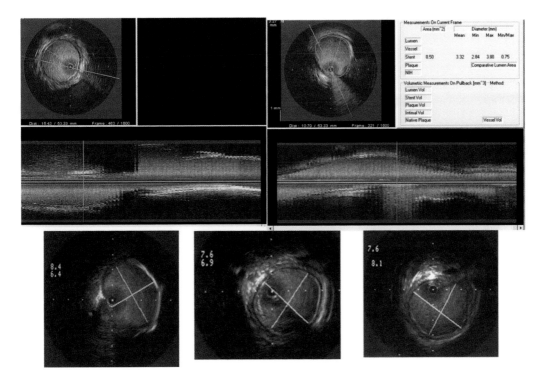

Figure 17 IVUS analysis of the iliofemoral vessels.

analysis of calcification (Fig. 17). In general, we see larger diameters with IVUS than with CT. In our experience, high-quality CT images are sufficiently good and we rarely use IVUS.

Percutaneous or Surgical Access Is Based On Preprocedure Assessment

The preprocedure assessment of the access vessels allows for the choice of the best technique. The femoral artery can be accessed percutaneously or by surgical cut down. Percutaneous access is an excellent choice in patients with large vessels and mild or no calcification, and by teams who have acquired significant experience with the percutaneous valve procedure. Preclosure using a single Prostar XL device (Abbott Vascular Devices, Redwood City, CA) (Fig. 18) is commonly used. Some operators have used two Prostar devices or three suture-mediated closure devices (6-F Perclose). Surgical exposure of the common femoral is preferred by many and provides an extra level of security especially when the preassessment showed vessels with challenging characteristics.

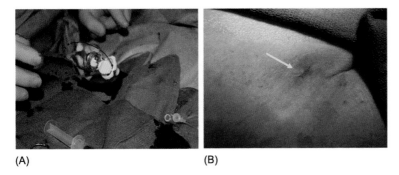

(A)   (B)

Figure 18 Femoral artery access by percutaneously Prostar XL device. (**A**) Prostar device for preclosure. (**B**) After procedure was completed with 24-F sheath.

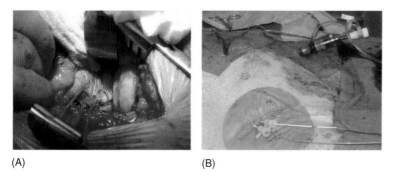

(A)   (B)

Figure 19   Retroperitoneal access with the (**A**) sheath tunneled from the inguinal entry site and (**B**) entering the common iliac tangentially.

We place the 22-F or 24-F delivery sheath from the start and proceed to cross the aortic valve, dilate the valve, and then deploy the prostheses. We find this method expedites the procedure greatly, as opposed to starting with a 6- to 8-F sheath to cross the valve, then placing a 12- to14-F sheath for valvuloplasty, then finally using the 22- to 24-F sheath.

If there is resistance advancing the dilators, never "push hard." Two signs are important to stop: patient having pain (in those not anesthetized), or the entire vessel "being rocked" on fluoroscopy as one tries to advance the sheath. Different lubricants have being tried to facilitate advancement of the dilators or sheaths without any clear advantage. If the dilators or the large sheath does not reach the common iliac, one could consider accessing the common iliac retroperitoneally. In this case, we do not use a conduit: the sheath is tunneled from the original inguinal access point and enters the common iliac tangentially, with minimal trauma to the vessel (Fig. 19).

ABDOMINAL AND THORACIC AORTA, ASCENDING AORTA, AND AORTIC ARCH

The abdominal aorta usually has adequate diameter for the large 22- to 24-F sheath. Occasionally CT has shown segments of significant narrowing with severe calcification in the abdominal aorta (Fig. 20), which exclude the patient for transfemoral access.

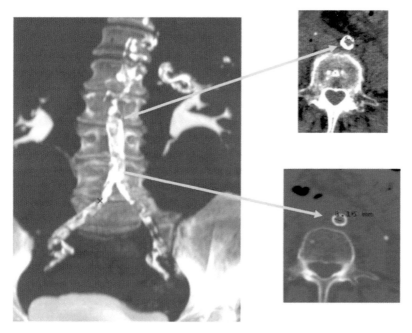

Figure 20   Concentric calcification in the abdominal aorta.

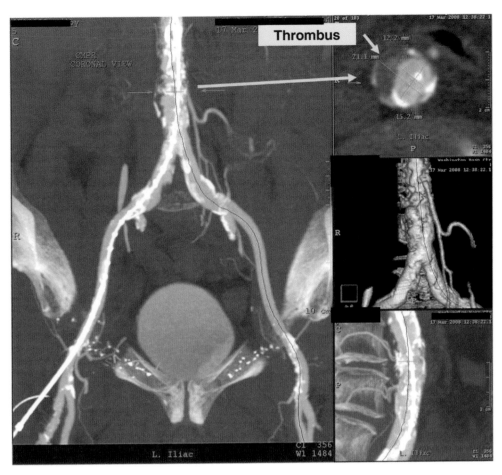

Figure 21 Extensive atherosclerosis of the aorta with thrombus.

Patients with extensive atherosclerosis of the aorta (Fig. 21) or large mobile protruding aortic atheromas are at high risk for neurological event during the procedure. Patients with porcelain aorta are in this group. Atherosclerotic material can also be displaced from the aortic valve itself or from the peripheral vessels and embolized to the brain, resulting in ischemic stroke (7). Careful advancement of the retroflex delivery system around the arch, and the new Retroflex II and III (with a cone at the tip) can help prevent the mobilization of aortic plaques.

Aortic aneurysms usually present no problem to advance the catheters and valve, but increase the risk of plaque or thrombus dislodgment. Thoracic or abdominal aortic grafts pose no problem to advance the delivery system, but aortoiliac grafts, especially with a long iliac limb do not allow for the large sheath to advance. Even if the diameter appears adequate, they wrinkle when the sheath is advanced and lock any movement. We do not recommend transfemoral approach in the presence of aortoiliac graft.

In case of severe peripheral disease or large atheroma in aorta it is better to change the strategy for transapical approach. CT images of the chest are helpful to plan the transapical procedure (Fig. 22).

AORTIC VALVULAR COMPLEX (AORTIC ROOT, AORTIC ANNULUS, AORTIC VALVE, AND CORONARY ARTERIES ORIGIN)

A very uncoiled aorta with the aortic valve in a vertical position (Fig. 23) precludes the ability to deliver the valve in the desired position. These cases are often excluded for the percutaneous aortic valve.

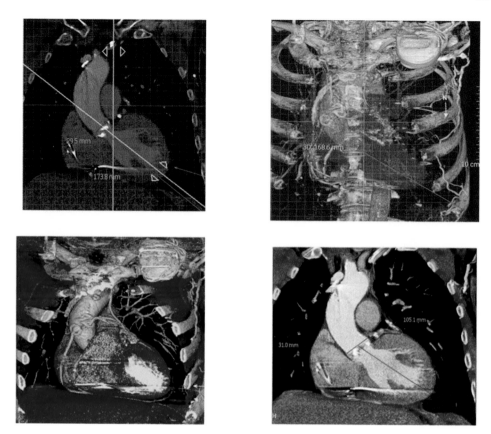

Figure 22   CT planning of transapical approach.

CT images of the aortic valve and root can be used to plan the best projection for valve delivery (Fig. 24). Heavy calcification of the aortic valve may cause problems for full and symmetric expansion of the valve.

Measurement of aortic annulus diameter before procedure is crucial especially in patients with borderline vascular access due to small iliac diameters. The annulus size will determine which valve size to use: 23- and 26-mm models are now available for annular size of 16 to 21 and 22 to 24, respectively. Measuring the annulus by transthoracic echocardiography usually underestimates the correct diameter. Transesophageal echo is now the standard for final determination of annular dimensions (Fig. 25). In cases that will possibly require a 26-mm valve and have borderline iliac size, one must do transesophageal echocardiography (TEE) before the percutaneous valve procedure to insure that the 23-mm valve will be sufficient. CT has not

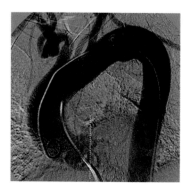

Figure 23   Uncoiled aorta with vertical orientation of the aortic valve.

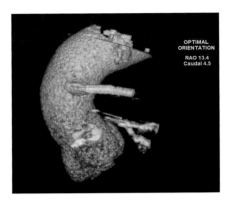

Figure 24   CT planning of the best projection for precise alignment of the aortic valve sinuses.

correlated well with TEE for this measurement, and further knowledge is required in this field before CT measurements are used for this purpose. We are beginning to acquire experience with echo imaging with intra-cardiac echocardiography (ICE) to have as an alternative to TEE.

The distance between aortic annulus and the coronary ostia showed a large variability and is independent of patient's height. The mean distance between the ostium of the coronary artery and the base of the sinus of Valsalva was reported to have a wide variation ranging from 7.1 to 22.7 with mean of 14.4 ± 2.9 mm. In almost 50% of the cases, the distance between the ostium and the annulus was smaller then the left coronary leaflet length and this may increase the risk of coronary occlusion during PAVR (8). It is important to evaluate the length between the inferior aspect of the annulus and the inferior aspects of the lowest coronary ostium for subsequent prosthetic aortic valve implantation (Fig. 26). The proximal one-third of the stent (aortic end) is uncovered to allow for coronary perfusion should the prosthesis stent cover the coronary ostia.

In a case of low left main coronary artery origin, it is recommended to do an aortogram during balloon valvuloplasty to determine if the aortic leaflet could obstruct the left main coronary artery ostium. Obstruction of coronary ostium can occur also during balloon valvuloplasty (Videos 5, 6, 7). The height of the Edwards SAPIEN valve is 14.5 mm and 16 mm for the 23 mm and 26 mm, respectively.

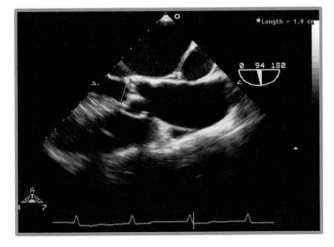

Figure 25   Annulus size measurement by TEE.

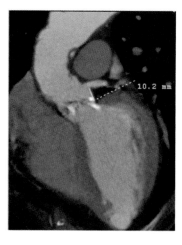

Figure 26 Measuring the length between the inferior aspect of the annulus and the inferior aspects of the coronary ostium.

LEFT VENTRICLE, CORONARIES, AND COEXISTENT CARDIAC CONDITIONS

Severe LV Dysfunction

Severe LV dysfunction may create a problem for PAVR. Immediately after balloon valvuloplasty or PAVR, the myocardium becomes transiently stunned and may have a serious drop in blood pressure and cardiac output. The presence of severe coronary disease may enhance the risk. Multiple preventive measures are used to address this issue (see following chapters).

In cases of very severe LV dysfunction, LV contractility reserve can be evaluated with Dobutamine testing. This is helpful to predict ability to survive the procedure as well as future LV function recovery.

Mitral Regurgitation

Severe organic mitral regurgitation should be an exclusion for PAVR. To evaluate how much the Mitral regurgitation (MR) could be secondary to critical aortic stenosis, one can perform aortic valvuloplasty and see the results through the next few weeks. In many patients the LV function improves and the MR diminishes significantly after valvuloplasty.

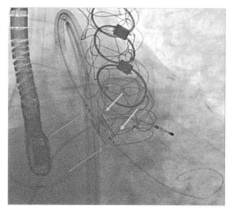

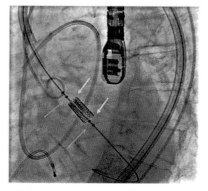

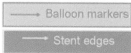

Figure 27 In case of patients with marked hypertrophy of the septum or sigmoid septum the valve is set lower in the balloon.

Patients with mild or moderate mitral regurgitation undergoing PAVR usually do well. In the majority of cases, MR grade stays the same; in a minority it may improve or worsen.

Left Ventricular Hypertrophy with Narrow Outflow Tract

In patients with marked hypertrophy of the septum or sigmoid septum accurate positioning of the percutaneous valve may be hampered: during inflation of the balloon the lack of space may squeeze the balloon toward the aorta before the stent/valve opens, and the valve will rise up with the risk of mal placement or even embolization. To avoid this we mount the valve lower in the balloon; this technique has resulted in less or no motion of the stent/valve during deployment (Fig. 27).

SUMMARY—PATIENT MATRIX

Detailed precise screening is the key for success in PAVR. Patients are selected based on their high surgical risk or inoperability. Because of the large delivery system, careful evaluation of the iliofemoral vessels is indispensable. Because this is the most common cause of morbidity/mortality, we recommend angio and high-quality CT in all patients. It is important to know the amount of atherosclerosis and plaque in the aortic arch and ascending aorta for potential risk of neurological events. Measuring the aortic annulus diameter is also important for valve sizing and avoiding paravalvular leak. The relation between the annulus, left coronary leaflet, and left coronary exists is important. Assessment of all these components is necessary for preprocedural planning of access approach, valve sizing, and deployment.

ACKNOWLEDGMENT

We are grateful to Nelson Puig, Senior CV Technician in the WHC Cath Labs, for generating most of the images presented in this chapter.

REFERENCES

1. Dewey TM, Brown D, Ryan WH, et al. Reliability of risk algorithms in predicting early and late operative outcomes in high-risk patients undergoing aortic valve replacement. J Thorac Cardiovasc Surg 2008; 135:180–187.
2. Osswald BR, Gegouskov V, Badowski-Zyla D, et al. Overestimation of aortic valve replacement risk by Euro SCORE: Implications for percutaneous valve replacement. Eur Heart J 2009; 30: 74–80.
3. Brown ML, Schaff HV, Sarano ME, et al. Is the European System for Cardiac Operative Risk Evaluation model valid for estimating the operative risk of patients considered for percutaneous aortic valve replacement? J Thorac Cardiovasc Surg 2008; 136:566–571.
4. Purser JL, Kuchibhatla MN, Fillenbaum GG, et al. Identifying frailty in hospitalized older adults with significant coronary artery disease. J Am Geriatr Soc 2006; 54:1674–1681.
5. Jones DM, Song X, Rockwood K. Operationalizing a frailty index from a standardized comprehensive geriatric assessment. J Am Geriatr Soc 2004; 52:1929–1933.
6. Joshi SB, Mendoza D, Steinberg D, et al. ilio-femoral CT Angiography with ultra-low dose intra-arterial contrast injection—A novel imaging protocol to assess eligibility for percutaneous aortic valve replacement. J Cardiovasc Comput Tomogr 2008; 2:S5–S6.
7. Berry C, Cartier R, Bonan R. Fatal ischemic stroke related to nonpermissive peripheral artery access for percutaneous aortic valve replacement. Catheter Cardiovasc Interv 2007; 69:56–63.
8. Tops LF, Wood DA, DelgadoV, et al. Noninvasive evaluation of the aortic root with multislice computed tomography. JACC Cardiol Imaging 2008; 1:321–330.

6 | Patient Selection for the CoreValve ReValving System

Nicolo Piazza, Peter de Jaegere, Yoshinobu Onuma, Patrick W. Serruys
Department of Interventional Cardiology, Erasmus University Medical Center, Thoraxcenter, Rotterdam, The Netherlands

Ganesh Manoharan
Department of Interventional Cardiology, Heart Center, Belfast, U.K.

> *The magic behind every outstanding performance is always found in the smallest of details.*
> *Gary Ryan Blair*

INTRODUCTION

Patient selection plays a crucial role in the success of transcatheter aortic valve implantation (TAVI)—this cannot be overemphasized. It requires meticulous attention to the smallest of details and needs to be performed in a systematic manner in every patient. Becoming over "complacent" and "routine" in the patient selection process can presage failure. Every patient deserves a fresh start approach.

TAVI is currently reserved for patients with severe aortic stenosis deemed high or prohibitive surgical risk—but this may change in the future. Although not the focus of this chapter, identification of high or prohibitive surgical risk patient should rely on the clinical judgment of a Heart Team (specifically, interventional cardiologists and cardiac surgeons) in conjunction with information gleaned from surgical risk scores such as the STS Predicted Risk of Mortality and logistic EuroSCORE (1,2).

This chapter focuses on the anatomic boundaries for implantation of the 26- or 29-mm sized prosthesis using the third-generation 18-F CoreValve ReValving system. In particular, the chapter will focus on the peripheral arterial system, aortic root, aortic valvar complex, left ventricle, and mitral valve, which are important for TAVI (Fig. 1). In essence, the patient must be assessed from access to implantation site.

WHY IS PATIENT SELECTION IMPORTANT?

A conservative approach during the initial premarket approval process (e.g., excluding patients with complicated cardiac anatomy, severe left ventricular dysfunction, severe coronary artery disease, and combination of valvulopathies) maximizes the chances of demonstrating efficacy while minimizing the risk of death or procedural complications.

It is assumed that adherence to patient selection criteria will reduce the frequency of complications such as dissection of the aorta or arterial tree, cardiac tamponade, obstruction of the coronary arteries, device maldeployment or migration, and severe aortic insufficiency. However, the association between patient selection criteria and procedural complications still needs further elucidation (3).

A collection report form or checklist can be used to (*i*) ensure consistency and completeness of data collection, (*ii*) adherence to clinical practice guidelines, (*iii*) facilitate communication among team members, and (*iv*) serve research purposes.

RISK–BENEFIT ANALYSIS

The fact that a patient is deemed inoperable and has suitable anatomy does not necessarily imply that they are candidates for the procedure. In other words, feasibility does not necessarily imply safety. Anecdotal experience suggests that patients with other limiting comorbidities such as severe pulmonary disease or debilitating neuromuscular disease may not even benefit from TAVI. Indeed, approximately one-quarter of patients remain in New York Heart Association class III or IV (this includes patients who may have improved from class IV to III) (4).

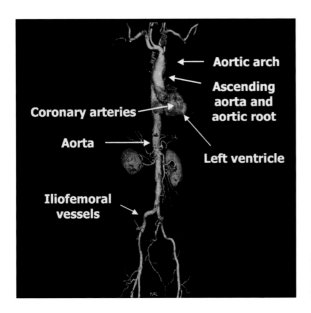

Figure 1 MSCT volume rendered anatomy of the arterial system. Patient Selection requires assessment of the patient from access to implantation site.

PERIPHERAL ARTERIAL SYSTEM

Assessment of the peripheral arterial system begins with a detailed history and physical exam. The history should evaluate for associated risk factors (e.g., diabetes, smoking, hypertension, and hypercholesterolemia), prior history of peripheral arterial bypass surgery, and symptoms of peripheral arterial disease.

Imaging techniques such as fluoroscopic angiography, computed tomographic angiography, and magnetic resonance angiography can provide objective information of the peripheral arterial system—salient features include vessel diameter, degree of calcification and atherosclerosis, obstruction, tortuosity, and ulceration.

Aortoiliofemoral Vessels

The iliofemoral artery remains the default approach for vascular access. To accommodate the 18-F vascular access sheath, the minimum requirement for vessel diameter is 6 mm (Fig. 2, Video 1). Subjective quantification of vessel calcification and atherosclerosis by using any of the

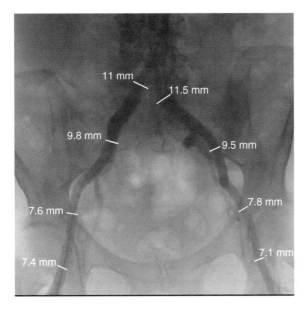

Figure 2 Iliofemoral angiogram demonstrating acceptable vessel diameter for accommodation of the 18-F vascular access sheath.

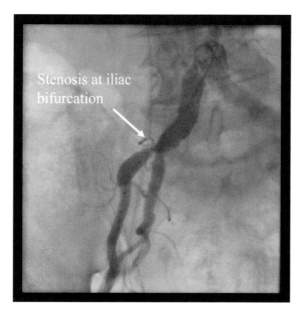

Figure 3 Iliofemoral angiogram consistent with severe atherosclerotic narrowing at the right iliac bifurcation point (white arrow).

aforementioned imaging modalities can help anticipate potential areas of dissection, rupture, or problems with advancing the delivery catheter system (Fig. 3, Video 2) (5). Furthermore, some physicians consider circumferential calcification observed on MSCT or severe atherosclerotic narrowing (>50%–70%) of the iliofemoral vessels to be contraindications to TAVI.

Although diseased peripheral vasculature is not an absolute contraindication to TAVI, it increases the risk for complications significantly. In these cases, two approaches can be considered: (*i*) attempt to cautiously advance the vascular access sheath and catheter delivery system across the diseased vasculature, implant the valve, and repair any complications such as dissections "on the way out" by percutaneous transluminal angioplasty/stent implantation or (*ii*) peripheral vascular interventions (percutaneous transluminal angioplasty or stent implantation) of the aortoiliofemoral vessels can be performed prior to valve implantation (Videos 3, 4, 5) (6). The former approach is generally advocated. Although the latter approach has been performed successfully in experienced centers, there is risk of dislodging the implanted stent during either (1) advancement of the vascular access sheath or delivery catheter or (2) in cases where the semideployed valve needs to be retrieved from the body (see Fig. 14 in chap. 17).

Significant tortuosity alone of the iliofemoral vessels is not necessarily a contraindication to TAVI as long as the vessels are otherwise healthy and compliant—gentle advancement of the stiff guidewire or vascular access sheath will tend to straighten the vessel.

Special precautions are necessary for patients with diabetes or on dialysis given their higher likelihood of significant peripheral vascular disease.

Patient Selection for Subclavian Access

In cases where the anatomy of the iliofemoral vessels is unacceptable, the second option for vascular access with the CoreValve system should be the subclavian artery. Possible options include both the right and left subclavian with a number of important caveats. First, similar to the transfemoral approach, the minimum acceptable artery diameter is 6 mm. Second, the left subclavian artery is preferred over the right. In most cases, the approach from the left subclavian is straightforward irrespective of the aortic root angulation. In contrast, if the angulation between the plane of the annulus and a horizontal reference line is more than 30 degrees (suggesting a horizontal aorta or vertical annulus plane), an approach from the right subclavian will be technically challenging (see Fig. 1 from chap. 10); it is virtually impossible to accurately position and deploy the prosthesis. Other possible options for vascular access include (*i*) direct access thoracotomy and (*ii*) retroperitoneal vascular access.

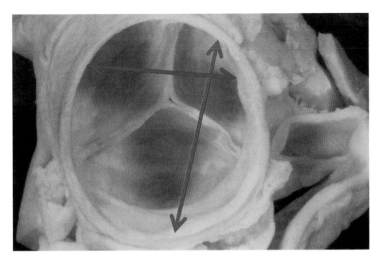

Figure 4 This short-axis basal view of the aortic valve highlights the potential hazard of two-dimensional imaging in measuring the "aortic valve annulus" (or any structure of the aortic root for that matter). Measurements made with two-dimensional imaging represent a tangent cut across the root and do not necessarily transect its full diameter. The blue and red arrows represent two conceivable tangents.

Some physicians view the presence of an internal mammary artery graft as a contraindication to the subclavian approach. Other physicians believe that the subclavian approach can be safely performed in the presence of an internal mammary graft if some criteria are met. In particular the minimum acceptable artery diameter should be 6.5 to 7.0 mm. Furthermore, to reduce the risk of retrograde dissection of the internal mammary artery graft, the segment of the subclavian artery proximal to the internal mammary should be free of atherosclerotic disease.

Aortic Arch

Due to the flexible nature of the Nitinol prosthesis, it is unusual to encounter resistance during advancement of the delivery catheter system across the aortic arch unless atherosclerotic plaques or calcium deposits get in the way (Videos 6 and 7). Nonetheless, note can be taken of the angulation of the aortic arch (e.g., large-radius turns or sharp bends) evaluated by contrast aortography, multislice computed tomography (MSCT), or magnetic resonance imaging (MRI).

Aortic Root and Ascending Aorta

By definition, the aortic root extends from the most basal attachment line of the aortic valvar leaflets within the left ventricle to their peripheral attachment at the level of the sinotubular junction. It follows that the ascending aorta extends from the level of the sinotubular junction to the take-off of the right subclavian artery.

It is our preference to describe the various components of the valve and describe the variable diameter of the root at its different parts rather than nominating any single component as the annulus. From a clinical standpoint, the diameters of the root measured by echocardiography, contrast aortography, MSCT, or MRI can vary markedly. The measurements of the aortic root obtained by echocardiography and contrast aortography are limited by their two-dimensional nature. These measurements correspond to some tangent cut across the root (Fig. 4) (7). The root is not particularly circular at any level. The "annulus," for instance, is more like an ellipse with a maximum and minimum diameter (8). Measurements of this structure, therefore, will depend on the plane or angulation selected. Three-dimensional imaging modalities (3-D echocardiography, MSCT, and MRI) on the other hand may provide more accurate measurements of the aortic root at any desired level or plane (Video 8—slicing of the aorta).

Figure 5 demonstrates the key measurements of the aortic root and ascending aorta for implantation of the CoreValve device. The maximum acceptable diameter of the ascending aorta is 40 and 43 mm for implantation of the 26- and 29-mm device, respectively (Fig. 6). The outflow portion of the prosthesis positions itself within the ascending aorta and functions to

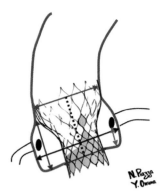

1. **AV Annulus diameter**

2. **Sinus of Valsalva diameter**

3. **Sinus of Valsalva height**

4. **Ascending aorta diameter**

5. **Height of the coronary ostia**

······· Ascending aorta diameter
measured 45 mm above AV
annulus

Figure 5   Pictorial representation of the aortic root and ascending aorta with a CoreValve prosthesis in-situ. Key measurements for CoreValve implantation are shown.

orient itself perpendicular to the direction of blood flow. Keeping in mind both the height of the prosthesis (~50 mm) and depth of implantation (~6–8 mm), the diameter of the ascending aorta is measured at a level 40–45 mm from the basal attachment line of the aortic valve leaflets (Fig. 5). A relatively large ascending aorta can run the potential risk of causing valve embolization if the inflow portion of the prosthesis is not well anchored.

   If the prosthesis is to be properly accommodated without impinging on the orifices of the coronary arteries, a number of anatomical factors should be taken into consideration: (*i*) the width and height of the sinus of Valsalva; (*ii*) height of the coronary artery orifice measured from the base of the native aortic leaflet to the inferior rim of the coronary ostia [Figs. 7(A) and (B)]; (*iii*) bulkiness of aortic valve calcification. During percutaneous balloon aortic valvuloplasty or valve deployment, the native aortic valve leaflets are displaced toward the coronary artery ostia. A narrow sinus of Valsalva (<27 mm and <29 mm for the 26- and 29-mm device, respectively), a short sinus of Valsalva (<15 mm), low-lying coronary artery (<10 mm height), large aortic valve leaflet, and/or severe leaflet calcification can act in concert to increase the risk of compromising the coronary artery ostia during CoreValve implantation (Fig. 6). Contrast aortography during preimplantation balloon aortic valvuloplasty can be helpful to understand how the native aortic valve leaflets and calcium deposits may become displaced and possible occlude the coronary arteries [Fig. 8, Videos 9, 10, 11].

Aortic Valve Annulus
The base of the aortic root formed by joining the basal attachment points of the aortic leaflets within the left ventricle is clinically, albeit confusingly, known as the "aortic valve annulus."

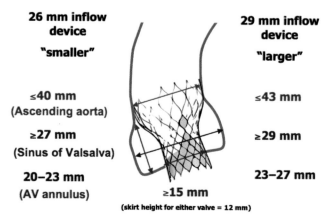

Figure 6   Anatomical prerequisites for implantation of the 26- and 29-mm CoreValve device. Minimum requirement of height of coronary artery ~10 mm (not shown in the figure).

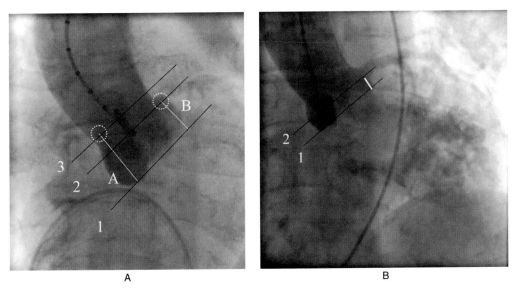

A   B

Figure 7 The take-off height of the coronary artery ostium is measured from the inferior rim of the ostium of the coronary artery to the most basal attachment point of the corresponding left or right native aortic valve leaflet. (**A**) First, we need to identify the ostium of the left and right coronary artery (dotted circles). Second, we need to identify the plane of the aortic valve annulus (line 1) that represents the most basal attachment point of the native aortic valve leaflets. Third, we need to identify the inferior rim of the coronary artery and draw a plane (line 2) parallel to the plane of the aortic valve annulus (line 1). In this example, the take-off height of the left and right coronary artery represents the distance between line 1 and 2, and line 1 and 3, respectively. Both heights were considered acceptable, i.e., >10 mm. (**B**) In this patient, the take-off height of the left coronary artery was 7.9 mm (distance between line 1 and 2). Although implantation of the CoreValve device was considered contraindicated, the patient nevertheless underwent successful valve implantation (see Videos 10–12 for further discussion and follow-up).

The diameter of this ring has played a crucial (and confusing) role in the selection of the size of prosthesis to be inserted. The 26- and 29-mm devices are intended for aortic valve annuli measuring 20 to 23 mm and 23 to 27 mm, respectively—the device was purposely oversized to create enough radial force to help anchor itself within the aortic root. If measurements of the "aortic valve annulus" fall within borderline limits of a 26- or 29-mm device, the following

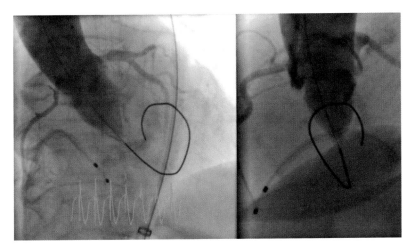

Figure 8 Contrast aortography performed during balloon aortic valvuloplasty can be used to examine the potential relationship between the coronary ostia and displacement of the aortic valve leaflets and calcium prior to valve implantation.

points should be kept in mind to facilitate selection of the appropriate-sized prosthesis: (*i*) measurements obtained from multiple imaging techniques (transthoracic or transesophageal echocardiography vs. MSCT vs. contrast aortography) and (*ii*) relative dimensions of the sinus of Valsalva and ascending aorta.

Issues such as "which imaging method should I use to measure the aortic valve annulus" and the implications of oversizing and undersizing the device relative to the aortic root will be discussed in other chapters.

Coronary Artery Disease
Coronary atherosclerosis is a common finding in patients with severe aortic stenosis; both conditions are associated with similar risks such as coronary atherosclerosis such as older age, hypertension, diabetes, hypercholesterolemia, and smoking. Although initial safety and efficacy trials excluded patients with severe coronary disease (>70% proximal stenosis), with increasing operator experience and CE mark approval there is a growing trend to perform either staged or concomitant percutaneous coronary interventions (PCI) in association with the valve procedure (Videos 12, 13, 14, 15) (9).

Patients with untreated severe proximal left and right coronary artery disease may not tolerate the stress associated with balloon aortic valvuloplasty or valve deployment. This may be even truer in those patients with left ventricular dysfunction. In our experience, PCI of at least the left main or proximal left anterior descending artery in patients with multivessel disease may provide enough cardiac reserve for a successful outcome. This may be performed either in a staged manner or concomitantly just before valve implantation. Temporary circulatory support using the TandemHeart® peripheral left ventricular assist device (pLVAD) is recommended for patients with left ventricular dysfunction. As an aside, the significant reduction of left ventricular stroke volume while on TandemHeart support can virtually eliminate migration of the balloon during aortic valvuloplasty and obviate the need for rapid bursting pacing.

Only a minority of patients with coronary disease (~10%) require PCI specifically in preparation for TAVI (10). The majority of these elderly patients have sufficient relief of their angina by valve replacement alone. On the other hand, approximately one-quarter of patients are in NYHA III or IV after valve implantation and factors such as residual coronary disease, pulmonary disease and/or physical deconditioning may be the limiting factors.

Left Ventricle
Four features of the left ventricle require evaluation: (*i*) left ventricular ejection fraction, (*ii*) left ventricular wall thickness, (*iii*) presence/absence of left ventricular thrombus, and (*iv*) presence/absence of subaortic stenosis.

Knowledge of left ventricular function can provide useful insight into the severity and duration of the valvular stenosis. Pertinent to the implantation procedure, the degree of left ventricular dysfunction can help gauge the hearts' ability to tolerate the stress of the procedure. Stress with the procedure can be encountered during induction anesthesia, rapid-pacing preimplantation balloon aortic valvuloplasty or procedural complications associated with hypovolemia and hypotension.

In patients with severe left ventricular dysfunction (especially <20%), the procedure should be facilitated by circulatory support systems (pLVAD, peripheral extracorporeal membrane oxygenation) (11). These devices may also be used in high-risk patients with complex coronary disease, undergoing concomitant PCI during the index valve procedure.

The in-hospital mortality rate of patients with low flow, low-gradient aortic stenosis (i.e., mean transaortic pressure gradient ≤40 mm Hg, left ventricular ejection fraction ≤35%) undergoing surgical aortic valve replacement can range from 6% to 33%, depending on the presence or absence of contractile reserve (12). Whether patients with low flow, low-gradient aortic stenosis undergoing TAVI have an elevated risk for short-term mortality and if this is related to contractile reserve is not yet known.

Patients with severe left ventricular hypertrophy are at relatively higher risk for cardiac perforation. Although this may appear counterintuitive, a small ventricular cavity and stiff guidewire can combine to increase this risk (Fig. 9).

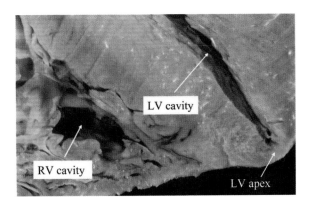

Figure 9 This specimen shows severe left ventricular hypertrophy associated with a small ventricular cavity. Note the thinness of the left ventricular apex despite the severity of left ventricular wall hypertrophy. *Abbreviations*: LV, left ventricle; RV, right ventricle.

Echocardiography, MSCT, or MRI can be used to assess for the presence or absence of atrial or ventricular thrombus. The presence of thrombus is a contraindication to perform TAVI.

Mitral Regurgitation

A complete preprocedural evaluation should include echocardiographic assessment of the mitral valve apparatus for regurgitation or stenosis. The clinical implications of the severity of mitral regurgitation and patient selection for TAVI are currently unknown. In our experience of 79 consecutive patients, mitral regurgitation was mild, moderate, and severe in 57%, 18%, and 1% of the patients, respectively. Of those with mitral regurgitation, 27 patients (50%) had organic and 27 patients (50%) had functional mitral regurgitation. After CoreValve implantation, the degree of mitral regurgitation remained unchanged in 61% of patients, improved in 17%, and worsened in 22% (13).

Carotid Duplex Ultrasonography

Symptomatic carotid or vertebral artery disease should be documented preprocedure to better appreciate the patients' atherosclerotic burden. Although patients identified with carotid artery stenosis (>50–70%) prior to cardiac surgery are at increased risk for stroke (14), similar findings are yet to be confirmed in patients undergoing TAVI.

Electrocardiography

Aortic stenosis is known to be associated with abnormalities of cardiac conduction. Following implantation of the CoreValve ReValving system, new onset left bundle branch block can be observed in up to 40% of patients. This may not be surprising considering the close anatomical proximity between the aortic valvar complex and conduction system. In almost all cases, the left bundle branch block develops during the procedure (in these cases, approximately 45% before valve deployment and in 55% after valve deployment). New conduction abnormalities, however, can also develop in the postprocedural period [Fig. 10(A)–(D)]. Patients with preexisting right bundle branch block may be at increased risk for complete heart block and need of pacemaking.

Up to one-third of patients undergoing surgical aortic valve replacement can develop intraventricular conduction defects (15,16). Furthermore, a permanent pacemaker is required in about 3% to 8% of these patients (17).

CURRENT EXCLUSION CRITERIA

Typical exclusion criteria comprise any of the following: known hypersensitivity or contraindication to antiplatelet or anticoagulant therapy, Nitinol, or contrast media that could not be adequately premedicated; any sepsis; uncontrolled atrial or ventricular arrhythmia; bleeding diathesis or coagulopathy; creatinine clearance <20 mL/min; and life expectancy less than 1 year.

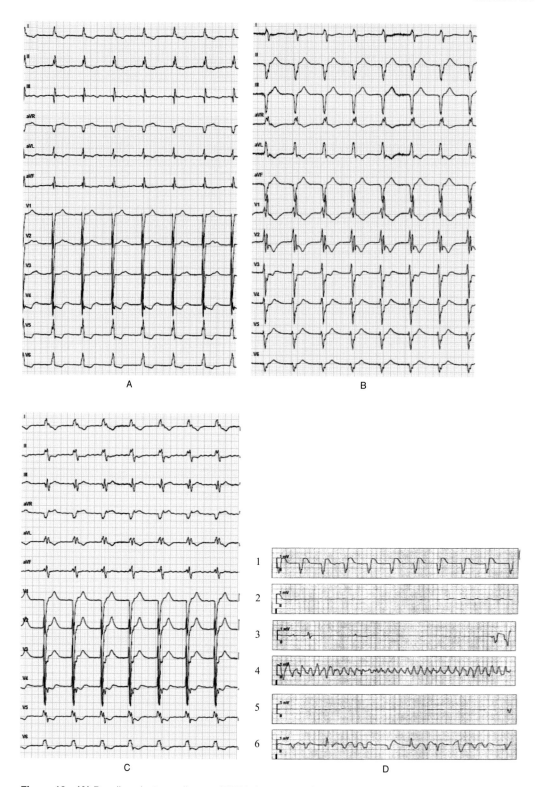

Figure 10   **(A)** Baseline electrocardiogram (ECG) demonstrated preexisting left bundle branch block. **(B** and **C)**
On postprocedural day 2 and 3, the patient developed alternating left and right bundle branch block, respectively.
(D) Continuous rhythm strip. On postprocedural day 5, the patient died from sinus arrest and complete AV block.
This case highlights the importance of continuous telemetry monitoring after the procedure and the consideration
for permanent pacemaking.

Elements below reflect Indications for Use according to the CE Mark

Diagnostic Findings	Non-Invasive			Angiography			Selection Criteria	
	Echo	CT/MRI	LV	Ao Root	CAG	Vascular	Recommended	Not Recommended
Atrial Ventricular Thrombus	X						Not Present	Present
Sub Aortic Stenosis	X	X	X				Not Present	Present
LV Ejection Fraction	X		X				≥20%	<20% without contractile reserve
Mitral Regurgitation	X						≤Grade 2	>Grade 2 Organic Reason
Vascular Access Diameter		X				X	≥6 mm Diameter	<6 mm Diameter
Aortic and Vascular Disease		X				X	None to Moderate	Sever Vascular Disease
Indications for 26 mm CoreValve Device								
Annulus Diameter	X	X					20-23 mm	<20 mm or >23 mm
Ascending Aorta Diameter		X		X			≤40 mm	>40 mm
Indications for 29 mm CoreValve Device								
Annulus Diameter	X	X					24-27 mm	<24 mm or >27 mm
Ascending Aorta Diameter		X		X			≤43 mm	>43 mm

General medical guidance for use CoreValve*

Diagnostic Findings	Non-Invasive			Angiography			Selection Criteria	
	Echo	CT/MRI	LV	Ao Root	CAG	Vascular	Recommended	Moderate-High Risk
LV Hypertrophy	X	X					Normal to Moderate 0.6 - 1.6 cm	Severe ≥ 1.7 cm
Coronary Artery Disease		X			X		None, Mid or Distal >70%	Proximal Lesions >70%
Aortic Arch Angulation						X	Large Radial Turn	Sharp Turn
Aortic Root Angulation		X				X	≤30 degrees	30-45 degrees
Aortic and Vascular Disease		X				X	No or Light Vascular Dosease	Moderate Vascular Disease
Vascular Access Diameter		X				X	>6 mm	Calcified and elongated >7 mm
Anatomic Considerations for 26 mm CoreValve Device								
Sinus of Valsalva Width	X	X		X			≥27 mm	<27 mm
Sinus of Valsalva Height	X	X		X			>15 mm	<15 mm
Anatomic Considerations for 29 mm CoreValve Device								
Sinus of Valsalva Width	X	X		X			≥29 mm	<29 mm
Sinus of Valsalva Height	X	X		X			>15 mm	<15 mm

*-General medical guidance reflects the experience to date with the product, but final judgment remains with the implanting physicians(s).

Consult with a certified proctor to determine if your patient is Moderate-High Risk

INTERNATIONAL
CAUTION: The CoreValve System is not currently available in the USA for clinical trials for sale.
CoreValve is a registered trademark of Medtronic CV Luxembourg S.a.r.l.

Figure 11 Medtronic CoreValve patient evaluation criteria.

SPECIAL CONSIDERATIONS

Transcatheter Aortic Valve Implantation for a Failing Surgical Bioprosthetic Aortic Valve (Transcatheter Aortic Valve in Surgical Aortic Valve (TAV-in-SAV) or REDO™)

The first successful implantation of a transcatheter aortic valve for a failing surgical bioprosthesis was reported in 2007; using the CoreValve device (18–19). Since then, numerous case reports have been published describing transcatheter aortic valve implantation for failing stented or stentless bioprosthetic valves or homografts (20–25). This is currently an off-label indication for the CoreValve device although feasibility studies are currently ongoing. There have been over 40 cases performed worldwide on compassionate basis.

CONCLUSION

Patient selection is a time-consuming process—it requires a systematic team approach best accomplished in a dedicated outpatient referral clinic. Adherence to the patient selection matrix should in theory minimize the risks of failure and complications. Figure 11 shows the patient evaluation criteria that provides general medical guidance based on the experience to date with the 18-F CoreValve System. It is important to realize that clinical judgment should not be reduced to simple algorithms or flow charts—final judgment remains with the implanting physician.

REFERENCES

1. Rankin JS, Hammill BG, Ferguson TB Jr., et al. Determinants of operative mortality in valvular heart surgery. J Thorac Cardiovasc Surg 2006; 131(3):547–557.
2. Nashef SA, Roques F, Michel P, et al. European system for cardiac operative risk evaluation (EuroSCORE). Eur J Cardiothorac Surg 1999; 16(1):9–13.
3. Piazza N, Otten A, Schultz C, et al. Adherence to patient selection criteria in patients undergoing transcatheter aortic valve implantation with the 18F CoreValve ReValving System – Results from a single center study. Heart 2009 Sep 10 [Epub ahead of print]
4. Serruys P. The CoreValve Expanded Evaluation Registry. The Rotterdam CoreValve Training Course. December 15, 2008.
5. Jilaihawi H, Spyt T, Chin D, et al. Percutaneous aortic valve replacement in patients with challenging aortoiliofemoral access. Cath Cardiovasc Interv 2008; 72(6):885–890.
6. Piazza N, Schultz C, de Jaegere PP, et al. Implantation of two self-expanding aortic bioprosthetic valves during the same procedure-Insights into valve-in-valve implantation ("Russian doll concept"). Catheter Cardiovasc Interv 2009; 73(4):530–539.
7. Piazza N, de Jaegere P, Schultz C, et al. Anatomy of the aortic valvar complex and its implications for transcatheter implantation of the aortic valve. Circ Cardiovasc Interv 2008; 1:74–81.
8. Tops LF WD, Delgado V, Schuijf JD, et al. Nonivasive evaluation of the aortic root with multi-slice computed tomography: Implications for transcatheter aortic valve replacement. JACC Cardiovasc Imaging 2008; 1:321–330.
9. Piazza N, Serruys PW, de Jaegere P. Feasibility of complex coronary intervention in combination with percutaneous aortic valve implantation in patients with aortic stenosis using percutaneous left ventricular assist device (TandemHeart). Cath Cardiovasc Interv 2009; 73(2):161–166.
10. Webb JG. Strategies in the management of coronary artery disease and transcatheter aortic valve implantation. Catheter Cardiovasc Interv 2009; 73(1):68.
11. de Jaegere P, van Dijk L, Laborde JC, et al. True percutaneous implantation of the CoreValve aortic valve prosthesis by the combined use of ultrasound guided vascular access, Prostar XL and the TandemHeart. Eurointervention 2007; 2:500–505.
12. Subramanian H, Kunadian B, Dunning J. Is it ever worth contemplating an aortic valve replacement on patients with low gradient severe aortic stenosis but poor left ventricular function with no contractile reserve? Interact Cardiovasc Thorac Surg 2008; 7(2):301–305.
13. Tzikas A, Piazza N, van Dalen BM, et al. Changes in mitral regurgitation after transcatheter aortic valve implantation. Catheter Cardiovasc Interv 2009; [Epub ahead of print].
14. D'Agostino RS, Svensson LG, Neumann DJ, et al. Screening carotid ultrasonography and risk factors for stroke in coronary artery surgery patients. Ann Thorac Surg 1996; 62(6):1714–1723.
15. El-Khally Z, Thibault B, Staniloae C, et al. Prognostic significance of newly acquired bundle branch block after aortic valve replacement. Am J Cardiol 2004; 94(8):1008–1011.
16. Thomas JL, Dickstein RA, Parker FB Jr., et al. Prognostic significance of the development of left bundle conduction defects following aortic valve replacement. J Thorac Cardiovasc Surg 1982; 84(3):382–386.

17. Kolh P, Lahaye L, Gerard P, et al. Aortic valve replacement in the octogenarians: Perioperative outcome and clinical follow-up. Eur J Cardiothorac Surg 1999; 16(1):68–73.
18. Webb JG. Transcatheter valve in valve implants for failed prosthetic valves. Cath Cardiovasc Interv 2007; 70(5):765–766.
19. Wenaweser P, Buellesfeld L, Gerckens U, et al. Percutaneous aortic valve replacement for severe aortic regurgitation in degenerated bioprosthesis: The first valve in valve procedure using the Corevalve Revalving system. Cath Cardiovasc Interv 2007; 70(5):760–764.
20. Attias D, Himbert D, Brochet E, et al. 'Valve-in-valve' implantation in a patient with degenerated aortic bioprosthesis and severe regurgitation. Eur Heart J 2009; 30(15):1852.
21. Attias D, Himbert D, Hvass U, et al. "Valve-in-valve" implantation in a patient with stentless bioprosthesis and severe intraprosthetic aortic regurgitation. J Thorac Cardiovas Surg 2009; 138(4):1020–1022.
22. Kelpis TG, Mezilis NE, Ninios VN, et al. Minimally invasive transapical aortic valve-in-a-valve implantation for severe aortic regurgitation in a degenerated stentless bioprosthesis. J Thorac Cardiovas Surg 2009; 138(4):1018–1020.
23. Klaaborg KE, Egeblad H, Jakobsen CJ, et al. Transapical transcatheter treatment of a stenosed aortic valve bioprosthesis using the Edwards SAPIEN Transcatheter Heart Valve. Ann Thorac Surg 2009; 87(6):1943–1946.
24. Schmoeckel M, Boekstegers P, Nikolaou K, et al. First successful transapical aortic valve implantation after aortic allograft replacement. J Thorac Cardiovas Surg 2009; 138(4):1016–1017.
25. Ussia GP, Mule M, Tamburino C. The valve-in-valve technique: transcatheter treatment of aortic bioprothesis malposition. Catheter Cardiovasc Interv 2009; 73(5):713–716.

7 | CoreValve ReValving System for Percutaneous Aortic Valve Replacement

Rob Michiels

CONSILIUM Associates LLC and Consultant to Medtronic-CoreValve, Irvine, California, U.S.A.

The CoreValve ReValving system for percutaneous aortic valve replacement (PAVR) consists of three components: the self-expanding multilevel support frame with a trileaflet porcine pericardial tissue valve, the catheter delivery system, and a disposable loading system. Design conception and iterative prototyping took place during 1997 to 2002 and first-generation device technical preclinical, animal, and cadaver work was completed by early 2004. A first-in-man clinical feasibility study was conducted during 2004 with the first-generation 25-F device. Safety and efficacy studies were conducted during 2005 and 2006 with two subsequent device generations, which saw the diameter of the PAVR delivery catheter dramatically reduced. Prior iterations are described in the literature and this chapter focuses on the current, third-generation 18-F device, which received CE Mark during 2007.

SUPPORT FRAME AND BIOPROSTHESIS

At the center of the system is a multilevel self-expanding and fully radiopaque Nitinol frame with a diamond cell configuration that holds the tissue valve and anchors the device in the native anatomy. This noncylindrical frame design incorporates varying levels into a single construct and exhibits three different diameters and three totally different degrees of radial and hoop strength (Figs. 1–3). An important benefit of self-expansion of the bioprosthesis frame is the elimination of the risk of trauma to the leaflets that may result from balloon inflation inside the prosthesis and that could affect long-term durability of the valve.

The (lower) inflow level of the memory shaped frame exerts high radial force for secure intra-annular anchoring. Its constant outward force eliminates the possibility of recoil and also allows the frame to adjust to the native annulus size and shape within its size design limitations. As a result, the self-expanding design contributes to mitigation of the risk of paravalvular leak.

The center portion of the frame is "constrained" to resist size and shape deformation (features high hoop strength). This section contains the valve (leaflets) to achieve supra-annular function. Its concave apposition to the sinus avoids the coronaries and allows both unimpeded coronary blood flow and coronary catheter access post implant. As such, the hourglass frame design avoids the need for rotational positioning since the upstroke of the valve commissures at all times remain removed from the coronaries.

The (upper) outflow level features the largest frame diameter to accommodate the ascending aorta size and exerts only low radial force. Its primary function is to assure optimal alignment of the prosthesis to the blood flow. The very top of this section also features two loops that serve to load the valve into the delivery catheter.

The porcine pericardial valve was specifically engineered for transcatheter delivery and thus features a number of unique characteristics to respond to the primary design requirement of saving space in the compressed state of the device so that it can fold into smaller catheters without the risk of tissue damage. While the valve retains a traditional three-leaflet configuration, its construct features only a single layer of pericardial elements that are first sewn together and then sewn to the frame. The valve leaflet pattern and the attachment geometry are keys to the valve's flow and durability characteristics.

The valve is constructed of six individual pieces (three skirt elements and three leaflet elements) of carefully selected porcine pericardium treated with standard tissue fixation and sterilization techniques (Fig. 4). Porcine tissue is a common material used in other implantable devices and was chosen for very specific design engineering reasons. First, while yielding identical or superior density, elasticity consistency, flexibility, and tissue strength characteristics,

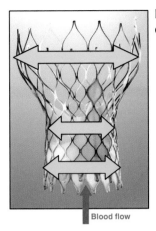

Differing circumferential dimensions:

– Largest dimension for ascending aorta contact

– Smallest dimension to preserve coronary blood flow and avoid coronary jailing

– Flared intra-annular dimension adapting to a range of annulus sizes

Blood flow

Figure 1 Self-expanding multilevel frame—dimensions.

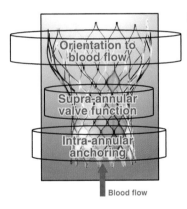

Different radial forces & hoop strengths:

– Orients the valve to blood flow regardless of angle of delivery

– Optimal valve geometry and valve function regardless of annular anatomy

– Intra-annular anchoring and adaptation to different annulus sizes and shapes

Blood flow

Figure 2 Self-expanding multilevel frame—functions.

Radial force (*R*): Physical property that has the ability to bring about change in shape/diameter of structure

$R > H$

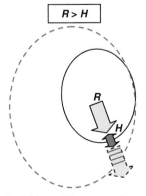

Hoop strength (*H*): Physical property that has the ability to resist change in shape/diameter of structure

$R < H$

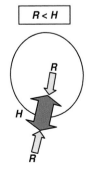

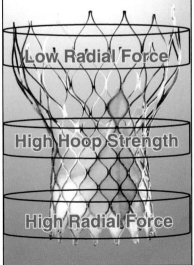

Radial force (*R*) overcomes hoop strength resulting in changed structure

Hoop strength (*H*) overcomes radial force resulting in no change to structure

Figure 3 Radial force and hoop strength.

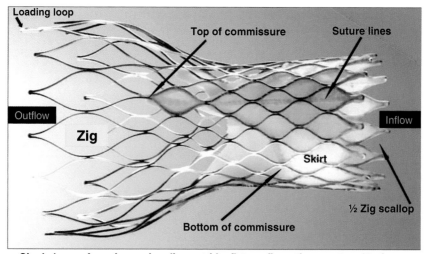

Single layer of porcine pericardium – tri-leaflet configuration – sutured to frame

Figure 4 CoreValve bioprosthesis.

it is much thinner than bovine pericardial tissue. This minimal tissue thickness leads to a substantial "space savings" in the folded configuration. In addition, the porcine pericardium exhibits superior homogeneous stretch, which is a key element required for the "suspension bridge type" design of the valve itself. Finally, the choice of porcine pericardium mitigates the risk of bovine spongiform encephalopathy.

It is important to note that the CoreValve design cannot be compared to traditional bio-prosthesis designs contained in stents/frames, which flex or bend to accommodate the loading forces encountered when the valve closes. Such traditional tissue valve designs absorb the majority of the loading forces at the top end of the stent posts and valve commissures, which is why they typically feature a very squat profile with multiple layers of sutured or folded tissue to provide the needed strength required for long-term durability.

In contrast, the CoreValve constrained part of the frame that contains the functional valve elements remains grossly static during the cardiac cycle and does not contribute meaningfully to load absorption. The engineered load absorption solution is contained in the valve construct itself. It combines the structural cable concept of a suspension bridge combined with angled commissural take-off points from the widening frame shape (Figs. 5 and 6). This translates in a much higher total functional valve height where the load is distributed evenly over the entire

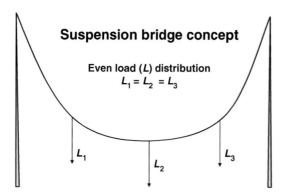

- **Load absorbed equally by each point on leaflet commissures**
- **NO frame flexing under load: static frame**

Figure 5 CoreValve design element 1.

Angled commissure take-off

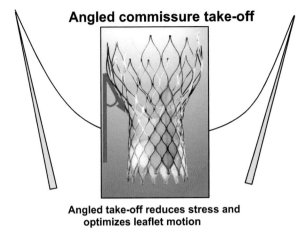

**Angled take-off reduces stress and
optimizes leaflet motion**

Figure 6 CoreValve design element 2.

length of the valve commissures without the need for tissue stacking. This single-layer construct also contributes significantly to space saving in the folded configuration of the device.

Substantial additional space saving was accomplished by uncoupling the anchoring (skirt area) and functional (leaflets) elements of the valve (Fig. 2). This has resulted in a bioprosthesis that is *implanted intra-annularly* but *functions supra-annularly*. The supra-annular function is also an important contributor to superior hemodynamic function of the valve.

The CoreValve bioprosthesis is currently available in two sizes. The 26-mm inflow model is intended for patient annulus between 20 and 23 mm and the 29 mm inflow model is intended for patient annulus between 24 and 27 mm. In the near future (estimated 2010) a 31-mm inflow model will be added for patient annulus between 27 and 29 mm and this valve will still fit in the 18-F delivery catheter.

Eighteen French Delivery Catheter System
The CoreValve delivery system (Fig. 7) is an over-the-wire catheter and accommodates a 0.035″ wire. The distal part of the catheter features an 18-F housing capsule that accommodates the bioprosthesis. This size allows true percutaneous femoral access with preclosing. Both the small and the large valve fit into this 18-F size catheter.

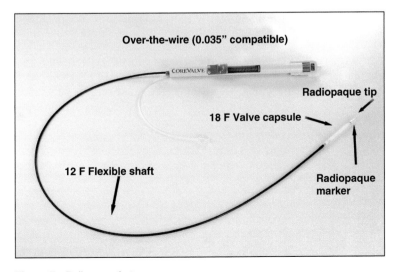

Figure 7 Delivery catheter.

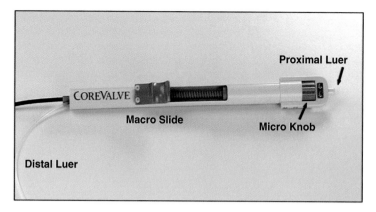

Figure 8 Delivery catheter handle.

The proximal part of the catheter shaft steps down to 12-F immediately behind the valve-housing capsule and provides enhanced interventional handling characteristics that assure easy navigation through the vasculature and access into the native aortic valve without the need for steerability elements.

The proximal catheter handle features two control elements (Fig. 8). A rotating knob for slow progressive sheath movement and slide knob for rapid sheath movement. Both controls are able to make the sheath move backward or forward and are interchangeably used during valve loading and valve delivery; however, optimal delivery technique avoids the use of the rapid slide.

The catheter tip is radiopaque and the distal part of the housing capsule features an additional positioning marker. The bioprosthesis frame is at all times fluoroscopically visible during the valve delivery procedure (both inside and outside the catheter).

Catheter-Loading System
CoreValve's third-generation loading system is fully disposable (Fig. 9, Video 1). It serves to load the bioprosthesis *into* the catheter housing cone in a consistent and nontraumatic manner. It comprises five individual elements (inflow cone, inflow tube, outflow cone, outflow cap, and outflow tube), which are applied in sequence by a single loader-operator.

During the loading procedure, the bioprosthesis must be precompressed to be loaded into the 18-F housing cone of the delivery catheter. The compression procedure is performed with the loading system and the framed bioprosthesis under temperature conditions of approximately 0°C to 8°C by immersion in cold saline. While loading, the bioprosthesis and the tip of the delivery catheter must be kept submersed at all times. Rinsing and loading of the valve must occur under strictly sterile conditions.

The detail manipulation sequences of this rinsing and loading procedure is beyond the scope of this resume and is explained in detail in the training materials provided by the company. For basic clarification, an animation of the loading sequence is provided on the DVD that accompanies this textbook.

Site and Training Requirements for Performing the CoreValve PAVR Procedure
After obtaining CE Mark during 2007, the product was only made available for expanded clinical evaluation to a predetermined number of carefully selected centers in Europe. The company

Model - CLS-3000-18 F

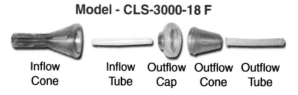

Inflow Cone   Inflow Tube   Outflow Cap   Outflow Cone   Outflow Tube

Figure 9 Disposable loading system.

decided to pursue this restrictive clinical strategy to assure successful maturing of this new technology, to assure appropriate training of physicians, and to gather additional clinical data. By the close of 2008, about 100 sites in 20 countries were active and well over 2,000 patients have been treated since the CE Mark.

While there is a tremendous amount of interest from centers across the world to be involved early with transcatheter heart valve therapy, candidate sites for use of the CoreValve PAVR technology continue to be carefully screened for a demonstrated strong clinical commitment by both the medical team and hospital administrators. A functional and cooperative heart team comprising members of the interventional cardiology, cardiac/cardiovascular surgery, anesthesiology, echocardiography, postprocedural care and nursing departments is essential to the success of the program. Also, on site back-up cardiac surgery facilities are mandatory.

While balloon aortic valvuloplasty (BAV) was largely abandoned during the late 1990s because of its poor long-term outcomes, it is clear that the past few years have seen a resurgence of the procedure in elderly patients as a short-term nonsurgical option. More importantly, when treating aortic stenosis with transcatheter technologies, BAV will always precede PAVR to assure an optimal landing zone for the bioprosthesis. As such, candidate sites should have extensive recent BAV experience before attempting PAVR.

The physician team should also acquire large access site preclosing experience before attempting PAVR. Furthermore, because some patients may require hemodynamic assistance, it is recommended that centers have access to and experience with temporary assist devices.

While a spacious and well-ventilated cardiac catheterization laboratory is acceptable for performing the PAVR procedure, the preference is for a fully hybrid operating room. It should be noted that a standard cardiac operating room with C-Arm equipment is deemed unacceptable for performing the CoreValve procedure.

Treating structural heart disease percutaneously represents a totally new challenge in the catheterization laboratory, and, the learning curve on PAVR procedures is steep for the entire hospital team. Some of the elements of the structured training and certification program that is controlled by the company are as follows.

CoreValve expects the hospital to identify and commit a specific CoreValve PAVR technical/clinical team. This team includes primary and secondary physician operators and a dedicated nurse/technician loading operator who will need to complete the separate physician and technician certification programs. Physician operators complete two half days of didactic sessions and attend cases at experienced sites. Subsequently they receive extensive case proctoring under the supervision of CoreValve assigned physician proctors and company clinical specialists. Patient selection is a crucial element of procedure success. During the training period and for a period after certification, all case files undergo a pre–case-scheduling review by an assigned CoreValve clinical expert team. Patient selection training is the subject of separate didactic sessions. Finally, there is an expectation that the hospital PAVR team re-qualify for strict sterile procedures.

Final certification is determined by the CoreValve physician proctor and qualifies only the designated physicians to perform unmonitored CoreValve implantations at the referenced hospital. Operator certification does not qualify the designated physician to proctor other operators at their or other hospitals, and certification as a proctor requires completion of a distinctly separate training program. At present, training is restricted to physicians/sites that have been cleared by the company for start-up.

Basic Overview of the CoreValve PAVR Procedure

The CoreValve PAVR ReValving system is designed to replace the native aortic heart valve in high-risk and inoperable elderly patients without open heart surgery and without concomitant surgical removal of the failed native valve (Video 2). The technology aims to transform open heart surgical aortic valve replacement into a beating heart percutaneous interventional procedure performed under fluoroscopy in the catheterization laboratory. While specific patient conditions may dictate an alternate protocol, these procedures are intended to be performed under local anesthesia, without the use of surgical cut-down/repair (with preclosing), without hemodynamic support, and without artificially accelerating the heart rate during the valve delivery.

There are two distinct schools of thought with regard to procedure sequence for the CoreValve PAVR procedure. The standard method for training purposes is the one that places the 18-F sheath at the last possible moment. The rationale behind this is to minimize occlusion time of the femoral artery. This being the case, initial crossing of the native valve is done through the 9-F introducer. Then the 18-F introducer is placed, and the subsequent BAV and valve implantation are performed. An acceptable alternate method (based on patient anatomy considerations) is to first focus exclusively on vascular access, then focus on the heart and finish with vascular closure.

The following enumeration describes the basic procedural steps but is not meant to be all inclusive. Also, with a rapidly increasing experience base, these sequences are being constantly monitored, analyzed, and refined.

Maintain strict sterile conditions.
Antibiotics to be administered as per the local hospital's surgical aortic valve replacement protocol.
Local or general anesthesia as determined by physician's preference and as per hospital protocol.
Heparin: 50 U/kg so that ACT is around 200 (between 200 and 300 is considered high), or appropriate alternate protocol (e.g., Angiomax) as per physician's discretion or hospital protocol.
Graduated pigtail catheter in the ascending aorta via radial or brachial artery.
Jugular access with a balloon-tip pacing lead for the procedure.
Prepare the vascular site according to standard hospital practice.
Predilate the native aortic valve with appropriate size balloon valvuloplasty catheter (rapid burst pacing to minimize balloon movement, as per physician's preference).
The bioprosthesis should only be loaded in advance (of the BAV) when annulus size and disposition are adequately and clearly established and final responsibility for approval to begin the loading process must remain with the implanting physician.
Backload CoreValve delivery catheter onto the guidewire while maintaining guidewire position across aortic valve.
Advance the delivery catheter over the guidewire to the aortic annulus under fluoroscopic guidance (*caution*: maintain constant visualization of the guidewire tip).
Position the catheter so that the first complete cells of the inflow portion of the frame are level with the valve annulus (the pigtail catheter in the sinus serves as a guidance marker).
Under fluoroscopic guidance, *slowly* release the bioprosthesis with microknob while constantly monitoring wire position (it is not recommended to use the macroslide during any portion of the deployment).
If necessary, proximal and distal repositioning of a partially deployed bioprosthesis (before annulus contact) can be achieved by careful manipulation of the catheter.
Once the frame is completely engaged on the aortic annulus, continue releasing bioprosthesis by using the microknob only.
Once the frame is completely engaged on the aortic annulus, proximal repositioning can still be achieved by careful manipulation of the catheter (step deployment technique).
At end of deployment, ensure that both frame loops have completely detached from the catheter tabs (confirm with fluoroscopy using orthogonal views).
Withdraw the delivery catheter to the descending aorta under fluoroscopic visualization as per the company-specified protocol (*caution*: avoid hooking catheter tip on frame or dislodgement of the bioprosthesis could occur).
Close the catheter sheath with the microknob or the macroslide under fluoroscopic guidance.
Avoid excessive catheter manipulation that could cause damage to the bioprosthesis leaflets;
Maintain guidewire position.
Perform aortogram (and echo, if desired) to assess proper expansion and positioning of the bioprosthesis.
If paravalvular leak is observed after full release: do not immediately attempt frame remodeling by means of balloon dilation but wait 5 minutes and reassess.
If paravalvular leak persists, consider alternate repositioning techniques and reserve frame remodeling by means of balloon dilation as a last resort.

Perform final aortogram.

Close access site.

If periprocedural echo has not been used, perform postprocedural echo before discharge to assess valve function.

Immediate post-PAVR care should be identical to the hospital's postsurgical aortic valve replacement protocol with special attention to rhythm disturbance (the temporary pacemaker should stay in place 48–72 hours postprocedure). Currently, there is no consensus on the methodology/rationale that determines pre- or postprocedural permanent pacemaker implantation (PPI). Substantial variability in PPI rates has been observed in certified sites and some physicians maintain a more liberal PPI determination than others. More research is being undertaken to understand possible predeterminants and/or clinical warning signs and to better understand the possible correlations between transcatheter aortic valve implantation and permanent pacemaker necessity.

Post-PAVR procedural Rx is similar to post-SAVR protocols. Plavix for 6 months is a requirement.

The above-mentioned procedure describes the basic percutaneous transfemoral technique for the CoreValve system and does not attempt to describe the numerous tips and tricks as well as established positioning, correction, and bail-out techniques that are part of the training process. Also, at the time of writing, the feasibility of a subclavian approach is being clinically demonstrated.

8 | The Edwards SAPIEN Transcatheter Aortic Heart Valve System

Jodi Akin and Pooja Sharma
Edwards Lifesciences, LLC, Irvine, California, U.S.A.

BACKGROUND

The *Edwards SAPIEN Transcatheter Aortic Heart Valve system* is the product of a collaborative and evolutionary process among physician pioneers, entrepreneurs, and industry leadership in heart valve therapy. The pioneering innovation of this stented aortic valve delivered by a catheter was first developed by Dr. Alain Cribier (Rouen, France). Together with a team of engineers led by Stanton Rowe and Stanley Rabinovich (percutaneous valve interventions, PVI), a prototype system was developed. Motivated by a dire, nonoperable patient with critical aortic stenosis, in April 2002, the first successful transcatheter aortic valve implantation in a human was performed using the antegrade approach. The valve performed well after successful transcatheter implantation, but the patient died of complications from peripheral arterial disease (1,2). Further experience with the antegrade approach proved its limitations due to technical complexities and risks.

In 2005, Edwards Lifesciences acquired PVI and the integration of nearly five decades of Edwards heart valve design and manufacturing processes were applied to the innovative stented valve platform. Concurrent delivery system programs for both transfemoral and transapical were in development. Dr. John Webb (St. Paul's Hospital, Vancouver) and colleagues refined the retrograde transfemoral approach, and in 2006, he reported the results from 18 patients who were deemed high surgical risk due to their comorbidities, and therefore underwent the transcatheter aortic valve replacement procedure. Implantation was successful in 14 patients and aortic valve area increased from 0.6 ± 0.2 to 1.6 ± 0.4 cm^2. Mortality at 30 days was 11% in this group with a mean age of 82 years. Iliac arterial injury, which occurred in the first two patients, did not recur with improvement in screening and access site management (3). In a follow-up publication in 2007 on 50 patients, Webb reported an improvement in procedural success from 76% in the first 25 patients to 96% in the second 25 ($p = 0.10$) and a decrease in 30-day mortality from 16% to 8% ($p = 0.67$). Successful valve implantation was associated with an increase in echocardiographic valve area from 0.6 ± 0.2 to 1.7 ± 0.4 cm^2 (4).

The transapical approach was also being concurrently developed. In 2007, Lichtenstein et al. (6) described the initial experience with the transapical approach in seven patients who were deemed high surgical risk due to their comorbidities. There were no intraprocedural deaths and 30-day mortality was 14%. The valve area increased from 0.7 ± 0.3 to 1.8 ± 0.7 cm^2 at 30 days, and there were no valve-related complications at follow-up. Later, Walter et al. described their experience from 59 patients with high operative risk. Good valve positioning was noted in 55 patients (93.2%) with 4 (6.8%) being converted to conventional sternotomy. Neither coronary artery obstruction nor migration of the prosthesis was observed, and all valves had good hemodynamic function. The average logistic EuroSCORE predicted risk of mortality was $27 \pm 14\%$ but the observed in-hospital mortality was 13.6% (5). The initial experience showed this approach to be a viable alternative for patients not considered to be good candidates for surgical valve replacement or transcatheter valve replacement via the transfemoral approach (6,7).

Ongoing Clinical Evaluations

Preclinical testing (bench and animal studies) as well as feasibility studies for both the transfemoral and transapical delivery system approaches were conducted in support of a CE Mark for each delivery system (same valve), which were conferred in August and October 2007 for the transfemoral and transapical delivery system, respectively. In total, nine discrete clinical trials and registries from first-in-man to randomized controlled clinical trials have been conducted to evaluate this platform with some still underway.

In addition to long-term follow-up on early feasibility studies and a postmarket registry (SOURCE), the PARTNER trial (an FDA-approved two-cohort, four-arm, multicenter trial) was initiated in April 2007 and is anticipated to complete enrollment in late 2009. The PARTNER trial is the first randomized controlled clinical investigation for THV therapy in the world. One-year follow-up is expected to be completed and published in 2010.

Today, more than 3000 implants with the Edwards SAPIEN THV system (transfemoral and transapical) have been completed via commercial access or clinical studies.

INDICATION AND CLINICAL SITE PREPARATION REQUIREMENTS FOR TRANSCATHETER HEART VALVE PROCEDURES

The Edwards SAPIEN THV is indicated for use in patients with symptomatic, severe aortic stenosis, requiring aortic valve replacement, who have a high risk for operative mortality, or are deemed nonoperable due to significant comorbidities. For these patients who are not able to undergo standard aortic valve replacement, a THV intervention for the treatment of their aortic stenosis is a less invasive option.

In preparation for the THV procedure, each hospital site participates in a robust and complete training program, sponsored by Edwards Lifesciences, which includes the following components:

- Simulator training
- Device demonstration
- Didactic sessions (taught by physicians experienced in the THV procedure)
- Training manual
- Live case observation
- Proctored THV cases

Along with extensive training, a high-quality imaging system is ideal for successful THV implantation, and the use of a fixed, mounted fluoroscopy system is ideal for the THV procedure.

According to a position statement on transcatheter valve implantation from the European Association of Cardio-Thoracic Surgery (EACTS) and the European Society of Cardiology (ESC), patient selection and risk assessment for this procedure should be performed by a multidisciplinary team including cardiologists, surgeons, imaging specialists, anesthesiologists, and other experts (8). Edwards Lifesciences encourages and supports this strong partnership, and recommends that each patient be carefully assessed to determine whether or not the patient is a candidate for transcatheter valve replacement.

PRODUCT OVERVIEW: EDWARDS SAPIEN™ TRANSCATHETER HEART VALVE

The Edwards SAPIEN valve is constructed of three bovine-pericardial tissue leaflets, which are hand-sewn and mounted on a balloon-expandable frame to offer high radial strength for uniform leaflet coaptation, excellent hemodynamics, and a large, consistent effective orifice area. The bioprosthesis is available in two sizes (23 and 26 mm) and is designed for implantation via either a transfemoral or transapical approach in patients with severe calcific aortic stenosis (AS) who require aortic valve replacement (AVR), but who are not good candidates for open-chest surgery due to extremely high operative risk or comorbid conditions.

Edwards SAPIEN transcatheter valve tissue is fabricated from bovine pericardial tissue. Valve leaflets are cut from specially selected areas of the bovine pericardial sac, and each leaflet is individually tested and sorted to ensure that the three leaflets of the Edwards SAPIEN THV are matched for similar material properties. Valve leaflets are preserved in a buffered glutaraldehyde to fully cross-link the tissue, while preserving its flexibility and strength. These leaflets then undergo the Carpentier–Edwards ThermaFix process, Edwards Lifesciences' third-generation of anticalcification technology. The Carpentier–Edwards ThermaFix process is the only tissue treatment that extracts two major calcium-binding sites (phospholipids and unstable/residual glutaraldehyde molecules).

The three leaflets are then hand-sewn and mounted onto a balloon-expandable stainless steel frame by using polytetrafluoroethylene (PTFE) sutures (Fig. 1). The frame undergoes

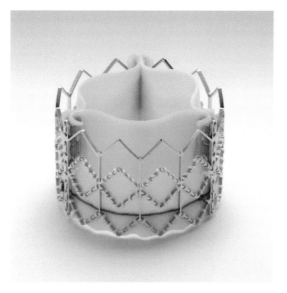

Figure 1 Edwards SAPIEN transcatheter aortic heart valve.

complete in vitro durability and fatigue testing and is also bench tested to ISO5840 standards. By using a discreet balloon-expandable design, the Edwards SAPIEN valve is designed to offer accurate placement of the bioprosthesis into the diseased area while minimizing the impact to surrounding structures.

The Edwards SAPIEN THV may be delivered via either a transfemoral or transapical approach. A brief overview of the transfemoral and transapical delivery systems, as well as valve delivery using each approach, is described in the following section.

PRODUCT OVERVIEW: EDWARDS SAPIEN THV DELIVERY WITH THE RETROFLEX TRANSFEMORAL KIT

The RetroFlex Transfemoral kit is used for transfemoral (retrograde) delivery of the Edwards SAPIEN THV, and includes the following components:

- Edwards SAPIEN THV
- RetroFlex Transfemoral Delivery System
- RetroFlex Introducer Sheath Set
- RetroFlex Dilator Kit
- RetroFlex Balloon Catheter
- Crimper
- Balloon Inflation Device

The following is a brief description of each component in the RetroFlex Transfemoral kit:

- Edwards SAPIEN THV (Fig. 1)
  - Built upon Edwards Lifesciences' more than 50 years of continuous refinement in surgical heart valve technology.
  - Designed to provide excellent hemodynamics, uniform leaflet coaptation, and a large consistent effective orifice area.
  - Incorporates the same manufacturing processes used on premier Carpentier–Edwards PERIMOUNT Magna Pericardial valves.
    - Bovine pericardial tissue.
    - Carpentier–Edwards ThermaFix process.
    - Leaflet thickness and elasticity matching.
  - Discreet balloon-expandable valve mounted on a stainless steel frame.

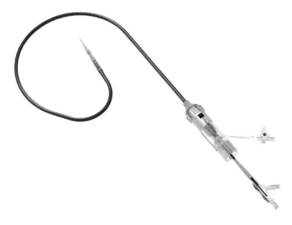

Figure 2   RetroFlex transfemoral delivery system.

- RetroFlex Delivery system (Fig. 2)
  - ○ 23- and 26-mm valve delivery.
  - ○ 0.035 in. guidewire compatibility.
  - ○ Articulating delivery system for smooth aortic arch tracking.
  - ○ Tapered distal end to improve native valve crossability.
- RetroFlex Introducer Sheath Set (Fig. 3)
  - ○ 22-F (23-mm valve) or 24-F (26-mm valve) sheath.
  - ○ Custom-designed sheath designed for pushability and excellent hemostasis.
  - ○ Enhanced triseal valve technology.
- RetroFlex vessel dilator kit (Fig. 4)
  - ○ Set of flexible, atraumatic dilators for smooth arterial dilation.
  - ○ Hydrophilic coating and tapered distal segment.
  - ○ 0.035 in. guidewire compatibility.

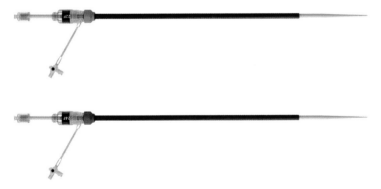

Figure 3   RetroFlex introducer sheath set: 23- and 26-mm valve delivery.

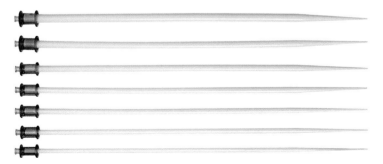

Figure 4   RetroFlex dilator kit.

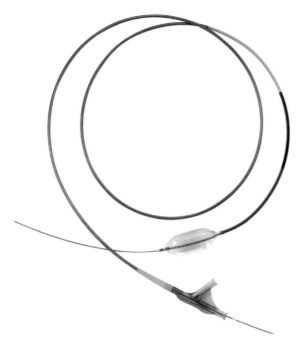

Figure 5   RetroFlex balloon catheter.

- RetroFlex Balloon Catheter (Fig. 5)
  - ○ Custom-designed large diameter balloon for predilatation of the native stenotic aortic valve.
  - ○ 0.035 in. guidewire compatibility.
- Edwards SAPIEN THV Crimper (Fig. 6)
  - ○ 23- and 26 mm single-use crimpers.
  - ○ Provides concentric valve crimping.
  - ○ Edwards Lifesciences proprietary design.
- Balloon Inflation Syringes (Fig. 7)
  - ○ Volume-based indeflators.

PROCEDURAL OVERVIEW: TRANSFEMORAL APPROACH

This section describes the basic procedural steps for Edwards SAPIEN valve delivery via the transfemoral procedure (Video 1). For a detailed description on product preparation and the procedure, it is necessary to refer to the "Instructions for Use" provided by Edwards Lifesciences.

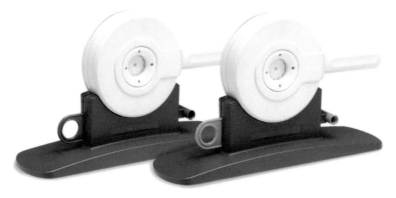

Figure 6   Edwards SAPIEN THV crimper.

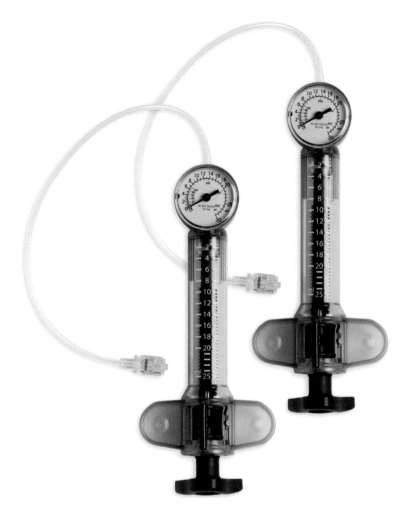

Figure 7   Balloon inflation syringes.

1. Edwards SAPIEN THV Preparation
    a. Prepare the Edwards SAPIEN THV separately, and crimp the valve onto the RetroFlex Delivery system by using the specially designed Edwards crimper.
2. Baseline Parameters
    a. Gain arterial access using standard catheterization techniques.
    b. Place a pigtail catheter into the aortic root for continuous blood pressure monitoring, and introduce pacing wires and position in the right ventricle.
    c. Perform selective supra-aortic angiograms in order to evaluate the height between the inferior aspect of the annulus and the inferior aspects of the lowest coronary ostium.
    d. Perform test pacing at 200 to 220 beats/min.
3. Predilatation of the native aortic valve
    a. Advance an 0.035 in. guidewire into the left ventricle and perform balloon valvuloplasty to prepare the native annulus for implantation of the Edwards SAPIEN valve.
4. Introduction of RetroFlex Delivery System
    a. Advance increasing sizes of Edwards specially designed dilators over the guidewire and used to dilate the arteriotomy. One femoral artery should be chosen for delivery system access, based on vessel size, tortuosity, and the presence (or absence) of calcification.
    b. Following dilation, place the RetroFlex Introducer sheath in the femoral vessel.
    c. Place the prepared Edwards SAPIEN THV through the valve loader, and advance the RetroFlex Delivery system through the sheath and upwards towards the descending

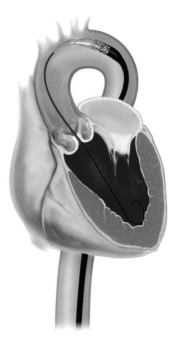

Figure 8   Articulating distal end facilitates guidance over the aortic arch.

aorta. Note: Guidewire position in the left ventricle should be verified prior to advancement of the RetroFlex Delivery system.
5. Positioning/Placement of the Edwards SAPIEN Valve
   a. Articulate the RetroFlex delivery system to track over the aortic arch, and using the tapered distal end, cross the native aortic valve and position the Edwards SAPIEN THV within the diseased annulus (Figs. 8 and 9).
   b. When accurate positioning is verified, begin rapid pacing and deploy the Edwards SAPIEN valve through complete balloon inflation (Fig. 10). After complete balloon deflation, stop rapid pacing.

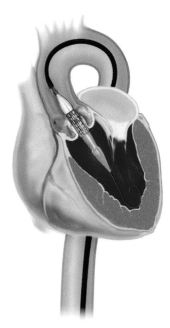

Figure 9   Tapered distal end aids in native valve crossing.

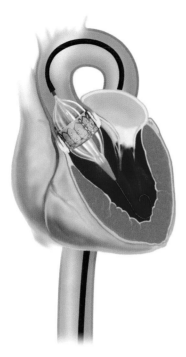

Figure 10   Balloon-expandable transfemoral valve deployment.

6. Removal of the RetroFlex Delivery system
   a. Following deployment, the RetroFlex Delivery system is dearticulated and removed from the sheath.
7. Postdeployment Assessment (Fig. 11)
   a. Perform a supra-aortic angiogram to evaluate device performance and coronary patency, noting transvalvular pressure gradients.

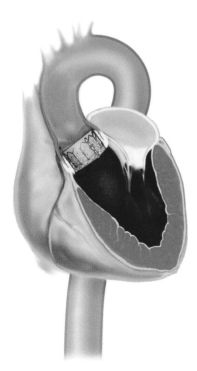

Figure 11   Edwards SAPIEN THV in situ.

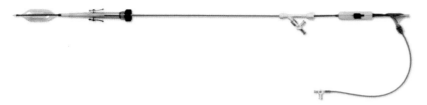

Figure 12   Ascendra transapical delivery system.

8. Closure
   a. Remove the sheath from the femoral vessel and close the access site using standard percutaneous closure techniques.

PRODUCT OVERVIEW: EDWARDS SAPIEN THV DELIVERY WITH THE ASCENDRA TRANSAPICAL KIT

The Ascendra Transapical kit is used for transapical (antegrade) delivery of the Edwards SAPIEN THV (study valve or bioprosthesis), and consists of the following components:

- Edwards SAPIEN THV
- Ascendra Transapical Delivery System
- Ascendra Introducer Sheath Set
- Ascendra Valvuloplasty Catheter
- Crimper
- Balloon Inflation Device

The following is a brief description of each component in the Ascendra Transapical kit:

- Edwards SAPIEN THV (Fig. 1)
  o Built upon Edwards Lifesciences' more than 50 years of continuous refinement in surgical heart valve technology.
  o Designed to provide excellent hemodynamics, uniform leaflet coaptation, and a large consistent effective orifice area.
  o Incorporates the same manufacturing processes used on premier Carpentier–Edwards PERIMOUNT Magna Pericardial valves.
    - Bovine pericardial tissue.
    - Carpentier–Edwards ThermaFix process.
    - Leaflet thickness and elasticity matching.
  o Discreet balloon-expandable valve mounted on a stainless steel frame.
- Ascendra Delivery System (Fig. 12)
  o 23- and 26-mm valve delivery.
  o Direct access to the native valve.
  o Designed with the surgeon in mind.
  o Controlled insertion through the apex.
- Ascendra Introducer Sheath Set (Fig. 13)
  o 26-F custom-designed introducer sheath.
  o Provides controlled insertion through the apex, and allows for smooth passage of the delivery system.
  o Enhanced triseal valve technology.

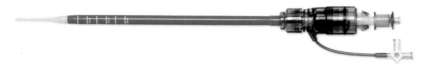

Figure 13   Ascendra transapical introducer sheath set.

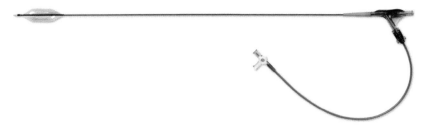

Figure 14 Ascendra balloon catheter.

- Ascendra Balloon Catheter (Fig. 14)
  - Custom-designed balloon for predilatation of the native stenotic aortic.
  - valve
- Edwards SAPIEN THV Crimper (Fig. 6)
  - 23- and 26-mm single-use crimpers.
  - Provides concentric valve crimping.
  - Edwards Lifesciences proprietary design.
- Balloon inflation syringes (Fig. 7)
  - Volume-based indeflators.

PROCEDURAL OVERVIEW: TRANSAPICAL APPROACH

This section describes the basic procedural steps for Edwards SAPIEN valve delivery via the transapical procedure. For a detailed description on product preparation and the procedure, it is necessary to refer to the "Instructions for Use" provided by Edwards Lifesciences.

1. Edwards SAPIEN THV Preparation
   a. Prepare the Edwards SAPIEN THV separately, and crimp the valve onto the RetroFlex Delivery system by using the specially designed Edwards crimper.
2. Baseline Parameters
   a. Gain arterial access using standard catheterization techniques.
   b. Place a pigtail catheter into the aortic root for continuous blood pressure monitoring.
   c. Perform selective supra-aortic angiograms in order to evaluate the height between the inferior aspect of the annulus and the inferior aspects of the lowest coronary ostium.
3. Apical Access
   a. Access the apex of the pericardium through a mini anterior thoracotomy at the fifth or sixth intercostal space. Incise the pericardium to expose the apex of the left ventricle. Place a reinforced double purse string on the left ventricular (LV) apex to access the left ventricle.
   b. Attach epicardial pacing leads to left ventricle and test pacing at 200 to 220 beats/min.
   c. Under image guidance, place a 14-F sheath through the purse string into the LV cavity and advance a 0.035 in. guidewire into the left ventricle, through the native valve into the descending aorta.
4. Predilatation of the native aortic valve (Fig. 15)
   a. Perform balloon valvuloplasty to prepare the native annulus prior to implantation of the Edwards SAPIEN valve.
5. Introduction of Ascendra Delivery system
   a. Position the tip of the Ascendra Introducer sheath in the LV outflow immediately below the aortic valve.
   b. Place the prepared Edwards SAPIEN THV through the valve loader, and advance the Ascendra Delivery system through the sheath and toward the ascending aorta.
6. Positioning/Placement of the Edwards SAPIEN Valve
   a. Cross the native aortic valve and position the Edwards SAPIEN THV within the diseased annulus (Fig. 16).

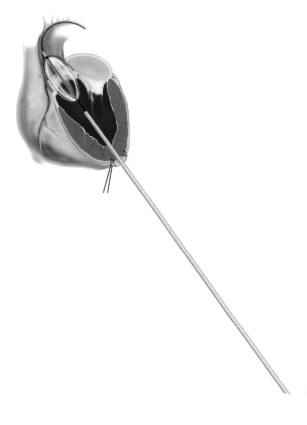

Figure 15 Edwards balloon catheter used for predilatation of the native valve.

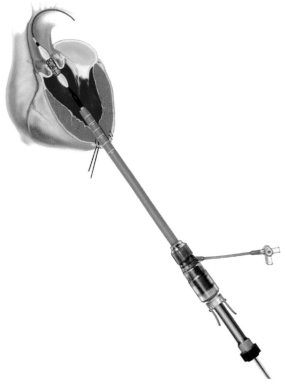

Figure 16 Direct access to native valve for accurate positioning.

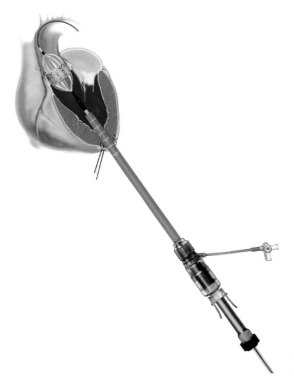

Figure 17   Balloon-expandable transapical valve deployment.

   b. When accurate positioning is verified, begin rapid pacing and deploy the Edwards SAPIEN valve through complete balloon inflation. After complete balloon deflation, stop rapid pacing (Fig. 17).
7. Removal of the Ascendra Delivery system
   a. Following deployment, the Ascendra Delivery system is removed from the sheath.
8. Postdeployment Assessment (Fig. 11)
   a. Perform a supra-aortic angiogram to evaluate device performance and coronary patency, noting transvalvular pressure gradients.
9. Closure
a. Remove the Ascendra Introducer Sheath from the apex and close the access site.

SUMMARY

The Edwards SAPIEN Aortic THV Valve (formerly Cribier–Edwards Valve) and delivery systems have developed through strong collaboration of physicians, entrepreneurs, and industry leaders in bioprosthetic heart valves. The devices have been well studied in rigorous clinical studies during pre- and postcommercial approval experiences in the European Union. The trials have demonstrated reasonable safety, effectiveness and iterative improvement in outcomes over time. The PARTNER trial, a currently enrolling US IDE randomized controlled clinical trial, will produce the first true clinical benchmarks for comparison of THV against conventional therapies. Product and procedural improvements including significant reduction in French size of the transfemoral and transapical delivery systems are in development and will soon be introduced. In August 2009, the PARTNER Trial completed enrollment.

The Edwards SAPIEN XT Valve and Delivery Systems: Edwards Lifesciences' Next Generation of Transcatheter Heart Valve Delivery

Building upon this transcatheter heart valve technology and clinical experience, Edwards Lifesciences continues to improve its product offering and has developed the next generation Edwards SAPIEN XT valve (Fig. 18). Like the Edwards SAPIEN Transcatheter Heart Valve, the Edwards SAPIEN XT valve also utilizes bovine pericardial tissue treated with the

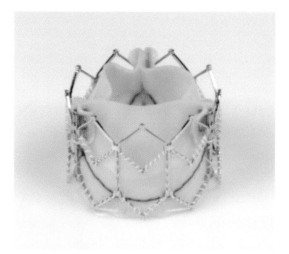

Figure 18 Edwards SAPIEN XT THV in situ.

Carpentier-Edwards ThermaFix process and proprietary leaflet matching technology. Along with these product features, this next generation balloon-expandable valve consists of a cobalt–chromium frame with a new geometry to allow for lower profile crimping and scallop-shaped leaflets to more closely mimic Edwards Lifesciences' leading surgical heart valves. In addition to 23 and 26 mm valve sizes, the Edwards SAPIEN XT valve offering will expand to include 20 and 29 mm valve sizes. Edwards Lifesciences has also developed two new delivery systems: the NovaFlex Transfemoral Delivery System and the Ascendra 2 Transapical Delivery System.

The Edwards SAPIEN XT with the NovaFlex Transfemoral Delivery System features an 18-Fr profile improving transfemoral valve delivery and expanding the treatable patient population. Building upon the RetroFlex Delivery System, NovaFlex continues to offer balloon-expandable deployment for accuracy and radial strength, a flexing delivery system for controlled navigation of the aortic arch, and a tapered distal end for enhanced native valve crossability. Similarly, the next generation Ascendra 2 Transapical Delivery System also offers a reduction in profile and continues to provide balloon-expandable valve delivery through straight and direct access to the native aortic valve.

For 50 years, Edwards Lifesciences has been a world leader in providing advanced treatments for cardiovascular disease. Combining technology breakthroughs with proven design and advanced manufacturing, our extensive tissue valve line continues to bring new treatment options to cardiac surgeons, cardiologists, and patients worldwide.

REFERENCES

1. Cribier A, et al. Percutaneous transcatheter implantation of an aortic valve prosthesis for calcific aortic stenosis: First human case description. Circulation 2002; 106(24):3006–3008.
2. Eltchaninoff H, Tron C, Cribier A. Percutaneous implantation of aortic valve prosthesis in patients with calcific aortic stenosis: Technical aspects. J Interv Cardiol 2003; 16(6):515–521.
3. Webb JG, et al. Percutaneous aortic valve implantation retrograde from the femoral artery. Circulation 2006; 113(6):842–850.
4. Webb JG, et al. Percutaneous transarterial aortic valve replacement in selected high-risk patients with aortic stenosis. Circulation 2007; 116(7):755–763.
5. Walther T, et al. Transapical minimally invasive aortic valve implantation: Multicenter experience. Circulation 2007; 116(11 suppl):I240–I245.
6. Lichtenstein SV, et al. Transapical transcatheter aortic valve implantation in humans: Initial clinical experience. Circulation 2006; 114(6):591–596.
7. Ye J, et al. Six-month outcome of transapical transcatheter aortic valve implantation in the initial seven patients. Eur J Cardiothorac Surg 2007; 31(1):16–21.
8. Vahanian A, et al. Transcatheter valve implantation for patients with aortic stenosis: A position statement from the European Association of Cardio-Thoracic Surgery (EACTS) and the European Society of Cardiology (ESC, in collaboration with the European Association of Percutaneous Cardiovascular Interventions (EAPCI). Eur J Cardiothorac Surg 2008; 34:18.

9 | Anesthesia for Transcatheter Aortic Valve Implantation

F. J. Orellana Ramos and J. Hofland

Department of Cardiothoracic Anesthesia, Erasmus University Medical Center, Thoraxcenter, Rotterdam, The Netherlands

Transcatheter aortic valve implantation (TAVI) represents a unique challenge for anesthesiologists in the Cardiac Catheterization Laboratory (CCL). A clear understanding of the pathophysiology together with the clinical implications of the diagnostic and therapeutic intervention of aortic valve disease is mandatory. Technical skills are not enough to ensure a successful outcome—special considerations include "How to provide safe service in an environment with a lack of space," "How to handle technical incompatibilities of machinery and danger of irradiation" and "How to deal with abnormal logistics, patient transport and so on" (1). Thus, factors like communication, good planning and preparation, availability of adjacent services as Cardiothoracic Surgery and Anesthesia, Vascular Surgery, Intensive Care, Diagnostic Laboratory, and even ancillary personnel are all of crucial importance. In this scenario, the anesthesiologist plays the role of a quality enforcer before, during, and after the intervention.

At present, patients undergoing TAVI are at a more advanced age and have more comorbidities than patients scheduled for conventional aortic valve replacement. This fact, together with peculiarities of the procedure and greater potential for complications, makes general anesthesia for TAVI, in our opinion, a first choice. Potential advantages of general anesthesia include appropriate level of hypnosis and analgesia, immobility, and control of the patients' cardiorespiratory status. In this way, the anesthesiologist can facilitate the job of the cardiologist during the procedure (2).

The key for successful outcomes, as with any invasive procedure, entails careful preoperative assessment, appropriate intraoperative monitoring and imaging, meticulous management of hemodynamics, and early treatment of expected side effects and complications (3).

In this chapter, we describe our approach to the anesthetic management of patients undergoing retrograde transfemoral TAVI and then briefly point out some of the similarities and differences for the management of patients undergoing antegrade transapical TAVI.

THE ANESTHESIOLOGIST IN THE CCL

The increasing number of new and sophisticated interventional techniques, in combination with the treatment of more complex patients makes the availability of an experienced anesthesiologist in the CCL mandatory (3). Although TAVI has been reported to be safe and effective for inoperable patients with aortic stenosis (AS) (4), there can be serious risks associated with the procedure: death, hypothermia, aspiration of gastric contents, hypovolemia, hemorrhage, severe hemodynamic instability, airway compromise, anaphylaxis, and various procedure-related complications (e.g., retroperitoneal bleeding, ventricular perforation, and aortic root rupture). The main goal for the anesthesiologist is to maintain a high level of patient care and reduce the potential for adverse events that could jeopardize an otherwise successful valve implantation.

The CCL provides unique challenges to the anesthesiologist: limited working area, lighting and temperature inadequacies (computerized radiology equipment requires a low temperature and the rooms are usually cooler than commonly set at the operating room [OR]), lack of skilled personnel, supplies and drugs, and high-radiation exposure. Despite these drawbacks, efforts must be directed to adopt those standards used in the ORs. A hybrid room would be the ideal environment to perform TAVI procedures as it combines the advantages of both locations (CCL and OR). On the other hand, the anesthesia care team should adopt special skills and attitudes: it's advisable to have experience with cardiothoracic anesthesia, knowledge of echocardiography and fluoroscopy, and participate regularly in the Interventional Cardiology program (must learn the procedure and how to best support the interventional cardiologist) (5).

PREOPERATIVE EVALUATION OF PATIENTS WITH AS

The ultimate goal of the preoperative risk evaluation is to optimize the medical condition of the patient and thereby reduce morbidity and mortality associated with TAVI.

The preprocedural evaluation is best conducted by a team of physicians (more specifically, a cardiologist, anesthesiologist, and a cardiothoracic surgeon). All previous surgical and interventional procedures should be well documented. At admission, signs of congestive heart failure and intercurrent diseases should be identified. A history of fatigability, shortness of breath, or cyanosis suggests a loss of cardiorespiratory reserve. For the anesthesiologist it is important to consider the interactions between a patient's physical condition, medication list, and the effects of anesthesia.

The severity of AS and adequacy of the iliac-femoral vasculature can be thoroughly studied with transthoracic echocardiography, multislice computed tomography, magnetic resonance imaging, and fluoroscopy. Because the standard of care in the CCL should equal that of the ORs, guidelines for preoperative testing should closely follow the recommendations of the National Institute for Clinical Excellence (6). Once a decision to perform TAVI has been made, the patient is typically admitted to the hospital one day before the intervention. Laboratory evaluations should include a complete blood count, electrolytes, renal function, and coagulation parameters. Added tests should be of importance, depending on the patient's current clinical status. Because anesthetic management needs to be tailored for individual patients, the anesthesiologist can now plan for the procedure along with the interventional cardiologist.

Global Perspective of Patient Preparation and Setup for TAVI

All patients receive antibiotic prophylaxis (first-generation cephalosporin or vancomycin) 1 hour before the procedure.

In patients with AS, chronic pressure overload results in increased left ventricular (LV) intracavitary pressures to overcome the impedance of the narrowed aortic valve orifice. Although muscular hypertrophy preserves systolic wall stress, blood supply to the thickened myocardium may become inadequate, inducing cardiac ischemia and impaired cardiac contractility. Later on, diastolic dysfunction may develop and preload takes great importance to maintain diastolic filling and adequate cardiac output (CO). The stenotic valve provides a narrow window for appropriate fluid loading, beyond which volume expansion produces increased filling pressures and may induce pulmonary edema. An unexpected decrease in systemic vascular resistance (SVR) can decrease mean arterial pressure and therefore coronary perfusion pressure (CPP). Thus, peri-interventional goals consist of maintenance of sinus rhythm (50–60 beats/min, higher rates with coexisting aortic insufficiency), adequate systemic resistance and vascular volume, and avoiding systemic hypotension with α-adrenergic agonists.

Sinus tachycardia and atrial arrhythmias may worsen LV-loading conditions and provoke heart failure—in these cases, cardioversion should be strongly considered. Defibrillator pads should be placed on the patient prior to positioning and before induction of anesthesia. If a patient becomes hemodynamically unstable secondary to a supraventricular tachyarrhythmia, cardioversion should be instituted without delay. In hemodynamically stable patients, a therapeutic diagnostic maneuver can be attempted (adenosine, vagal stimulation) before further treatment is administered (e.g., esmolol, amiodarone, and electrocardioversion). When ventricular tachycardia cannot be ruled out, amiodarone is the preferred drug of choice, especially with impaired cardiac function. Acute bradyarrhythmias, which may induce over distension of the left ventricle are best treated with combined α- and β-adrenergic agonists or with cardiac pacing; overshoot tachycardia should be avoided (atropine can have unpredictable effects).

Patients with severe AS usually have limited coronary flow and/or cardiovascular reserve that can negatively influence cerebral and pulmonary blood flow. Furthermore, coronary artery disease can be identified in approximately 50% of patients undergoing TAVI and can increase the complexity of the procedure. In approximately 10% of our patients, concomitant PCI is performed during the index procedure but before valve implantation. Occasionally, a percutaneous ventricular assist device (pVAD) can facilitate the procedure especially for patients with LV dysfunction. Our center commonly uses the TandemHeart, a left atrial-to-femoral artery bypass system, comprising a 22-F left atrial transseptal inflow cannula, 17-F femoral arterial

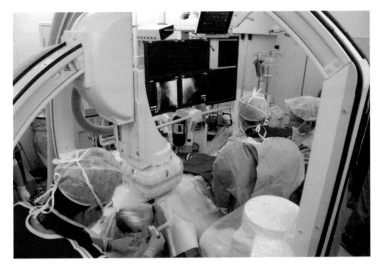

Figure 1 During a TAVR the anesthesia care team should be in close proximity to the patient and high doses of radiation are received.

outflow cannula, and an extracorporeal centrifugal pump. The TandemHeart device can deliver nonpulsatile flow rates of up to 4 L/min.

SETUP, EQUIPMENT, AND PREPARATION IN THE CCL FOR TAVI

Radiation exposure can be particularly high for both the patient and personnel in the CCL—appropriate protection, including thyroid shields and dosimeters are mandatory (Fig. 1). The anesthesia care team should follow a preventive and safety program for X-ray protection.

Adequate space for the anesthesia staff and equipment must be provided. Most of the time, we tend to use portable equipment (Figs. 2A and B).

Before starting the procedure, the anesthesia care team should ensure that all of the following items are present and are functioning correctly:

- Ensure that a source of oxygen and suction equipment reach the patient. A scavenging system should be available (although volatile agents may not be needed when using total intravenous anesthesia).
- Anesthesia workstation, emergency cart, and supplies equivalent to the OR setup.
- Immediate availability of a defibrillator and self-inflating (Ambu) resuscitation bag.
- Extensions both for the respiratory circuit and for IV lines. All equipment should be properly positioned in the CCL. The fluoroscopy equipment limits access to the patient, especially when the biplane c-arm is used and when the cardiologist moves the table to accommodate for better images (Fig. 3). Functioning intravenous lines of adequate length must be confirmed before the cardiologist begins with vascular puncture.
- Standard and invasive monitors.
- Adequate padding for patient comfort to prevent any tissue damage.
- A patient heating device to avoid hypothermia

ANESTHETIC TECHNIQUE AND PERIOPERATIVE CARE

The choice of the anesthetic technique (7, 8) varies among centers and is probably not associated with a significant difference in outcome but a common feature to all of the techniques is that they challenge the cardiovascular system. On the other hand, various pharmacological resources to manipulate heart rate, optimize preload, contractility, and systemic vascular resistance can be used to compensate for unwanted effects on the cardiovascular system.

During our initial experience, we used either local anesthesia and mild sedation promoting spontaneous respiration or deep IV sedation with insertion of a laryngeal mask. Because of the complexity of the patients and the duration of the procedures, we adopted a general anesthetic

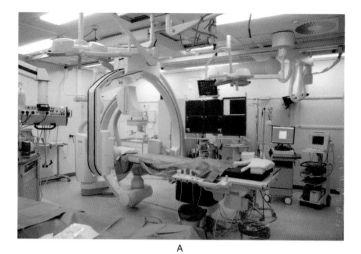

A

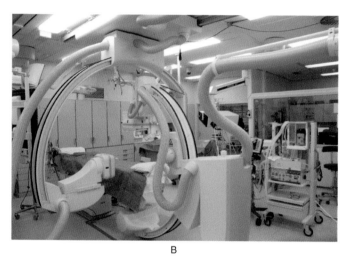

B

Figure 2   Set up of equipment in the CCL.

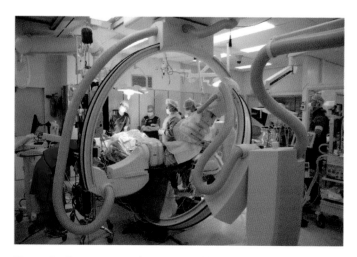

Figure 3   Fluoroscopy equipment in the CCL with the biplane c-arm deployed around the patient. Extensions for breathing circuit and IV lines are used.

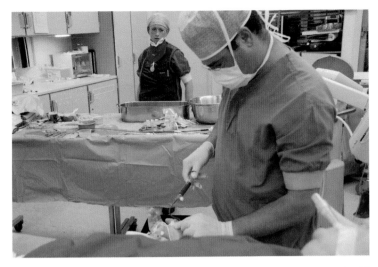

Figure 4 Right radial artery catheterization for blood samples and invasive blood pressure measurement.

approach. General anesthesia can provide physiological stability and can improve the tolerability of the procedure. Immobility of the patient may facilitate the delivery and deployment of the prosthesis and may allow for better control of complications should they occur.

In patients currently undergoing TAVI, anesthetic requirements are typically reduced because of advanced age and decreased cardiac output.

When patients arrive in the CCL, basic anesthetic monitoring is established (9). Large-bore peripheral venous access and a right radial/brachial arterial line are obtained (Fig. 4). The left radial artery remains free for insertion of a pigtail catheter by the cardiologist. Continuously transducing arterial blood pressure from a femoral arterial sheath is not useful and reliable because of damping of the signal by intra-arterial catheters and wires and its intermittent availability during the procedure. Therefore, we prefer to have a separate arterial catheter where blood samples can be obtained and continuity of an adequate signal is secured without disturbing the cardiologist.

We regularly use a point-of-care testing (i-Stat©, Abbott Point of Care Inc., UK) for certain laboratory tests; in this way, we can quickly assess a panel of critical tests such as blood gas samples, electrolytes, complete blood counts, and glucose levels. Significant blood loss can occur during TAVI because of the size and frequency of catheter and sheath changes. Routine hematocrit and hemoglobin monitoring will guide the necessity for red blood cell transfusions.

Before central-line placement, light sedation is administered. For this purpose, we prefer low doses of midazolam (1–2 mg IV) and occasionally low doses of fentanyl (25–50 mcg IV) is given in combination.

Central-line placement in the right internal jugular vein is performed under local anesthesia with the aid of ultrasound (Fig. 5). The use of ultrasound for central venous access has been reported to be safer and faster than traditional surface landmark guidance (10). Routinely, an introducer sheath (8.5–9 F) with a lateral access port and two extra lumens is used. This allows for the possibility to insert a temporary pacemaker or a pulmonary artery catheter during or at the end of the procedure.

Some patients may require inotropic and/or vasopressor support before induction of anesthesia. For this purpose, dobutamine, norepinephrine, and phenylephrine infusions are prepared in advance. Although dobutamine infusion in patients with AS is not generally recommended, our experience suggests that such administration may be considered for patients with LV dysfunction in the absence of coronary artery disease. Nonetheless, titration should be performed carefully to avoid arrhythmias and myocardial ischemia.

The choice of induction technique depends heavily on the preference of the anesthesiologist. A wide range of strategies can be used with success: it's more a question of *how* than *what* drugs must be used. In general, we prefer to use more cardiovascular stable drugs. Although

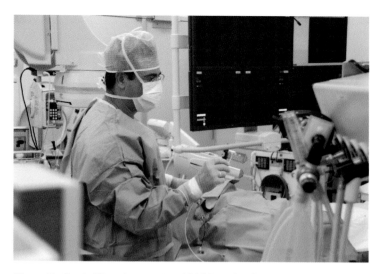

Figure 5 Central line placement and PAC insertion (under fluoroscopy). Patient is lightly sedated.

induction with a classical cocktail of midazolam and sufentanil/fentanyl is generally safe, this strategy may be less attractive when a fast-track approach is preferred.

To limit the duration of anesthesia and ensure prompt extubation of the patient, we usually prefer a "multimodal induction" approach. Etomidate has a rapid onset of action and is considered to be a cardiovascular stable induction agent. For this reason, we avoid the use of propofol and thiopental for intravenous induction. In addition to the use of midazolam as described, we administer glycopyrronium and titrate the dose of etomidate. Furthermore, S-ketamine (a bolus of 50 mg), fentanyl (100 mcg), and a neuromuscular blockade drug (cisatracurium 0.15–0.20 mg/kg) are administered before endotracheal intubation. This "multimodal induction" has some advantages: arterial pressure is well maintained and proper analgesia is established (i.e., opioid in combination with S-ketamine).

A single induction dose of a relaxant that undergoes organ-independent Hofmann elimination with nearly no side effects and/or drug interactions facilitates a fast track approach. On the other hand, use of low doses of S-ketamine, a noncompetitive antagonist of the NMDA receptor Ca^{2+} channel pore, does not interfere with Bispectral index (BIS) monitoring. BIS monitoring is a tool that can gauge the depth of anesthesia during the procedure.

Premedication is needed to avoid potential side effects of ketamine (e.g., hypersalivation and psychomimetic reactions). An outstanding and practical review of the use of ketamine during balanced anesthesia (propofol–ketamine technique for minimally invasive procedures) can be found in the book by Dr. Friedberg (11)—this has been our inspiration for dealing with high risk-patients in the CCL.

Maintenance with a continuous infusion of IV propofol at low doses (2–4 mg/kg/h), titrating to a BIS of around 60 to 65 with additional boluses of an opioid (fentanyl) and/or S-ketamine (25 mg, with a limit of 100 mg per case) has proved to enable a quick wake up with minimal cardiovascular effects. On the contrary, some patients receive an infusion of remifentanil at low doses (0.05–0.125 mcg/kg/min). In a selected number of patients we add sevoflurane as adjuvant, for its cardioprotective/preconditioning properties. All anesthetic drugs are titrated carefully with attention to maintaining SVR and CO and the balance between myocardial oxygen demand and supply in the presence of a hypertrophied ventricle and reduced coronary flow. Hypotension is treated immediately: a pure α-adrenergic receptor agonist is the preferred vasoconstrictor agent. Phenylephrine increases SVR and CPP without causing tachycardia or increase in oxygen demand. If needed, we start a continuous intravenous infusion of norepinephrine. However, a too aggressive treatment of hypotension may induce high arterial and filling pressures that may cause ischemia in the hypertrophied left ventricle (12).

After induction and hemodynamic stability secured, the cardiologist may begin the TAVI procedure. Using long acting local anesthesia to avoid discomfort and pain into the recovery period can be recommended. A mixture of lidocaine and bupivacaine with addition of epinephrine to obtain a concentration of 1:200,000 is cheap, easy to prepare, and ideal for prolonged analgesia at the puncture site, though other local anesthetics can also be used: for example, mepivacaine, levobupivacaine, and ropivacaine. In addition, we give intravenous paracetamol at the end of the procedure for pain management. Nonsteroidal anti-inflammatory drugs should be avoided in elderly patients with cardiovascular disease and renal dysfunction.

Common problems during TAVI are blood loss and hypothermia. The amount of blood loss is highly variable, depending on the integrity of the vasculature and technique of the attending cardiologist (Figs. 6A and B). Hypothermia may still be problematic even after warming devices are used. During TAVI all patients are actively warmed with air blanket warming systems (WarmAir, Cincinnati Sub-Zero Products, Inc., USA). The aim is to extubate the patient at the end of the procedure and therefore, a body temperature of $\geq35.5^{\circ}$C is obligatory.

Patients having preexisting renal insufficiency and/or diabetes mellitus are at risk of nephrotoxicity and the development of acute renal failure due to the use of radiocontrast media. Cautious prehydration and maintenance of stable hemodynamics can limit the extent of nephrotoxicity. In addition, adjuncts like furosemide, dopamine, and acetylcysteine (1,200 mg in 500 mL N/saline over 30 minutes) may be used but their effectiveness is less well established (13).

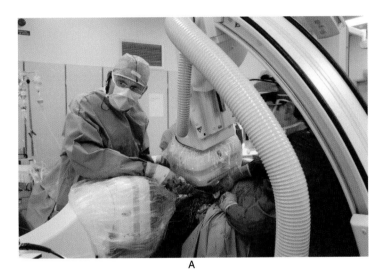

A

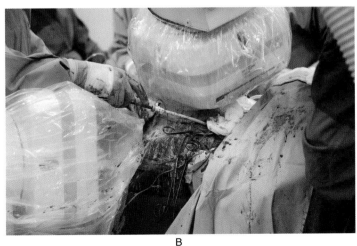

B

Figure 6 Blood loss during TAVR.

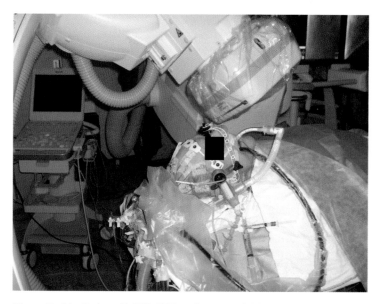

Figure 7   Monitoring with BIS, TEE, and transcranial Doppler.

SPECIAL INTRAPROCEDURAL MONITORING

Apart from the recommended basic and invasive monitoring (14), special intraoperative monitoring can be added (Fig. 7).

Transesophageal echocardiography (TEE) has nearly replaced pulmonary artery catheters (PACs) for intraoperative monitoring and is our standard, both in the OR and in the CCL. The anesthesiologist typically performs the TEE. TEE can provide useful information about aortic valve morphology, LV function, positioning of the prosthesis across the aortic root and can readily identify certain procedural complications.

Phases of TAVR with Potential Consequences for the Anesthesiologist (15)

Predeployment
By the cardiologist (Fig. 8), access is gained percutaneously through the femoral artery under ultrasound guidance while a pigtail catheter is inserted via the left radial or brachial artery.

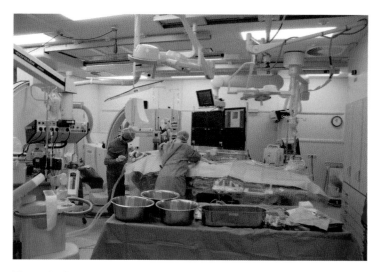

Figure 8   Patient is under general anesthesia and stable; cardiologist can start with TAVI.

A bipolar right ventricular transvenous pacing lead is introduced through the femoral vein for rapid ventricular pacing and is tested. In this phase maintaining hemodynamic stability and adequate hypnosis and analgesia needs extra attention. Compared to conventional surgery, "surgical stimulation" is limited to the vascular puncture. During the predeployment phase, serious problems can arise from the vascular access site (dissection, rupture, and hemorrhage) or perforation of the left or right ventricle by the extra-stiff guide wire or temporary pacing lead, respectively.

Valvuloplasty
Passage of stiff wires and large bore catheters across the aortic valve can induce arrhythmias and even conduction abnormalities. Balloon aortic valvuloplasty (BAV) allows for easier passage of the prosthesis and permits adequate cardiac output while the prosthesis is positioned across the stenosed aortic orifice. BAV is performed under rapid right ventricular pacing (180–220 beats per minute). The goal of BAV is to adequately dilate the aortic valve annulus to ensure proper seating of the prosthesis within the aortic root. Rapid pacing may induce cardiac ischemia or arrhythmias and therefore must be kept to a minimum. Between sequences of rapid pacing, it is imperative that hemodynamic parameters return toward "normal."

During BAV, we tend to administer a basal infusion of phenylephrine and if needed, additional bolus doses of 100 to 200 mcg. Ephedrine or norepinephrine may be alternatives. An infusion of norepinephrine is sometimes used. When resolution is delayed we prefer to administer low-dose boluses of epinephrine, 10 to 20 mcg, titrating to effect and repeated if needed. Arterial pressure must be completely recovered between sequences of rapid pacing.

Complications associated with BAV can include coronary ostial obstruction or embolization, aortic root rupture, myocardial depression, arrhythmias, conduction blocks, severe aortic regurgitation, and stroke. Electrocardiogram and TEE can be useful to rule out several of these complications.

Positioning and Deployment
Deployment of balloon-expandable devices requires rapid ventricular pacing to significantly diminish cardiac output and ensure stable position of the prosthesis during valve deployment. Deployment of self-expanding devices does not require rapid ventricular pacing. While positioning the prosthesis across the aortic root, the large diameter delivery catheters can obstruct blood flow and create hemodynamic instability. Similar pharmacological principles already discussed in "Valvuloplasty" section can be applied. In the setting of poor LV function and absence of coronary artery disease an infusion of dobutamine may be started just before positioning and deployment. In some instances, the only treatment is urgent deployment of the prosthesis, which immediately reduces LV afterload and myocardial oxygen demand. During this crucial phase, the cardiology team should be very pragmatic and avoid repeated aortograms and/or wasting of time.

Potential problems in this phase of TAVI can include incorrect placement (too high or too low), device embolization distally into the aorta or proximally into the left ventricle, central or paravalvular regurgitation, coronary ostial obstruction, arrhythmias, AV block, and impingement of the anterior mitral valve leaflet affecting its function. TEE can be helpful to diagnose and/or avoid these complications, assess LV function, degree and etiology of aortic regurgitation, and the need for further dilation or implantation of a second prosthesis (valve-in-valve).

Postdeployment
After final assessment of device position and function, the delivery system is removed and the vascular access site is closed percutaneously with the aid of a 10-F Prostar device. Integrity of vessel repair and the absence of vascular complications (perforation, dissection and occlusion) can be assessed with angiography. At this stage, some patients experience an increase in cardiac output and blood pressure requiring a decrease or discontinuation of vasopressor/inotropic agents.

Percutaneous Versus Transapical Approach

Patients with severe peripheral vascular disease need an alternative approach to the trans-femoral route. In these situations, a subclavian or transapical approach can be pursued depending on operator experience and device availability. With respect to the transapical approach in our center, the procedure is performed in the CCL by a heart team consisting of the interventional cardiologist and cardiac surgeon. The transapical approach is performed under general anesthesia and access is obtained via the LV apex through a small left anterior thoracotomy at the fifth or sixth intercostal space. Some surgeons may require double-lumen intubation but this is not obligatory. Both induction and maintenance of anesthesia are performed with similar considerations given to the transfemoral approach with the caveat that surgical stimulation is higher. Epicardial pacing wires are placed onto the left ventricle for rapid ventricular pacing and a pigtail catheter is introduced into the ascending aorta via the femoral artery. The femoral vessels are made accessible but not exposed for cardiopulmonary bypass in case a patient needs this support. The delivery system and prosthesis are brought through the apex across the aortic valve. The previously placed purse string sutures around the LV apex are secured after removal of the introducer. Left ventricular apical closure can be difficult and therefore cardiopulmonary bypass may be required for extensive repair. In anticipation to these difficulties, red blood cell salvage and a rapid infusion device should be immediately available for each transapical procedure. Recurrent pleural effusions are common in these patients so a thoracotomy drainage is left in place.

Pain management is best accomplished with the use of systemic opioids and intercostal nerve blocks. Because higher doses of opioids are used and hypothermia is often present, only a selected group of patients are extubated in the procedure room.

POSTANESTHESIA CARE

Patients undergoing general anesthesia should be transferred to an ICU facility. However, the stability and function of the temporary pacemaker lead should be verified before transferring of the patient. Vital signs and neurological status should be recorded immediately upon arrival in the ICU and followed at regular intervals. All access sites should be routinely checked for signs of bleeding. Blood loss may not be apparent in cases of retroperitoneal bleeding, pericardial effusions, or hemothorax. A peripheral vascular exam should confirm normal distal pulses and perfusion of the extremities.

Discharge criteria and management in the intensive care are discussed elsewhere in this book, but most often patients are transferred to the ward the morning after the procedure.

REFERENCES

1. Rupreht J, Hofland J, Leendertse-Verloop K. Anaesthesia and sedation outside the OR. In: Educational Issues 2005, University of Trieste, School of Anaesthesia and Intensive Care, APICE School of Critical Care Medicine, Trieste, Italy. Milan, Italy: Springer-Verlag, 2006:153–160.
2. Shook DC, Gross W, Offsite anaesthesiology in the cardiac catheterization lab. Curr Opin Anaesthesiol 2007; 20:352–358.
3. Ree RM, Bowering JB, Schwarz S. Case series: Anesthesia for retrograde percutaneous aortic valve replacement-experience with the first 40 patients. Can J Anesth 2008; 55:761–768.
4. Cribier A, Eltchaninoff H, Tron C, et al. Treatment of calcific aortic stenosis with the percutaneous heart valve. J Am Coll Cardiol 2006; 47:1214–1223.
5. Melloni C. Anesthesia and sedation outside the operating room: How to prevent risk and maintain good quality. Curr Opin Anaesthesiol 2007; 20:513–519.
6. Clinical Guideline 3: Preoperative tests. NICE Guideline. At: http://www.nice.org.uk/nicemedia/pdf/cg3NICEguideline.pdf. Accessed July 31, 2009.
7. Covello RD, Maj G, Landoni G, et al. Anesthetic management of percutaneous aortic valve implantation: Focus on challenges encountered and proposed solutions. J Cardiothorac Vasc Anesth 2009; 23:280–285.
8. Fassl J, Walther T, Groesdonk HV, et al. Anesthesia management for transapical transcatheter aortic valve implantation: A case series. J Cardiothorac Vasc Anesth 2009; 23:286–291.
9. ASA. Basic standards for preanesthetic care. At: http://www.asahq.org/publicationsAndServices/standards/03.pdf. Accessed July 31, 2009.

10. Orellana FJ, Ligthart JMR. Diagnóstico ecográfico de trombosis de la vena yugular interna. Rev Esp Anestesiol Reanim 2008; 55:650–651.
11. Friedberg BL. Anesthesia in cosmetic surgery. New York: Cambridge University Press, 2007.
12. Mittnacht A, Fanshawe M, Konstadt S. Anesthetic considerations in the patient with valvular heart disease undergoing noncardiac surgery. Semin Cardiothorac Vasc Anesth 2008; 12: 33–59.
13. Joe RR, Diaz LK. Anesthesia in the cardiac cath lab: Catheter and EPS, therapeutic procedures for pediatrics and adults. ASA Newsl 2003; 67:10.
14. Kotob F, Twersky RS. Anesthesia outside the operating room: General overview and monitoring standards. Int Anesthesiol Clin 2003; 41(2):1–15.
15. Cheung A, Ree R. Transcatheter aortic valve replacement. Anesthesiol Clin 2008; 26:465–479.

10 | Tips and Tricks During the Procedure: Options for Vascular Access (Femoral, Subclavian, Transaortic, and Transapical)

Jean-Claude Laborde
Cardiology Department, Glenfield Hospital, Leicester, U.K.

Rüdiger Lange
Clinic for Cardiovascular Surgery, German Heart Center Munich, Munich, Germany

INTRODUCTION

After the pioneering works (1) using a 25-F catheter and retroperitoneal surgical iliac access, transcatheter aortic valve implantation (TAVI) has rapidly evolved into smaller profile devices The Medtronic CoreValve now comes with an 18-F delivery system for both valve sizes and the Edwards SAPIEN system with a 22- and 24-F delivery system for the 23- and 26-mm prosthesis, respectively. More recently, the 18-F Edwards SAPIEN XT device has been introduced into clinical practice. Despite this rapid progress, the devices used presently still remain relatively bulky and this, coupled with the high incidence of peripheral vascular disease in cardiac and elderly patients, has driven transcatheter valve technologies to evolve alternative routes of delivery to treat a wider range of patients. Among the growing number of centers that are introducing the transcatheter aortic valve implantation procedure, associated surgical and cardiology teams developed other transvascular accesses for TAVI (axillary, subclavian, transaorta) to offer the most adequate treatment for the individual patient. In particular the transapical implantation technique with the Edwards SAPIEN system, using a 26-F delivery system has yielded promising results.

FEMORAL ARTERY VASCULAR ACCESS

The transfemoral access is the predominant route for implantation of both the CoreValve and the Edwards SAPIEN prosthesis. First, we review the vascular criteria that have to be carefully analyzed to insure a safe femoral approach for TAVI, and then we approach more complex anatomical situations and review the different "tips and tricks" that allow to extend the femoral approach to acceptable boundaries.

Imaging

It is beyond the purpose of this chapter to determine which imaging modality (peripheral angiography, CT scan, or MRI) provides the most accurate analysis of the diameter, tortuosity, and degree of calcifications of the arterial vessels. The daily choice reflects the experience and expertise in each center. Both of the respective imaging techniques have advantages and drawbacks in defining the above arterial vessel criteria. Today, it is only during the early phase of the development of this technique in new centers that a combination of two imaging modalities is recommended to insure an optimal analysis. However, this recommendation should also be the rule in all complex anatomies.

General Requirements for Transfemoral Access

For the femoral puncture site, as a minimum requirement, the common femoral artery should be ≥ 6.0 mm in diameter with ≥ 15 mm length between the superficial epigastric artery and the femoral bifurcation, avoiding all severe calcified vessels. Compliance to these criteria usually allows for a safe and successful puncture in addition to successful percutaneous closure with the 10-F Prostar device.

The second step is to assess the feasibility and safety of advancing the 18-F introducer through the iliac arteries. This step is more difficult and requires a complete analysis of the entire arterial vessel anatomy, including diameter, tortuosity, lesions, and the degree of calcifications. The latter plays a major role in the decision making. Ideally, the preoperative setting should include at least an angiogram of the aorto-iliac arteries with the use of a graduated pigtail. For more detailed information, a CT scan or MRI can be useful to assess circumferential calcifications, or a mural thrombus in relation to an unsuspected arterial aneurysm.

To which extent the femoral approach should still be considered an acceptable option in difficult anatomies in regard to the potential risk of iliac rupture is again a difficult question but some rules, tips and tricks, and technical aspects can be provided.

First of all, the risk of arterial rupture is directly related to a combination of three major features: small artery vessel diameter, severe tortuosity, and heavy calcifications. These features reemphasize the need to respect some basic rules that should lead to the exclusion of the femoral approach in case of the following:

- iliac artery diameter of <6.0 mm,
- external iliac artery loops,
- circumferential arterial calcifications, and
- severe kinking or tortuosity of the abdominal or intrathoracic aorta.

Assessing the feasibility and more importantly the safety of the femoral route is in general the first step in chronologic order when a patient is considered for TAVI. Relatively easy in case of simple anatomy, it can turn to a difficult decision in complex anatomies.

Before all, no simple algorithm or guidelines from the preoperative assessment can be given. Considering the different levels of expertise of the interventional cardiologist and the cardiac surgeon in peripheral vascular disease, a highly individualized and thoughtful approach is required. Assessing the feasibility and more importantly the safety of the femoral route requires a complete analysis of all the steps of the procedure with their respective pitfalls and potential complications:

- Assess peripheral artery vessels for the risk of distal ischemia. Patients with previous occlusion of the superficial femoral artery are at risk of acute ischemia if minor emboli in the profundis artery are present.
- Assess the common femoral artery for the puncture site and potential risk of occlusion or prolonged bleeding in the presence of severe calcifications or small vessel diameter.
- Assess the iliac arteries for the risk of arterial rupture in the presence of severe calcifications or diseased vessels.
- Assess the thoracic and abdominal aorta for risk of distal emboli in case of valve retrieval for malpositioning or migration.
- Assess the angulation and calcifications of the aortic arch and native aortic valve for the risk of valve misplacement, stroke, aortic dissection, and cardiac tamponade.

For the femoral puncture site, noncompliance to the fundamental anatomical criteria and techniques of puncture may increase the risk for complications:

- Potential retroperitoneal bleeding due to high puncture.
- Complete occlusion of the femoral artery favored by prolonged blood flow reduction with the 18-F catheter and use of 10-F Prostar in <6.0 femoral artery diameters.
- Prolonged bleeding following failure of the 10-F Prostar secondary to low puncture at the femoral bifurcation level.

The technique of arterial puncture, careful use of the 10-F Prostar device (described in details in the next chapter), and a thoughtful appraisal of the femoral artery anatomy are of equal value for a successful femoral approach.

TIPS AND TRICKS TO IMPROVE SAFETY OF THE FEMORAL PUNCTURE TECHNIQUE

The technique of femoral artery puncture using fluoroscopy represents an alternative approach to the use of echo-Doppler techniques.

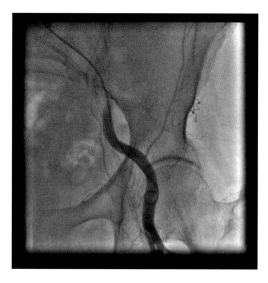

Figure 1 Contrast fluoroscopy of iliofemoral vessels showing the end of the pigtail catheter being used as a target for correct puncture site.

Technique of Femoral Artery Puncture

From the contralateral femoral approach, a 5-F pigtail catheter is advanced through the aorto-iliac bifurcation and the distal tip of the pigtail catheter positioned at the common femoral artery by using a regular 0.035 guidewire or a 0.035 Terumo guidewire if the iliac artery vessels are tortuous or calcified. If needed, contrast injection is performed using 5 mL of contrast medium to insure correct position of the distal pigtail position between the superficial epigastric artery and the femoral bifurcation. The distal tip of the puncture needle is then positioned under fluoroscopy guidance <1 cm below the pigtail and carefully advanced with a step (>70°) angle to minimize the path between the skin and the artery wall aiming at the center of the pigtail to enter the artery by the mid-portion of the anterior arterial wall of the common femoral   artery (Fig. 1) (Case 1).

Progression of the 18-F CoreValve Introducer

When the anatomical criteria (artery diameter, vessel tortuosity, calcifications) are favorable, progression of the 18-F introducer through the iliac artery is in general smooth and uneventful. However, a significant number of patients undergoing TAVI have severe peripheral obstructive arterial disease, which may raise concerns for the safety of the transfemoral approach.

Among the tips and tricks that could slightly improve the safety of the femoral access are the following:

- The 18-F introducer should be preshaped manually before introduction and carefully advanced using only gentle forward pressure into the artery with clockwise and counter-clockwise maneuvers to release tension on the arterial wall during advancement.
- Always advance the 18-F introducer into the femoral and iliac arteries by using the support of on a 0.035 stiff guidewire (Amplatz Extra-stiff).
- In challenging iliac anatomies with uncertainty about the success of the femoral approach, first advance the 18-F dilator on the Extra-stiff wire to test the feasibility prior to using the 18-F vascular access sheath.
- Consequently, if this maneuver is successful, the 18-F vascular access sheath can be advanced up to the abdominal aorta—the procedure subsequently follows the usual steps. If it is not successful and the 18-F vascular access sheath meets resistance during advancement in the iliac artery vessel, the procedure should be carried out with the introducer only partially inserted into the iliac artery instead of applying unreasonable force with the risk of dissection or rupture. To which extent one should apply force to advance the 18-F vascular access sheath is a matter of experience. However, one should always be ready to abort the procedure when excessive force is required. In these cases, the contralateral transfemoral, axillary, or transapical approach should be considered.

- Advancement of the 18-F dilator into the iliac arteries may also fail due to atherosclerotic plaques or significant arterial stenoses. In such instances, balloon angioplasty of the iliac artery can be considered to facilitate the way for the 18-F introducer. One potential consequence of not following this rule is the risk of dislodgment of the implanted stent by the 18-F delivery catheter when advanced forward through the iliac artery (Case 2). Stenting of the iliac artery, even if there is a dissection after balloon angioplasty for example, should only be discussed after valve implantation but before complete withdrawal of the 18-F vascular access sheath.

Others options while facing failure to advance the 18-F introducer or 18-F valve catheter in tortuous and calcified iliac arteries includes the exchange of the 0.035 extrastiff guidewire for a 0.038 "Back-up Meyer" wire to straighten the iliac vessel or eventually the contralateral femoral approach (Case 3).

Advancement of the 18 F-CoreValve Catheter

In standard iliac anatomies or when the iliac difficulties are overcome with the complete advancement of the 18-F introducer up to the abdominal aorta, the progression of the 18-F valve catheter up to the native aortic valve for the implantation of the CoreValve is almost always successful. In rare circumstances, severe angulation and calcifications of the horizontal part of the aortic arch eventually combined with a severely angulated aortic valve anatomy could compromise the progression of the 18-F valve catheter. This difficulty can be overcome with the use of a "goose-neck" catheter.

Technique of Using the Goose-Neck Catheter for the Progression of the 18-F Valve Catheter in Difficult Anatomy

This technique requires the withdrawal of the 0.035 Extra-stiff guidewire previously positioned into the left ventricle.

By using the contralateral femoral approach, a 7-F goose-neck catheter is then inserted and deployed at the abdominal aortic level. A 0.035 regular guidewire is then advanced through the goose-neck" catheter. The correct position of the guidewire into the "goose-neck" catheter is checked by closing and gently pulling on the 7-F goose-neck catheter. Then the usual steps of crossing the native aortic valve, exchange of the regular wire for an Extra-stiff guidewire and valvuloplasty if not previously performed are done. When advancing the 18-F valve catheter, the goose-neck catheter is then closed on the distal tip of the 18-F valve catheter and then advanced forward following the progression of the 18-F catheter into the aorta.

At the level of the aortic arch and/or of the native aortic valve, by pulling on the goose-neck catheter at the same time that the 18-F delivery catheter is pushed forward, facilitates the progression through the arch and the ascending aorta by releasing the tension on the distal tip of the 18 F-catheter.

This tricky technique increases the overall success rate of the femoral access by increasing the feasibility of this approach.

But at this stage when additional maneuvers are required to increase the feasibility of the femoral approach, one should question the safety of the procedure.

To correctly evaluate the safety of valve implantation, one should therefore remember the self-expandable characteristic of the CoreValve prosthesis that requires, at the time of valve implantation, a simultaneous and progressive retrieval of the 18-F catheter at the same time during release of the valve to insure a correct position of the valve. In heavily calcified and tortuous anatomies it becomes increasingly difficult to correctly position the prosthesis because of frictions on the 18-F delivery catheter. To some extent, the friction on the 18-F delivery catheter can compromise the smooth release of the valve during implantation. Such severe frictions can result from the following:

- Bending or plicature of the 18-F introducer into tortuous and calcified iliac arteries.
- Stiff angulation and severe calcifications on the aortic arch.
- Severe angulation of the native aortic valve (vertical annular plane).

These three aforementioned factors may increase the complexity of the transfemoral approach and lead to the following:

- Malpositioning of the valve due to frictions on the 18-F catheter not allowing a smooth release.
- Stroke from dislodgment of atherosclerotic plaques when crossing the aortic arch or the native aortic having required excessive pushing on the 18-F valve catheter.
- Type A aortic dissection for the same reasons.
- Cardiac tamponade from wire perforation more difficult to control due to increased friction into the 18-F valve catheter in severely angulated anatomies. Note that this risk also increases specifically when severe circumferential left ventricular hypertrophy is associated.

Finally, assessment of the safety of the femoral approach for TAVI requires an analysis of numerous anatomic parameters that go far beyond the simple analysis of the feasibility of femoral access.

Access Concerns in Complex Anatomy

Therefore, one should always consider three questions before final decision regarding the vascular access (Case 4):

1. Is the femoral route technically feasible and safe?
2. Does the femoral route insure a safe progression and implantation of the valve?
3. Finally, is there a better access option to insure the safety of the implantation?

SPECIAL CONSIDERATIONS FOR THE SAPIEN TRANSFEMORAL DELIVERY SYSTEM

The minimal vessel diameter for implantation of the Edwards SAPIEN should be not less than 8 mm. For both the sizes, the 21- and the 23-delivery system, either a Prostar or up to 3 Perclose systems may be used. Using a closure device for the Edwards delivery systems makes it almost paramount to perform an angiography of the puncture site at the end of the procedure. Vascular problems, such as dissection or vascular rupture occur considerably more often with the Edwards SAPIEN delivery systems than with the smaller CoreValve catheter. With the new generation of Edwards delivery systems this problem will be overcome.

Summary

If the percutaneous femoral approach continues to represent in the near future the access of choice for the vast majority of patients proposed for TAVI, others accesses will undoubtedly continue to expand with increased experience and knowledge.

AXILLARY/SUBCLAVIAN ACCESS

In contrast to the femoral/iliac vessels, the axillary artery is usually relatively free of atheroma and thus fulfils in most patients the anatomic and morphologic requirements. Therefore, it represents a potential alternative to the femoral route in patients with peripheral vascular disease involving the iliac arteries.

Imaging

As for the femoral route, angiogram, CT scan, or MRI provide accurate analysis of the diameter, tortuosity, and degree of calcifications of the subclavian and axillary artery vessels in relation to the aortic arch, mammary, and carotid arteries. Particular attention should be devoted to the debranching site of the subclavian artery from the aortic arch, where most frequently stenosing calcification is to be expected.

General Requirements

Today, little is known about the safety of this approach for the TAVI procedure compared with the femoral access that has been the usual route since the pioneering experience.

There are still some questions about the technique, and the specific safety of this access has already been the subject of investigation during this early stage. As a result, some anatomical criteria should lead to the exclusion of axillary/subclavian route:

- arterial vessel diameter of <6.0 mm
- severe tortuosity
- circumferential calcifications

SUBCLAVIAN/AXILLARY ACCESS ASSESSMENT

Left Subclavian/Axillary Access

Assessing the feasibility and safety of the axillary access requires a complete analysis of the route from skin to the aortic valve.

- First, a previous pacemaker poses an obstacle to the surgical approach, as it runs the risk of pacemaker-led damage and infection and should therefore be a contraindication to the axillary approach at the side of the pacemaker.
- In the presence of a functional right internal mammary artery (RIMA) or left internal mammary artery (LIMA) grafts, the risk of graft occlusion or injuries is to be evaluated carefully. The criteria that strictly contraindicate the axillary approach in regard to a potential risk of subclavian dissection or ostial graft occlusion in patients with patent LIMA are the following:
  - Diameter artery of <6.5 mm from origin of subclavian artery to the ostia of LIMA.
  - Severe tortuosity.
  - Circumferential calcifications or atherosclerotic disease of the subclavian artery proximal to the LIMA (risk of dissection).
  - Atherosclerotic lesions requiring peripheral balloon angioplasty (PTA).

If those anatomical criteria are present, transient obstruction of the blood flow through the patent LIMA or RIMA grafts during 18-F introducer sheath progression is acceptable and safe to a certain extent.

Some preventive strategies can help to avoid injury and obstruction of the LIMA graft:

- Control the progression of the guidewire through the axillary/subclavian vessels under fluoroscopic guidance to avoid graft injury with the wire. Perform balloon aortic valvuloplasty before valve implantation by using 12-F introducer sheath to allow blood flow perfusion through the LIMA during valvuloplasty.
- Advance preshaped 18-F introducer respectfully to the curve given to the introducer and have the valve catheter ready to be advanced to minimized time of graft obstruction.
- After progression of the valve delivery catheter through the 18-F introducer sheath and after crossing the native aortic valve, withdrawal of the 18-F introducer sheath distal to the ostia of the LIMA will allow reperfusion of the LIMA.
- Valve position and implantation proceeds as usual.

Right Subclavian/Axillary Access

When the right axillary access is discussed, the route of the innominate artery should be assessed using similar criteria and preventive strategies as previously described for the left axillary access with patent LIMA.

The last anatomical criterion to be integrated in the algorithm for the axillary access decision is the anatomy of the native aortic valve. Importantly, the anatomy of the native aortic valve has a discriminating role for the right axillary approach. As a matter of fact, from the right axillary approach, due to the stiffness of the guidewire and the valve catheter, the latter tends to be positioned in a more vertical angle to the native aortic valve. As a result, if facing a vertical anatomy of the aortic root (i.e., horizontal aortic valve annulus) valve implantation can be safely achieved. As the aortic root becomes more horizontal (i.e. aortic valve annulus becomes more vertical), valve implantation via the right axillary approach becomes almost impossible (Fig. 2). As a rule, angulation of the aortic valve annular plane greater than 30° from the horizontal, disqualifies the right axillary approach (Case 4). In contrast, the left subclavian/axillary access is feasible irrespective of the native aortic valve anatomy.

Finally, one question that regularly arises is surgical or percutaneous approach.

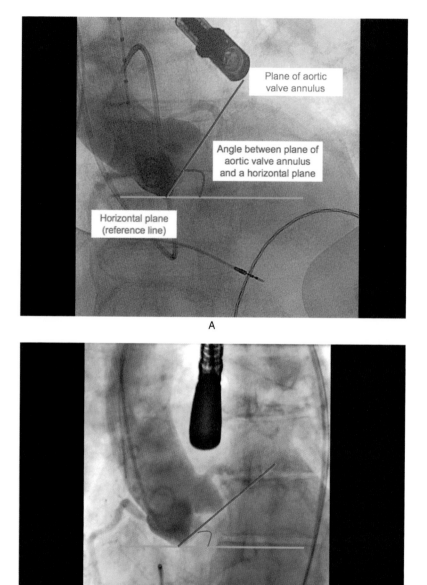

Figure 2 The aortic root angulation (**A**) is more horizontal than the aortic root angulation (**B**). Stated in other words, the plane of the aortic valve annulus (**A**) is more vertical with respect to the horizontal than the plane of the aortic valve annulus (**B**). Implantation via the right subclavian approach would be technically more challenging (if not impossible) in **A** than in **B**. The angulation of the aortic root poses no caveats when implanting via the left subclavian approach.

The use of the Prostar XL in closing large femoral access sites has revolutionized TAVI, making this technique eligible to be performed under local anesthesia. But the Prostar XL may eventually fail and manual compression is required to maintain hemostasis. Thus, percutaneous approach using the Prostar XL is not recommended for the subclavian approach because direct manual compression is not possible. Thus, surgical cutdown is required.

TRANSAPICAL ACCESS

Edwards SAPIEN

To date, only the Edwards SAPIEN prosthesis is available for the transapical access. Except for the presence of severe injury of the skin after radiation therapy of breast cancer, no true contraindication exists for the transapical access. Prior to thoracotomy, we inserted two guidewires in the right femoral artery and vein for percutaneous CPB connection in case of need. This is a safety measure that should be respected in any case. A 3 to 4 cm skin incision is performed below the left nipple. It is recommended to identify the apex of the left ventricle by using transthoracic echocardiography and mark the apex on the skin. Accordingly, the chest is entered through the fifth or sixth intercostal space. The mid-clavicular line should be in the center of the incision. A small size soft tissue retractor (Edwards, Cardiovation) is inserted. The pericardium is incised longitudinally or transversely and suspended. We recommend a transverse incision because this allows to lift the apex later by pulling on the pericardial stay sutures. In contrast, after a longitudinal incision the heart can only be moved from left to right. The apex is then identified and its position verified ideally by the distal course of the left anterior descending artery. Bipolar pacemaker wires are sewn to the epicardial surface and a rapid pacing test at 160 to 200 beats/min is performed that lowers the arterial pressure below 60 mm Hg. For the placement of the pacing wires it is recommended to look for a position on the left ventricular pericardium, because the right ventricular myocardium may be extremely soft and fragile, especially in very old, female patients. A slightly supra-apical position is usually chosen as the site for the introduction of the delivery system since the apex itself is normally covered by epicardial fat. For the placement of the sutures it is important to identify a location on the myocardium which is relatively free of epicardial fat. We strongly recommend using 2 to 0 instead of 3 to 0 Prolene (Ethicon Inc., Somerville, New Jersey) for the apex sutures, because 3 to 0 may cut through the fragile myocardium. There are two different techniques for placing the sutures: either two perpendicular sutures armed with big Teflon felts or two concentrical pursestring sutures armed with Teflon after each insertion into the myocardium. It is of utmost importance that these sutures go deep into the myocardium, meaning the needle should enter the epicardial surface in a right angle. These sutures should be placed by an experienced surgeon, because any technical failure may lead to severe bleeding problems or even death of the patient after an otherwise uneventful valve implantation. After 5000 IU of heparin have been administered the apex is punctured and a soft guidewire is advanced in the ascending aorta under fluoroscopic control. A 6-F angiocath is placed over the wire and, after measurement of the aortic and LV pressures, a right Judkins catheter (Cordis, Johnson & Johnson, Norderstedt, Germany) is inserted and advanced into the descending aorta. The Terumo wire is subsequently replaced with an Amplatz super stiff wire (Amplatz super stiff, 260 cm; Boston Scientific, Natick, Massachusetts), which is placed in the abdominal aorta at the level of the renal arteries. The 6-F angiocath is replaced with a 12-F sheath and a valvuloplasty of the aortic valve is performed under rapid pacing by using the 20-mm balloon supplied with the prosthesis. After hemodynamical recovery, which we find of utmost importance to wait for, the 12-F sheath is replaced by the 26-F valve delivery sheath. The catheter-mounted valve is then advanced at the level of the aortic annulus and the correct intra-annular position confirmed by aortography. After that the valve is deployed by controlled insufflation of the balloon, again under rapid pacing. Immediately prior to inflation contrast medium is injected into the aortic root. This technique allows for correction of the position of the prosthesis during inflation of the balloon and is extremely helpful. After the prosthesis has been checked for any paravalvular leakage, all wires and introducer are removed. The sutures are tight consecutively, again by an experienced surgeon.

Medtronic CoreValve

Very limited experience has been reported about the transapical implantation of the CoreValve prosthesis and the device is no longer available on the market. With the first-generation delivery system, the release of the valve from the upper notches posed a serious problem. After full deployment of the valve, the upper part of the valve frame and the retracted introducer sheath were tilted toward the aortic arch, especially in the case of a relatively short ascending aorta. Therefore, unhooking the introducer from the frame was compromised. The second generation was extended by a guiding catheter that was supposed to be placed in the descending aorta to allow for a straighter line between the introducer sheath and the valve frame. However, also with this device, unhooking of the valve frame was difficult. Furthermore, since the guidewire extension pushed against the upper part of the aortic arch, manipulation of the valve during implantation was severely limited. With this experience further attempts were abandoned and the valve implantation only considered for vascular access.

TRANSAORTIC ACCESS

In very rare instances neither of the above-described accesses may be accomplishable with the currently available technology. Typically, a patient presents with severely calcified, tortuous femoral/iliac arteries with multiple stenoses <6 mm in diameter. The left subclavian access is consequently evaluated and shows severe calcifications and high-degree stenosis at the debranching site off the arch. The right innominate artery exhibits a severe stenosis and furthermore, the angle between the ascending aorta and the native aortic valve is unfavorable for implantation. The transapical access is not feasible because the size of the native valve ring is 26 mm and thus far, too big for an Edwards SAPIEN prosthesis. For this constellation, an alternative approach may be considered, which is the transaortic access.

A partial, upper median mini-sternotomy is performed under general anesthesia and the ascending aorta exposed. Two, full-bite Teflon-armed pursestring sutures are placed as close as possible to the innominate artery, to gain length for the introducer sheath. Subsequently the 18-French introducer is advanced into the aorta via Seldinger technique under fluoroscopic control. Since the CoreValve introducer is not designed for this access and thus, much too long, care must be taken not to damage the aortic wall or even pierce the left ventricle. BAV is then performed under rapid pacing and the valve subsequently advanced. When releasing the valve only the top 2 to 3 cm of the introducer sheath should be inside the aorta to give the valve enough length to be deployed.

The transaortic access is considered an "ultima ratio," but has been performed by the authors in three patients without any complications and with an excellent result. The mini-sternotomy does not seem to incriminate the aged and rather sick patients profoundly, as long as extracorporeal circulation and open-heart surgery with cardioplegic arrest is avoided. As soon as larger valve prostheses enter the market, the need for this approach, however, may even be further reduced.

DECISION TREE FOR TRANSCATHETER VALVE IMPLANTATIONS

There is no simplified algorithm for access decision. Optimal decision making comes from the interdisciplinary team, respectful of their knowledge and expertise regarding the different approaches and techniques of TAVI. A group that implants both prostheses currently available and masters all potential access sites may use the following decision tree for the primary planning of the procedure (Fig. 3). This algorithm may be applied for all patients considered for TAVI in the following manner: As a first step the *transfemoral* approach is considered and investigated. If this access is feasible, according to the criteria described in this chapter, the choice of the valve type is based on clinical preference, the vessel diameters and the size of the aortic annulus. For small annulus sizes between 18 and 20 mm, to date, only the Edwards SAPIEN prosthesis is acceptable, for very large sizes, between 25 and 27 mm, only the Medtronic CoreValve. Furthermore, if the peripheral vessel diameter does not exceed 6 mm at the narrowest site, only the 18-F Medtronic CoreValve delivery system may be considered. On the other

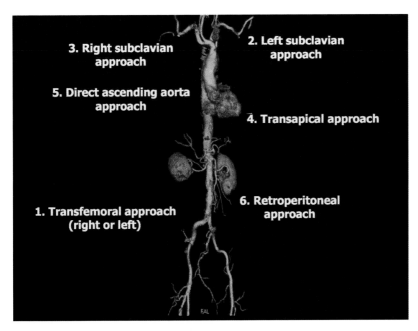

Figure 3 Volume rendered multi-slice CT scan of the arterial vascular tree. Options for vascular access during transcatheter implantation of the aortic valve: (1) femoral artery (right or left); (2) left subclavian artery; (3) right subclavian artery; (4) transapical; (5) direct ascending aorta; (6) retroperitoneal access.

hand, an increased diameter of the sinotubular junction beyond 42 mm precludes a Medtronic CoreValve and an exceptionally short distance between the coronary arteries and the aortic valve ring the Edwards SAPIEN prosthesis. If the transfemoral access has to be disregarded for anatomical reasons, the second step is to evaluate the left *trans-subclavian* access. In regard to the vessel diameter and morphology, the same selection criteria exist as for the femoral approach. A previously implanted pacemaker on the same side is a contraindication. For the choice of the valve prosthesis the same parameters have to be considered as for the transfemoral approach. The right subclavian artery should be used only in highly selected cases where no other access is possible, because the delivery system enters the ascending aorta from the innominate artery perpendicularly, which puts the prosthesis in an improper angle to the plane of the native valve ring (Fig. 2). If the subclavian access is not feasible, the next step will be to evaluate the *transapical* approach. Since the transapical access is very safe, it should also be considered in cases where the transarterial access might be possible, but where it seems unreasonably dangerous. The only contraindication for the transapical access might be severe previous skin injury following radiation therapy for breast cancer. However, since only the Edwards SAPIEN is available for this approach to date, the respective exclusion criteria given by the valve ring diameter have to be respected. If for different reasons no other access seems feasible the *transaortic* approach should be considered as an ultima ratio. Although less preferred by the authors, a retroperitoneal approach can also be used as a last resort.

Among the different measurements and assessments to be performed before patient approval for TAVI, the analysis of the entire vascular anatomy is a prerequisite, because it determines the procedural success and the complication rate. For the ultimate decision process advanced knowledge in peripheral vascular disease is mandatory to better evaluate the potential risk of complications when manipulating with large introducers and stiff wires in elderly patients with frequently calcified and tortuous vessels. Therefore, careful screening and analysis of the entire vascular tree from the access site to the aortic valve anatomy should be a systematic part of the preoperative analysis and its importance is not to be underestimated. Optimal decision comes from a heart team mastering all different approaches and techniques of TAVI. The decision is not to be based on what the team may be able to perform, but on what is best for the patient.

REFERENCE

1. Grube E, Laborde JC, Gerckens U, et al. Percutaneous implantation of the CoreValve self-expanding valve prosthesis in high-risk patients with aortic valve disease: The Siegburg first-in-man study. Circulation 2006; 114:1616–1624.

11 | Percutaneous Placement and Removal of Large Diameter Femoral Artery Sheaths with the Prostar XL Device

Lukas C. van Dijk and Peter M. T. Pattynama
Department of Radiology, Erasmus University Medical Center, Thoraxcenter, Rotterdam, The Netherlands

Peter de Jaegere, Jurgen M. R. Ligthart, and Patrick W. Serruys
Department of Interventional Cardiology, Erasmus University Medical Center, Thoraxcenter, Rotterdam, The Netherlands

Joke M. Hendriks
Department of Vascular Surgery, Erasmus University Medical Center, Thoraxcenter, Rotterdam, The Netherlands

INTRODUCTION

For successful transcatheter aortic valve implantation (TAVI) as well as endovascular abdominal aneurysm repair (EVAR), and thoracic endovascular aneurysm repair (TEVAR), the insertion of large diameter arterial sheaths is necessary. Because of the necessary caliber of the sheaths, usually between 18 and 24 F (6–8 mm), the access is almost exclusively chosen via the femoral–iliac arteries. In the past years we gradually changed our technique from a surgical cut-down to a percutaneous technique in all patients. The advantages of this less invasive technique are increased patient comfort immediately after the procedure and a diminished requirement for anesthetic drugs during and after the procedure. In most patients, the percutaneous technique of placement and removal of large diameter femoral arterial sheaths can be performed under local anesthesia only. In other words, the need for the presence of an anesthesiological team is dictated by the condition of the patient only and, to some extent, to the length of the procedure and not by the necessity to perform an open-surgical cut-down in the groin.

To achieve an optimal result and avoid complications a careful approach is mandatory. In this chapter, we describe the technique we employ in our institution.

METHODS

Patient Selection

Two aspects are essential for the selection: (*i*) The femoral artery wall must be free of calcified plaque at the area of puncture and (*ii*) the diameter of the femoral and iliac arteries must be large enough to accommodate the necessary sheath. Usually a minimal lumen diameter of 6, 7, and 8 mm is considered necessary for the insertion of an 18-, 22-, and 24-F sheath, respectively. We use CT angiography to reliably and noninvasively judge the femoral artery wall for tortuosity, calcification, and to measure lumen diameters [Fig. 1 (A) and 1(B)] (Video 1).

Materials

The following materials are needed beside the standard materials for an interventional procedure via femoral artery access (Video 2):

Prostar XL device set (Abbott, Abbott Park, Illinois)
Ultrasound machine with linear array probe (5–10 MHz)
Introducer sheath 10 F
Artery puncture needle
Guidewire 0.035" soft type
Guidewire 0.035" extra-stiff type
Diagnostic angiography catheter straight 65 to 80 cm

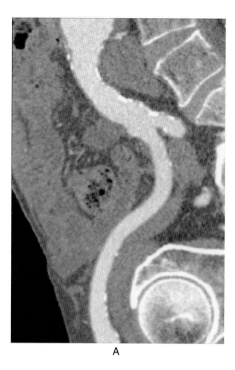

A

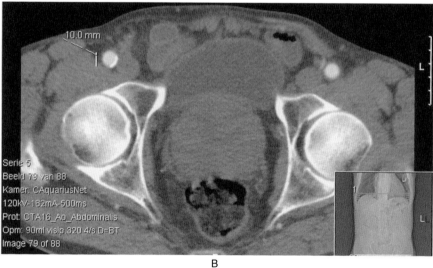

B

Figure 1 Longitudinal (**A**) and cross-sectional (**B**) view delineating the anatomy and dimensions of the femoral and iliac artery (Figure 1A) and of the femoral artery (Figure 1B) by MSCT.

Local anesthetic (Lidocaine)
Needle holder
Small dissecting forceps
Scalpel

PREPARATION
Before we prepare the patient's groin we carefully mark the preferred puncture place in each groin with an ink marker and the aid of ultrasound. This allows accurate placement of the wholes of the drapes on the groins. This is necessary because we need an acoustic window at

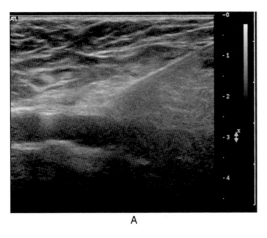
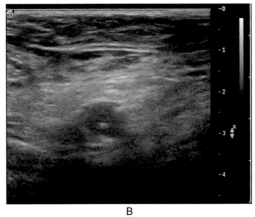

A   B

Figure 2   Longitudinal (**A**) and cross-sectional (**B**) view of the common femoral artery by ultrasound. In Figure 2A, the punctures needle that is advanced toward the femoral artery is clearly seen in the right upper quadrant part of the picture.

the puncture site for the ultrasound guidance. The wholes in the drapes are sealed of with thin sterile foil to prevent fluid contact of the groin puncture site with unsterile areas. It is possible to use ultrasound through this foil.

Ultrasound-Guided Puncture

Puncture
Local anesthesia: With the aid of the ultrasound Lidocaine 2%, 10 to20 mL is deposited in the skin, subcutis, and around the femoral artery [Fig. 2(A) and (B); Video 3].

To allow reliable closure of the arterial puncture site it is essential to enter the arterial wall of the common femoral artery exactly through the front wall (12-o'clock position), in a plaque-free area with an angle of 45° cranio-caudal. The most reliable way to achieve this is to use ultrasound guidance. Typically with a sterile packed 5 to 10 MHz linear array transducer. We also use the ultrasound guidance to accurately deposit the local anesthetics. After the (single-wall) puncture, a 10-F introducer sheath is placed over a standard J-tip guidewire.

Preparation and Introduction Prostar XL

Placement of the Sutures
To allow the placement of the two suture wires with the Prostar XL (Video 4), a transversal incision at the puncture site with a length 1 cm is necessary. With the aid of a blunt surgical preparation clamp a subcutaneous channel with a diameter of approximately 1 cm around the 10-F introducer sheath is made from the skin to the arterial wall.

Over a standard guidewire the introducer sheath is removed and the Prostar device is inserted. The device is advanced up to the arterial wall, if necessary with a twisting motion of the device to facilitate this.

Only if a pulsatile drainage of arterial blood is seen through marker tube the next step— retrieval of the four needles with the two suture wires attached—should be performed. The needles are removed and the suture wires are packed in gauzes with a 1% chlorhexidine in 70% alcohol solution, to keep them clean and aseptic.

Over a guidewire the Prostar XL device is removed and the 10-F introducer sheath replaced.

If one or more of the four needles are deflected, for instance by a calcified plaque, three or less needles will appear. In this case the needles should be repositioned in the Prostar device. This can be done with aid of surgical needle holder. At that point one can decide to convert to open-surgical preparation, or a second attempt—using a new Prostar device—is possible.

Placement of the Large Diameter Sheath
Over a standard 0.035" guidewire a straight 4-F angiography catheter is positioned in the abdominal aorta. The standard guidewire is replaced by an extra-stiff guidewire (Back-up Meier or Lunderquist). The large diameter sheath (usually 18 F) is placed over the extra-stiff guide-wire.

Closing After Removal of Sheath
Removal of the sheath with closure of the puncture hole (Video 5). After the endovascular procedure has been finished the suture wires are unpacked from the antiseptic gauzes and a sliding knot is prepared in each of the two wires. The knots are placed with the aid of a knot pusher directly following the removal of the large sheath. The skin incision can be closed by glue (cyano-acrylate), foil, or a skin suture.

DISCUSSION
The results of Starnes et al. (1) show technical success in 94% of the cases in which a sheath of 12 F or larger was used Success rate was 89% with sheaths of 18 F and larger.

In the only prospective randomized study published so far Torsello et al. (2) found an overall reduction in procedure costs despite the costs of the Prostar device due to the shortened procedure time compared to surgical cut-down.

Recommendations
Patient selection is probably important for the success rate. The obvious selection criterion is the diameter of the access arteries: this must be large enough for the required sheath. Furthermore calcifications on the ventral wall of the artery can be problematic, because they can cause deflection of the suture needles of the Prostar device.

We recommend preprocedural CT-angiography of the iliac and femoral arteries. In case of iliac narrowing it can be necessary to perform a pre-TAVI iliac stenting procedure (3). In these cases we prefer the use of the Wallstent (BSC, Maple Grove, Minnesota) or the Fluency-covered stent (BARD, Tempe, Arizona) because their structure is less likely to catch the large sheath compared to balloon-expandable stents or Nitinol self-expandable stents.

Meticulous Technique
Apart from experience with the technique of using the Prostar device, we strongly feel that the location of the femoral artery puncture is an important determinant for success. As well as the group of Arthurs et al. (4) we recommend ultrasound-guided puncture enabling exact localization of a calcium-free area of the ventral wall of the common femoral artery. Instead of the Prostar XL, other closure devices have been proposed such as the use of the Perclose (Abbott, Abbott Park, Illinois) with good results (5).

Complications To Be Anticipated
The complications are not indifferent from the usual femoral access complications: bleeding or thrombosis. Therefore it is mandatory to have "on the spot" vascular surgery available in case of failure.

REFERENCES
1. Starnes BW, Andersen CA, Ronsivalle JA, et al. Totally percutaneous aortic aneurysm repair: Experience and prudence. J Vasc Surg 2006; 43:270–276.
2. Torsello GB, Kasprzak B, Klenk E, et al. Endovascular suture versus cutdown for endovasculair aneurysm repair: A prospective randomized study. J Vasc Surg 2003; 38:78–82.
3. de Jaegere PP, van Dijk LC, van Sambeek MR, et al. How should I treat a patient with severe and symptomatic aortic stenosis who is rejected for surgical and transfemoral valve replacement and in whom a transapical implantation was aborted? Percutaneous reconstruction of the right ilio-femoral

tract with balloon angioplasty followed by the implantation of self-expanding stents. EuroIntervention. 2008; 4(2):292–296.

4. Arthurs ZM, Starnes BW, Sohn VY, et al. Ultrasound-guided access improves rate of access-related complications for totally percutaneous aortic aneurysm repair. Ann Vasc Surg. 2008;22 (6): 736–741.

5. Kahlert P, Eggebrecht H, Erbel R, et al. A modified "preclosure" technique after percutaneous aortic valve replacement. Catheter Cardiovasc Interv 2008;72 (6): 877–884.

12 | Intraprocedural Imaging: Percutaneous Aortic Valve Replacement

Samir R. Kapadia and E. Murat Tuzcu

Department of Cardiology, Heart and Vascular Institute, Cleveland Clinic, Cleveland, Ohio, U.S.A.

Percutaneous aortic valve replacement, like any other structural heart disease intervention, depends on accurate imaging before, during, and after the procedure (1). Role of imaging during percutaneous procedure can be equated to adequate exposure and visualization in open-surgical valve replacement. Adequate visualization makes the procedure faster, safer, and more predictable. Further, imaging during the procedure plays a key role in identifying, preventing, and treating the complications (2).

BASICS OF IMAGING

X-Ray Imaging

Fluoroscopy is the cornerstone of imaging in the cardiac catheterization laboratory. It allows accurate visualization of radiopaque structures with excellent temporal and spatial resolution, which is especially necessary for mobile cardiac structures. However, for the visualization of nonradiopaque structures like arteries and noncalcified valves, iodinated contrast is necessary. Fluoroscopy collects information from the entire path of X-ray beam as it traverses from the source to the detector. All structures in the path of the X-ray beam contribute to the final attenuation and hence the image. Typically, a two-dimensional (2-D) image is created on the screen with each X-ray pulse. Three-dimensional reconstruction is not possible unless imaging is performed with rotational angiography. Fluoroscopic imaging allows excellent visualization of the devices to allow proper and safe manipulation of the instruments. Orientation of the device in space is created by visualizing images in more than one plane and also seeing the response to torquing the device in the same projection. Typically, RAO (right anterior oblique) projection allows anterior–posterior distinction whereas LAO (left anterior oblique) projection makes left–right distinction possible. Turning the device to see whether it turns anteriorly or posteriorly with clockwise or counter-clockwise rotation can help with orientation in space.

Ultrasound Imaging

Transesophageal echocardiography (TEE) is the main stay for ultrasound imaging. On the other hand, experience with intracardiac echocardiography (ICE) is rapidly expanding and may become the ultrasound imaging modality of choice in aortic valve replacement.

2-D TEE allows tomographic imaging of the heart where the echogenic structures are seen with great temporal and spatial resolution. TEE under conscious sedation is very safe and effective in the catheterization laboratory. Proper sedation and suctioning of the posterior pharynx makes it reasonably comfortable for the patients. Anatomical visualization of the valves, aorta, and cardiac chambers provides the "eye" to the interventional procedures. Unlike open surgery, the valve replacement is done in beating heart and real-time functional assessment provided by the echocardiography is essential complement to invasive hemodynamic monitoring. Assessment of regurgitation, wall motion abnormalities, changes in right or left ventricular function, etc. can provide insight into the causes of hemodynamic changes. There are a number of limitations of TEE and echocardiography, in general. Tomographic imaging does not allow one to see the trajectory of devices. This is somewhat better with 3-D or biplane TEE but the field of view is quite limited compared to fluoroscopy. Calcium is the major impediment to ultrasound imaging. Aortic wall or at times valvular calcification prevents accurate measurements and visualization of the anatomy. It is sometimes difficult to evaluate the Edwards SAPIEN valve and balloon complex or CoreValve prosthesis with echocardiography. Reflective characteristics of the balloon and stent may be difficult to differentiate particularly when the aortic valve is heavily calcified. This may limit the role of TEE in guiding the positioning of the valve. Perpendicularity of the imaging planes is operator dependent and sometimes dependent on the anatomy of the heart and esophagus.

ICE imaging has clear advantages in terms of the ease of the procedure and control of imaging by a single operator. Visualization of the aortic valve is particularly clear in longitudinal and horizontal axis with ICE imaging. ICE imaging has several limitations. The cost of the probe is not trivial. This probe is still not optimal for the assessment for the left ventricular wall motion and mitral valve (MV). Although echocardiographic interrogation by ICE is not routinely required, it can be an important in case of a complication. Further, with manipulation of the probe there can be displacement of temporary pacing wire. Securing the pacing wire with temporary screw-in lead can be a solution, but again this increases procedural time and expense.

ANATOMY OF IMAGING

X-Ray Imaging
Anatomic definition of the left ventricle, aortic valve, coronary arteries, ascending aorta, aortic arch, abdominal aorta, pelvic arteries, and femoral arteries is the first and foremost requirement for successful percutaneous aortic valve procedure. Biplane assessment of the anatomy, if feasible, is probably the best to save dye-load and procedural time (3).

Left Ventricle Anatomy
Left ventriculogram to see the left ventricular (LV) cavity size and the relation of left ventricular outflow tract (LVOT) to ascending aorta can be helpful. RAO view helps one to determine the "useable length" of the LV cavity from the aortic valve to the apex [Fig. 1(A)]. It is not uncommon to place the stiff wire in the lateral part of the apex to maximize this usable length of the ventricle. LAO view allows one to see the lateral span of the left ventricle as well as the angle of entry from the ascending aorta to the LVOT [Fig. 1(B)]. LV angiography is not necessary if the wire can be placed comfortably in the ventricle with a nice loop. If there is any doubt, a small injection (even hand injection) in the left ventricle with a pigtail placed close to the apex can provide most useful information.

Aortic Valve Anatomy
Aortic valve apparatus consists of the leaflets, annulus, and sinuses to the sinotubular (ST) junction. Visualization of each sinus is critical to understand the plane of aortic orifice. Typically in the LAO view (enough to see the valve away from the spine, i.e., 30–40 degrees), left coronary

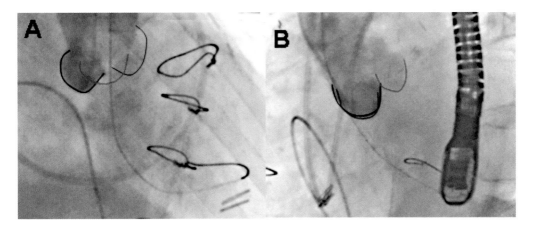

Figure 1 The position of the stiff wire is seen in the (**A**) RAO and (**B**) LAO projection (Video 1, Video 2). It is important to have adequate wire loop in the left ventricle. Note that the wire is away from the septum in the lateral part of the apex of the heart. Also note that the wire falls in the commissure between the right and noncoronary cusps (*upper panel arrows*). Noncoronary cusp is black, right coronary cusp is blue and left coronary cusp is red.

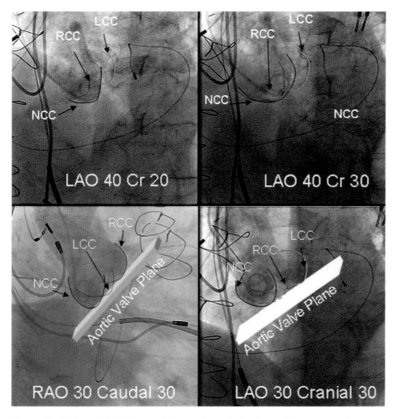

Figure 2 LAO and RAO views of the aortic root injection to demonstrate the coronary cusps. Note that the NCC is typically lower in this view. When the aortogram is performed in the cranial angulation, one can align the leaflets to properly visualize aortic valve plane. RAO caudal view is another common view for aortic plane. *Abbreviations*: LCC, left coronary cusp; RCC, right coronary cusp; NCC, noncoronary cusp.

cusp (LCC) is seen to the left whereas the right coronary cusp (RCC) and noncoronary cusps (NCC) are overlapped to the right half of the aortic diameter [Fig. 2(A)]. Aorta is tilted such that the noncoronary sinus is usually the lowest sinus in this view. Typically the pigtail catheter tends to enter this sinus and can be easily counter-clocked in the left or clocked in the right coronary sinus. Cranial angulation allows one to line up the fluoroscopic plane to the aortic orifice. Camera can be angulated until the bottom of NCC lines up with the bottom of RCC in this view. In RAO projection, the RCC is in the front and the NCC is in the back. LCC overlaps both these leaflets but mainly the NCC [Fig. 2(B)]. The tilt of the aorta makes the LCC higher than the RCC and NCC in this view. Caudal angulation (20–30 degree) can help to make the X-ray beam parallel to the aortic orifice. Motion of each cusp is important to appreciate as it helps one to cross the valve in an organized manner and also identify exact location of calcification when the coronaries, annulus are also calcified along with the leaflets.

The extent of calcification should be carefully assessed. Typically, the mitral annular calcification extends from the part of the annulus supporting the LCC and the NCC, which can be seen in the LAO view. The pattern of calcification may be an important determinant of adequate apposition of the stent/frame and paravalvular leak. ST junction calcification is another important factor that needs to be evaluated before the procedure (Fig. 3). Although not a concern with the CoreValve ReValving system, circumferential calcification of the ST junction can cause restriction of the balloon and "watermelon seeding" of the stent in the left ventricle at the time of deployment. This is particularly relevant if diameter of the ST junction is small. Careful assessment of balloon shape and motion at the time of valvuloplasty can help one to predict the problem. Mounting of the stent somewhat proximally on the balloon can decrease the overhang of balloon in aorta at the time of deployment.

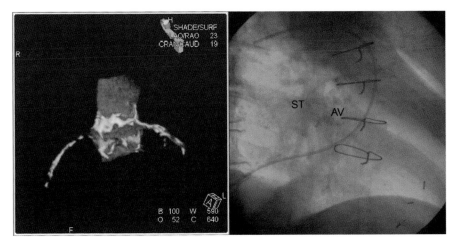

Figure 3 Severe calcification of the sinotubular junction is seen in LAO and RAO projection. This is seen on CT (*left panel*) and fluoroscopy (*right panel*). If the diameter of sinotubular junction is less that the balloon size, "watermelon seeding" is possible.

Coronary Anatomy

The location of the left and right coronary artery origins should be carefully assessed. The height of LCA origin can be judged in the LAO cranial view (Fig. 4). It is also important to note the origin in relation to the aortic commissures. This can be potentially assessed on the RAO view, although CT and TEE allow easier determination. Although compromise of the RCA has not reported with valve deployment, careful assessment of its origin and height is warranted.

Ascending Aorta and Arch

The angle between the ascending aorta and LVOT determines the ease of crossing the aortic valve. Although the LAO angle is the most important angle, RAO angulation is also important. The wire, as it sits across the aortic valve, delineates the path with which the device will take as it crosses the aortic valve. The horizontal length of the arch is another area where the system can have a considerable slack that may lead to motion in the critical step of valve deployment. Calcification of the ascending aorta and arch vessels need close attention for atraumatic manipulation of these large devices in the aorta.

Abdominal Aorta and Pelvic Vasculature

Careful assessment of the anatomy of descending aorta, pelvic bifurcation, and ileo-femoral system during preprocedure evaluation can make the procedure safer Femoral puncture site should be in the common femoral artery before the bifurcation but below the inferior epigastric artery (Fig. 5). Avoidance of calcified plaque by assessing the puncture site with fluoroscopy or ultrasound can be helpful. Careful attention should be paid to the tortuosity and its interaction to the wires and sheath. It is not uncommon for the artery to kink with devices and stiffer wires may be necessary to better track the larger sheath. Special attention should be paid to the common iliac artery bifurcation. The iliac system has a large curve at this point and the artery is relatively immobile as the internal iliac artery fixes the system to the posterior abdominal wall. The angle and calcification of the aortic bifurcation should be inspected to predict how the large sheath will sit in relation to the aortic wall.

Ultrasound Imaging

Anatomy on TEE

The aortic valve annulus should be assessed and measured at the time of the procedure. Many of the patients do not have TEE assessment prior to procedure, although if there is any question regarding the morphology (bicuspid or tricuspid) or annular size, TEE should be done in the preparatory phase of the procedure. The aortic annulus is crown shaped and not necessarily

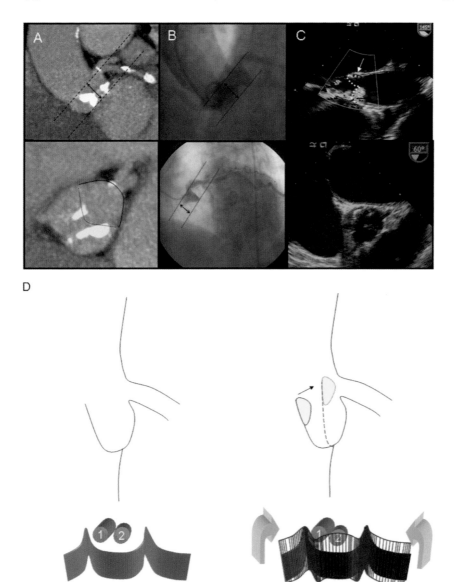

Figure 4 (**A–C**) This picture shows the height of the LMT ostium in relation to the aortic valve annulus. Proper angulation of the camera to align aortic cusps is necessary for accurate measurement. (**D**) Although the measurement of height can be made in this manner, LMT may not get jeopardized if the origin is posterior and near the commissure.

symmetrical. One practical approach to annular measurement is to try and predict where the stent will appose and measure that diameter. Efforts to align the TEE imaging plane to the center of the aorta should be done. The aortic outflow view commonly measures the diameter between the RCC and LCC. A biplane assessment may allow one to measure annulus perpendicular to this measurement although reliable measurements may not be possible in these other views. Baseline assessment of aortic regurgitation, mitral regurgitation, and LV wall motion should be systematically performed.

ICE Imaging
Long-axis view of the valve is obtained by advancing the probe in a neutral position in the right atrium to the level of aortic valve calcification. The probe can be turned counter-clockwise

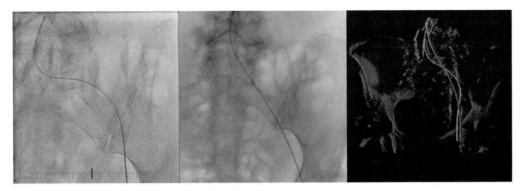

Figure 5 Illustration of iliac curvature as a soft wire is introduced via left femoral artery. The middle panel shows how a stiff wire can be helpful to demonstrate whether the vessel will straighten. The right panel shows the superimposed DYNACT runs of the soft (white) and stiff (red) wires. This can be very helpful to see where and how the artery confirms to stiff wire.

after the tricuspid valve is visualized. Dorsal flexion can help to enlarge the field of vision. This typically visualizes the aorta from NCC to RCC in a plane somewhat different from that seen in outflow view on TEE (Fig. 6). Manipulation of the probe to align ultrasound beam to long axis of aorta should be performed for accurate measurement. To see the aortic valve in short axis, the probe can flexed in to tricuspid valve as the ultrasound beam points superiorly to see the aorta in cross-section. Calcification of leaflet, aortic insufficiency (AI), and left coronary artery (LCA) origin in relation to commissures can be assessed in this view.

PROCEDURAL IMAGING

Crossing of Aortic Valve
Fluoroscopy is primarily used for this step. The aortic valve is frequently crossed with an AL-1 catheter and a straight 0.035 in. wire. The LAO projection is safer because it allows clear separation of coronary ostia from the aortic orifice. The catheter should be placed in the jet as seen by systolic rapid motion. The wire is then advanced slowly out of the catheter in systole. If the wire turns to the left, the catheter is likely directing the wire in the LCC and counter-clock rotation of the catheter will redirect the wire in the center (Video 3). If the wire goes to the right, it can be in NCC or RCC (which can be determined by RAO view) and clocking or counter-clocking, respectively, will redirect the wire in the center. Adjusting the height of the catheter will alter the trajectory and help with crossing. The RAO view is helpful in patients where right and left leaflets are immobile and the opening is facing anteriorly (common for bicuspid valves). A supra-aortic angiogram may be necessary, in some patients, to further define the anatomy—especially when the anatomy is altered or distorted, for example, prosthetic valve or root enlargement.

Balloon Valvuloplasty
Once the aortic valve is crossed, a stiff wire is advanced in the left ventricle. Proper positioning of the wire is essential to prevent complications like MV injury or LV perforation during BAV or valve deployment. A gentle loop in the stiff wire involving the part of the wire proximal to the transition prevents ventricular irritation and provides support to keep the devices from injuring the left ventricle.

Entry of the balloon in the ventricle predicts the ease with which the valve will cross. Motion of the balloon as it is inflated with rapid pacing is important to monitor (Video 4, Video 5). The reason for balloon motion should be determined. It can be improper positioning, slack in the system, short balloon in a tight valve, inadequate response to pacing, etc. (Video 6, Video 7). Leaflet motion with balloon inflation should be inspected. If there is any concern of LMT (left main trunk) obstruction, injection of contrast at the time of balloon inflation can help to determine this (Fig. 7). The pigtail catheter should be carefully placed in the left sinus to

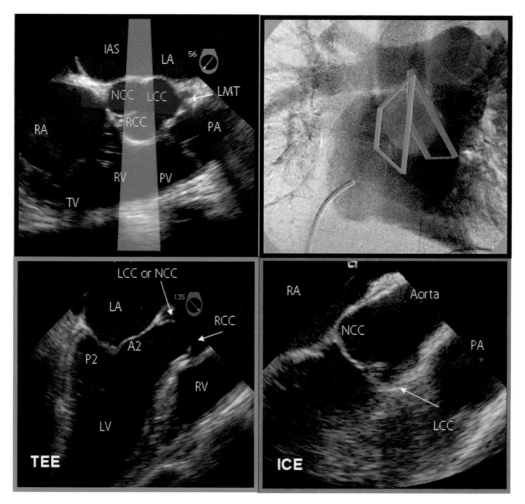

Figure 6 This ICE image shows a longitudinal view of ascending aorta (Video 8, Video 9). As shown in the inset, the sections are not identical in TEE and ICE. The blue color defines TEE plane and the orange color shows ICE imaging plane. ICE can also help to monitor the procedure like TEE (Video 10, Video 11).

adequately visualize coronary flow through the LMT. TEE can help to monitor LMT flow during balloon inflation. After BAV, the severity of aortic regurgitation should be judged with TEE and hemodynamic changes (hypotension, decrease in aortic diastolic pressure, and increase in LV end-diastolic pressure).

Introduction of the Sheath
Serial dilations should be performed under fluoroscopic guidance. Careful monitoring of the motion of arteries and aorta during the introduction of dilators can help decide how much force can be safely exerted. Sheath introduction is done with fluoroscopic guidance while also monitoring the position of the wire in the left ventricle.

Advancement of the Valve
The valve is introduced in the sheath, carefully without inadvertently advancing the sheath. Valve exit is monitored with fluoroscopy to ensure that the valve does not damage the aortic wall as it comes out of the sheath. Fluoroimaging helps to prevent pushing the device against the wall or calcified plaques in the arch. With regard to the Edwards SAPIEN delivery catheter, clockwise rotation may help to align the valve to the center of aortic orifice, which can be confirmed by imaging in LAO and RAO projections.

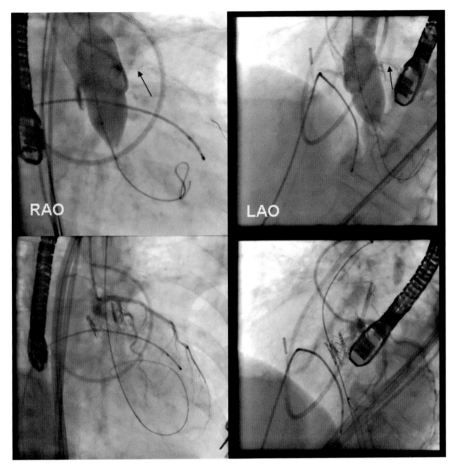

Figure 7 Biplane demonstration of the injection of aortic root with balloon inflation to identify if the LMT is at risk of closure with valve deployment. In this picture, flow is seen in the LMT although it is not very brisk (*arrows*) (Video 12, Video 13). We did use wire in LMT at time of AV deployment (Video 14, Video 15) there was no compromise of the LMT with AV deployment (Video 14, Video 16). Lower panels show selective coronary angiogram after AV deployment (Video 17, Video 18).

Crossing of the Valve

As the device is advanced across the valve, buckling should be avoided. Careful watch on the wire allows one to put enough tension to provide adequate rail. Maximum care should be given not to withdraw the wire from the left ventricle. Device is then placed in the aortic orifice and proper positioning is confirmed by fluoroscopic and imaging.

Positioning of the Valve

Edwards SAPIEN Prosthetic Heart Valve

This is the most crucial step in percutaneous aortic valve replacement with the current system because the valve is not repositionable. The stent is 14 to 16 mm long depending on the size of the valve. The stent is positioned such that 60% of the stent is ventricular and 40% aortic prior to balloon inflation. One has to take several situations into consideration while positioning (4). The valve tends to follow the direction of ascending aorta into the ventricle and does not confirm to the curve due to its extreme stiffness (Fig. 8). In situations where ascending aorta makes a sharp angle with LVOT, the stent will be at a steep angle in the aortic orifice. In this situation, there will be "realignment motion" of the valve as balloon inflation brings the system in the center of the aortic orifice. This motion typically moves the stent in the aortic direction in

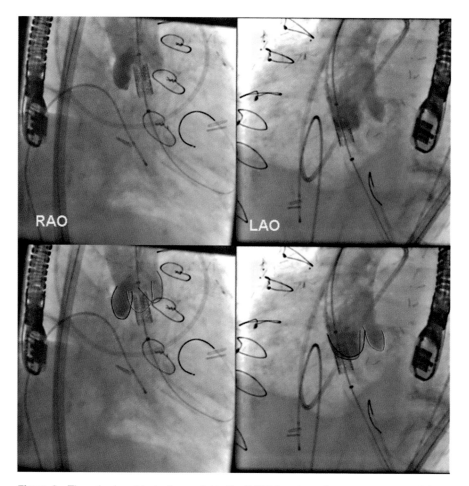

Figure 8   The valve is not typically parallel to the LVOT. It rests on the outer curvature of the aorta where in the commissure between the right and the noncoronary cusps (Video 19, Video 20).

the transfemoral cases because the valve moves from posterior to anterior and right to left as it centers itself. Therefore, a slightly ventricular position is justifiable in patients with a horizontal ascending aorta. It is also important to assure that the aortic edge of the stent extends to the tip of aortic leaflets to prevent overhanging of the native leaflets over the stent, which can lead to severe aortic regurgitation because it prevents proper closure of the prosthetic valve leaflets. Motion of the balloon at the time of valvuloplasty also gives an indication whether the stent is likely to move ventricular or aortic with inflation. This may also push one to err on the side of a slightly more aortic or ventricular positioning to counter the possible motion. It is important to note that these are very fine adjustments that are repeatedly confirmed by aortic root injection.

Aortic root injection is made with 5 to 10 cc dye injected with power or hand injection within 0.5 seconds. Patient's kidney function should be kept in mind and contrast load should be limited in patients with impaired renal function. Careful attention to the calcium landmarks is also very helpful. Respiratory motion is minimized by holding the respirator. It is extremely helpful to do rapid pacing, breath hold and injection of the root to confirm that the desired position is achieved.

Although fluoroscopy provides the majority of guiding during positioning, echocardiographic assessment is critical to corroborate the fluoroscopic findings. The relation of the aortic edge of the stent to the valve tips is investigated by TEE or ICE. The angle of the prosthetic valve to LVOT is well appreciated on TEE but not so much by ICE. Central or eccentric crossing of the valve can be confirmed by obtaining the short-axis view of aortic valve. Movement of the stent with pacing or breath-hold can also be monitored by echocardiography. Sometimes it is very difficult to clearly identify the stent edges distinct from the balloon folds. It is reasonable to measure the stent length to confirm that the identification of the edges is reliable.

CoreValve ReValving System
By using fluoroscopic guidance, the CoreValve prosthesis is positioned approximately 6 to 8 mm below the basal attachment of the aortic leaflets (i.e., aortic valve annulus). A pigtail catheter positioned in the base of the noncoronary sinus is used a reference marker; radiopaque calcium deposits and repeated contrast aortograms can be used as aids to refine valve positioning. Positioning can also be verified using TEE. Although rarely, if ever, a problem, impingement of the anterior MV leaflet by the inflow portion of the CoreValve prosthesis can be ruled out by TEE.

Valve Deployment

Edwards SAPIEN Prosthetic Heart Valve
Once proper positioning is confirmed by fluoroscopy and ultrasound, pigtail catheter is slowly withdrawn, carefully watching and confirming that the stent does not move. With breath-hold and rapid pacing, the stent is then deployed if no inadvertent displacement is seen by fluoro landmarks and ultrasound imaging.

CoreValve ReValving System
The CoreValve prosthesis is released from the delivery catheter in a stepwise manner. Valve positioning can be verified at any time with respect to its position to the pigtail catheter or even more precisely by contrast aortography. After the valve is released by more than one-third, the obstruction is relieved and the leaflets begin to function. Very importantly, once the valve is thought to be completely released, detachment of the loading hooks of the prosthesis from the delivery catheter must be verified in at least two orthogonal views. If both loading hooks are not completely released, pulling on the delivery catheter may result in valve embolization.

Assessment of Valve
The most important indicator of success is adequate hemodynamic recovery after valve deployment. Aortic pressure wave form along with the systolic and diastolic blood pressure provides most useful insight into the valve function. Proper positioning and adequate deployment of the valve is confirmed by echocardiography and fluoroscopy. Typically there is some flaring of the ends of the stent when the valve is properly sized and adequately deployed. Quick assessment of severity and mechanism of AI and LV function in cases of hemodynamic instability is crucial to identify and treat complications (see later).

Removal of Sheath
The next very important step is to remove the sheath and obtain hemostasis. If there is any doubt that vasculature is traumatized, placing a catheter from the contralateral groin to obtain and angiogram as the sheath is removed can be helpful. Most of the times the sheath is occlusive in the iliac arteries and therefore, suctioning from the sheath as the contrast is injected from the catheter placed from the contralateral groin artery is necessary to visualize the iliac artery with the larger sheath. Rupture or significant dissections of the iliac arteries have to be rapidly identified for expeditious management.

IMAGING TO PREDICT, IDENTIFY, AND RESOLVE COMPLICATIONS
Identifying and treating complications is one the most important roles of the procedural imaging. Cardiac perforation and ascending aortic dissection are typically seen while attempting to cross the aortic valve or advancing the cone of the RF2 system to uncover the balloon. LMT occlusion and aortic regurgitation are seen soon after aortic valve deployment, although severe AI after aortic valvuloplasty is also possible. Aortic and iliac trauma is caused at the time of sheath insertion but it is not evident until the sheath is being removed. Some of these complications are detailed in the following sections.

Embolization

Embolization of the valve typically happens in few cardiac cycles. Late embolization is rare (5,6). Most commonly there is distal embolization where the valve can be recaptured on the balloon and deployed in the descending aorta. Proximal embolization in the ventricle requires surgery to remove the valve. Attempt to stabilize a valve that is deployed ventricularly is possible by deploying another valve in the first valve (7,8).

Aortic Insufficiency

Aortic insufficiency can result form paravalvular leak or central AI. Paravalvular leak typically occurs due to non uniform expansion of the stent leading to malapposition between the valve and the native aortic leaflets. When the valve is placed at a correct height, the most common location of the aortic insufficiency is the posterior location along the NCC and LCC (Fig. 9). Severity of AI is judged by the width of the regurgitant jet along with hemodynamic assessment. If the stent is not properly expanded, and there is no central AI then post dilating stent with additional 1 to 3 cc of contrast can help to achieve better apposition. Central AI can result when the aortic annulus is larger and smaller size valve is placed or when the stent is postdilated with a larger balloon. In many occasions the central AI is caused by the stiff wire across the valve. Removal of wire from the left ventricle will help to eliminate this type of AI. Rarely the AI is from nonclosure of one of the leaflets of the prosthetic valve. This happens when the native leaflets overhang on the stent resulting in inadequate pressure generation required for the closure of the prosthetic valve. This causes severe AI with hemodynamic instability. Another valve deployment inside of the first valve may be necessary to overcome this problem. Rarely, postdilatation with a larger balloon can help to reorient the native leaflets enough to result in proper functioning of the prosthetic valve. If the AI is moderate by echocardiography but is not causing any hemodynamic changes (very low aortic diastolic pressure with steep increase in LV end diastolic pressure, ST changes suggestive of global ischemia, hypotension, pulmonary hypertension, etc.), it is best to be conservative and not do anything else.

LMT Occlusion

This is a catastrophic complication in the absence of bypass grafts. Severe ST changes, inability to recover blood pressure after the valve deployment and severe wall motion abnormalities are the key manifestations. Injection of dye in the aortic root can confirm this diagnosis. TEE can also be helpful to confirm lack of flow in the LMT. Rapid support of the circulation by femoral cannulations for cardiopulmonary bypass or the use of TandemHeart can help to prevent end-organ damage while the coronary perfusion is reestablished. Percutaneous revascularization is probably the best option because urgent CABG in these high-risk patients can be catastrophic. Importantly, the time it takes for the bypass operation can lead to meaningful myocardial damage. Prevention is the best solution for this problem. If the LMT origin is thought to be low and is likely to be compromised as documented by dye injection in the aortic root while inflating aortic valvuloplasty balloon, a coronary wire should be placed in the LAD prior to valve deployment. This will prevent total occlusion of the LMT and will provide rapid access in case of LMT compromise.

Aortic Dissection

Ascending aortic dissection has been reported when multiple attempts are made to cross the stenotic aortic valve with the stent. This situation is less likely to occur with the use of RF2 delivery system. However, careful monitoring of the ascending aorta with TEE is necessary to recognize this complication early. Excessive force is never a good solution when the stent has difficulty crossing the stenotic valve. Reorientation of the stent with torquing and flexion of the flexor sheath solves the problem in many cases. RF2 system is really helpful in these situations.

LV Perforation

This catastrophic complication is seen with the use of RF2 system when the cone is advanced in the ventricle to uncover the balloon prior to valve deployment. Development of pericardial effusion, hemodynamic and electrical instability points to this complication. Prevention is again

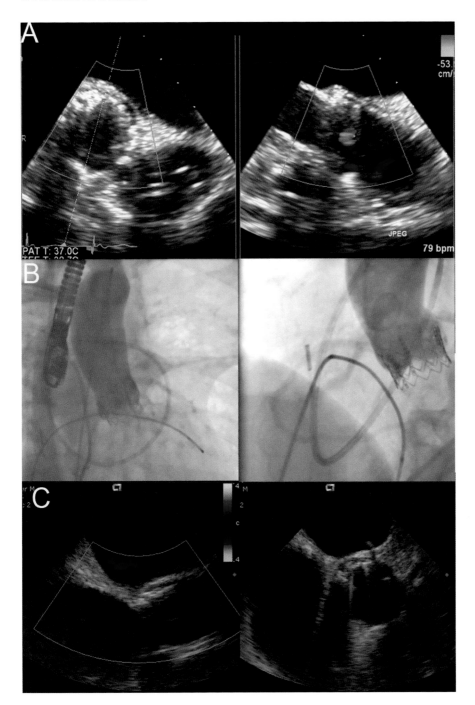

Figure 9 (**A**) TEE to show good deployment of valve without significant AI (Video 21). (**B**) Aortogram can be also helpful to assess the severity of AI (Video 15, Video 22). (**C**) Valve can be well visualized on ICE (Video 23, Video 24).

the best cure for this problem. Proper wire positioning and careful manipulations of the devices can help in prevention. This is particularly likely in patients with small LV cavity without severe hypertrophy. Management depends on the extent of the perforation along with hemodynamic consequences. It frequently requires putting pt on cardiopulmonary bypass and repairing the perforation surgically. TEE is very helpful in the diagnosis of these complications.

Iliac and Femoral Complications

Trauma to the ilio-femoral system with the large sheath, resulting in serious vascular complication increases the hospital mortality. Anticipation of the problem is necessary for expeditious management (9). Aortography and selective injections are used to define the nature and extent of the problem. Perforation, dissection, and stenosis can happen and are managed with mostly endovascular techniques.

FUTURE

DynaCT in the catheterization laboratory has taken us to the new level of imaging. It is no longer required to reconstruct in mind the location of device in space, but it is actually possible to do reconstruction in the three dimensional space with rapid acquisition of images with rotational angiography (Video 25). It is also possible to overlay the fluoroimages on the previous acquisitions, which may help to minimize contrast and time with increased safety in the future (10). These acquisitions do require considerable radiation and contrast in many situations, but the progress in the field may ultimately help to reduce both of these in near future (11).

REFERENCES

1. Block PC. Transcatheter aortic valve replacement: Here and now, but lots to learn. J Invasive Cardiol 2009; 21(3):99–100.
2. Tops LF, Kapadia SR, Tuzcu EM, et al. Percutaneous valve procedures: an update. Curr Probl Cardiol 2008; 33(8):417–457.
3. Aregger F, Wenaweser P, Hellige GJ, et al. Risk of acute kidney injury in patients with severe aortic valve stenosis undergoing transcatheter valve replacement. Nephrol Dial Transplant 2009; 24(7):2175–2179.
4. Webb JG, Lichtenstein S. Transcatheter percutaneous and transapical aortic valve replacement. Semin Thorac Cardiovasc Surg 2007; 19(4):304–310.
5. Clavel MA, Dumont E, Pibarot P, et al. Severe valvular regurgitation and late prosthesis embolization after percutaneous aortic valve implantation. Ann Thorac Surg 2009; 87(2):618–621.
6. Al Ali AM, Altwegg L, Horlick EM, et al. Prevention and management of transcatheter balloon-expandable aortic valve malposition. Catheter Cardiovasc Interv 2008; 72(4):573–578.
7. Tuzcu EM. Transcatheter aortic valve replacement malposition and embolization: Innovation brings solutions also new challenges. Catheter Cardiovasc Interv 2008; 72(4):579–580.
8. Ussia GP, Mule M, Tamburino C. The valve-in-valve technique: Transcatheter treatment of aortic bioprothesis malposition. Catheter Cardiovasc Interv 2009; 73(5):713–716.
9. Jilaihawi H, Spyt T, Chin D, et al. Percutaneous aortic valve replacement in patients with challenging aortoiliofemoral access. Catheter Cardiovasc Interv 2008; 72(6):885–890.
10. Plass A, Schepis T, Scheffel H, et al. Multimodality Preoperative Planning and Postoperative Follow-up of a Hybrid Cardiac Intervention. Heart Surg Forum 2008; 11(6):E375–E377.
11. Garcia JA, Bhakta S, Kay J, et al. On-line multi-slice computed tomography interactive overlay with conventional X-ray: A new and advanced imaging fusion concept. Int J Cardiol 2009; 133(3):e101–e105.

13 | Tips and Tricks for Crossing the Aortic Valve with a Guidewire (Retrograde Approach)

Alain Cribier and Hélène Eltchaninoff

Department of Cardiology, Hôpital Charles Nicolle, University of Rouen, Rouen, France

For many years, crossing the stenotic aortic valve to measure the transvalvular gradient has been a part of the invasive evaluation of aortic stenosis (AS). The need for crossing the valve was further reinforced in the 1980s (1) by the onset of retrograde transfemoral balloon aortic valvuloplasty (BAV). However, as the accuracy of hemodynamic assessment by echocardiography was proven, the need for invasive assessment was progressively limited to patients with discordant clinical and echocardiographic findings. A limited number of operators continued to perform BAV, modifying the technique. Over the last couple of years, the onset of transcatheter aortic valve replacement brought back the absolute need of crossing the native aortic valve, and each operator had to refamiliarize or learn the technique, which often was considered a challenging and time-consuming task. However, with the appropriate material and adequate technique the clinician may negotiate the stenotic valve within minutes.

This chapter describes the retrograde technique to cross the aortic valve currently used in our institution, which has been validated by our large experience and pioneering work of BAV (>1000) and transcatheter aortic valve implantation. With this technique, there have been no failures to cross the aortic valve.

EQUIPMENT

Catheters

A variety of catheters can be used for crossing the aortic valve (Fig. 1). The best ones are those that allow an easy orientation of the catheter tip to direct the guidewire toward the aortic orifice. Although we primarily used the multipurpose or the Sones catheters for many years (2), currently we preferentially use a 5- or 6-F left coronary Amplatz catheter (3). Other catheters (Aortic Stenosis Catheter; Cook Inc., Bloomington, IN) have been designed specially for the purpose of crossing the aortic valve, offering various shapes and curve lengths adapted to the size and angulation of the aortic root (4). In our hands, the Amplatz left 2 is usually chosen in patients with an enlarged or a horizontal aortic root whereas the Amplatz left 1 is preferred in cases with a small and vertical aortic root (Fig. 2).

Guidewires

The catheter is advanced to the ascending aorta over a regular 0.035 in. J wire, through an arterial introducer one size larger than the catheter size to assess accurately the left ventricle/femoral pressure gradient after crossing. The guidewire is then removed and exchanged for a straight-tip, fixed-core, 0.035 in. guidewire that is used to cross the aortic valve.

Hydrophilic or Teflon-coated straight-tipped guidewires (Fig. 3) are currently available. Our preference is to use a Teflon-coated wire (ex: Medtronic PTFE guidewire, Medtronic Vascular, Danvers, Massachusetts), which appears to be more stable and easier to control while facing the stenotic jet. The hydrophilic properties of the Terumo guidewire (Radiofocus, Terumo, Tokyo, Japan) do not facilitate in any way the crossing of the calcific aortic valve. Other investigators prefer using a moveable core straight guidewire for crossing (4).

After the valve is crossed, the straight guidewire must be exchanged for a long extra-stiff guidewire that will provide adequate support for advancing the balloon dilatation catheter and the aortic bioprosthesis. We recommend using the 260-cm long, 0.035 in. Amplatz Extra Stiff J Guidewire (COOK, Bjaeverskov, DK), which offers optimal support and whose flexible distal end is easy to preshape.

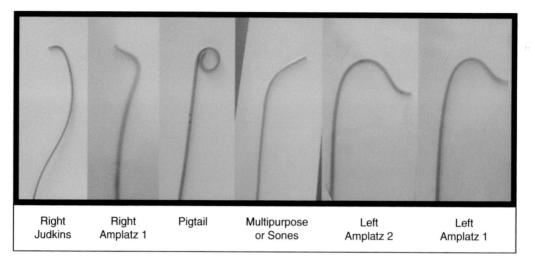

Right Judkins	Right Amplatz 1	Pigtail	Multipurpose or Sones	Left Amplatz 2	Left Amplatz 1

Figure 1 Catheters frequently used for crossing the aortic valve.

Preshaping the Extra-Stiff Wire

Before use, it is recommended to preshape the flexible distal 3 to 4 cm of the extra-stiff guidewire in a large curve over the end of a hemostat (Fig. 4) in a way one would make a paper ribbon. In addition to the rapid pacing, this helps considerably to stabilize the balloon across the aortic valve during balloon inflation and diminishes the risk for wire perforation of the left ventricular apex.

SPECIFIC MANEUVERS TO CROSS THE AORTIC VALVE (VIDEO 1)

Unfractionated heparin (50 IU/kg) must be administered before starting the crossing maneuvers. Formation of thrombi must be further avoided by flushing the catheters and cleaning the wires regularly. Continuous measurement of systemic arterial pressure is made throughout the procedure using the side arm of the femoral sheath. A supra-aortic angiogram may be previously obtained that will help to determine the distribution of calcium over the valve and the appreciative site of valve opening.

The recommended technique for crossing the valve is as follows:

1. The best working position is the left anterior oblique (LAO) projection, from 20° to 40° depending on the angle of the aortic root.

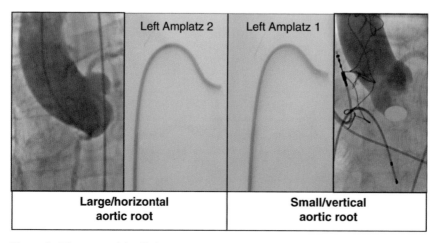

Left Amplatz 2	Left Amplatz 1
Large/horizontal aortic root	**Small/vertical aortic root**

Figure 2 The two models of left coronary artery Amplatz catheters used for crossing the valve in our institution.

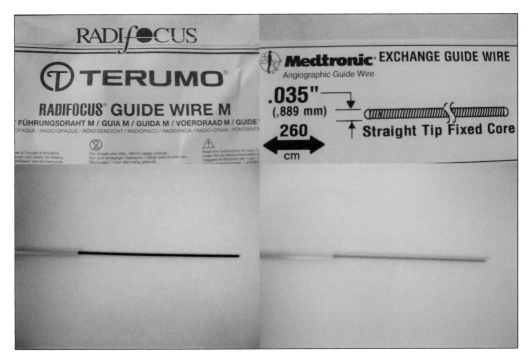

Figure 3   The two models of straight tip guidewire frequently used for crossing the valve.

2. The tip of the catheter is initially positioned at the upper limit of the valve, which is most often clearly delineated by the valvular calcific deposits. The catheter is then slowly retracted (using the left hand) while firm clockwise rotation is maintained to direct the catheter tip toward the center of the valve plane. During the pull back, the straight guidewire is sequentially advanced (<3 cm) and retrieved inside the catheter (using the right hand) (Fig. 5). With experience, it is usually possible to advance it in systole and retrieve it in diastole, following the heart rate. During this maneuver, the valve area is meticulously mapped with the wire until the orifice is crossed (Fig. 6).

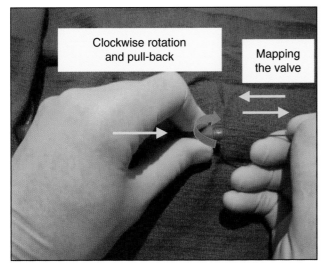

Figure 4   Catheter and wire manipulation for crossing the valve.

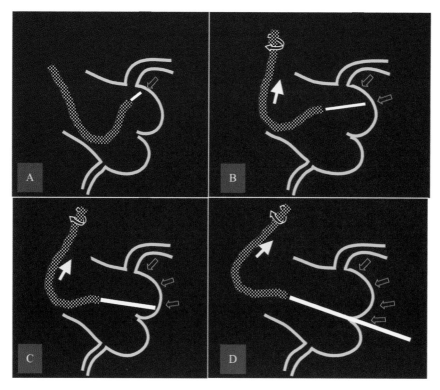

Figure 5 Technique of aortic valve mapping for crossing the valve. (**A**) Initial position and (**B**) to (**D**) stepwise mapping of the aortic valve until crossing (LAO 40° view).

3. Once the wire crosses the valve, it is recommended to use the right anterior oblique (RAO) projection for introducing the catheter inside the left ventricle to decrease the risk of trauma to the left ventricular wall (Fig. 7). The Amplatz catheter does not have to be advanced deeply inside the left ventricle. Its distal end is often in contact with the left ventricle's anterior wall and may cause an artifactual pressure waveform after the guidewire is removed. In many cases, it may thus be advised to exchange the straight wire for a long exchange guidewire, and then to exchange the Amplatz catheter for a single or dual lumen pigtail catheter before recording the left ventricular pressure and measure the transvalvular gradient. Using a pigtail catheter will also facilitate the safe introduction and optimal placement of the extra-stiff guidewire within the left ventricle.

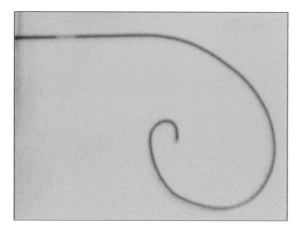

Figure 6 Preshaping of the flexible extra-stiff guidewire.

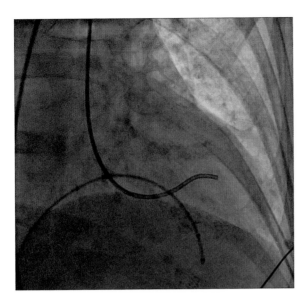

Figure 7   The left coronary Amplatz 2 catheter inside the left ventricle after crossing (RAO view).

4. The preshaped extra-stiff guidewire can then be advanced into the pigtail catheter. Its placement inside the left ventricle should be done in the RAO 30° position. Attention should be placed to obtain an optimal position of the curved extra-stiff guidewire's flexible end: the superior concavity should rest in the left ventricular apex (Fig. 8). This will improve the stability of the wire during balloon valvuloplasty and bioprosthesis delivery, while decreasing the risk of left ventricular wall injury and ventricular arrhythmias.

COMPLICATIONS

With experience, complications are rare during these maneuvers (3) and most of them may be easily prevented by maintaining an adequate technique.

– Ventricular arrhythmias (ventricular extra-systolic beats or nonsustained ventricular tachycardia) can often be observed after the valve has been crossed with wires and catheters that can generally be controlled by changes in the equipment's position in the left ventricle.

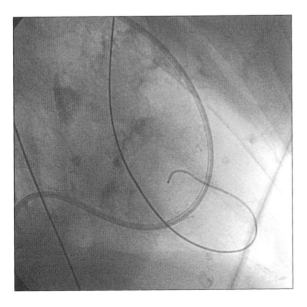

Figure 8   Optimal position of the extra-stiff guidewire inside the left ventricle.

– Acute coronary occlusion by dissection of the proximal segment of the right or left coronary artery is exceptional. This is generally due to the accidental introduction of the straight guidewire in the coronary artery leading to dissection of the vessel wall. ST segment elevation, hypotension, and chest pain are indications of acute coronary occlusion during the crossing maneuvers and require urgent coronary angiography and angioplasty. The LAO projection recommended for crossing the valve facilitates keeping the wire away from the coronary artery ostia. The risk of accidental catheter insertion in the right coronary artery is much higher in the RAO projection.

– Cardiac perforation from wires and catheters can be easily prevented by following the technical precautions given above. However, the complication should be suspected if hypotension occurs. Echocardiography in the cardiac catheterization laboratory is critical to detect and then promptly treat pericardial effusion.

– Left bundle branch block can result from contact between the septum and the wires and catheters. Complete heart block may more occur in patients with underlying right bundle branch block that may require prophylactic placement of a temporary pacemaker. However, when the technique is performed in the course of transcatheter valve implantation, a transvenous pacing catheter is systematically placed in the right ventricle at the beginning of the procedure that will be used for both prevention of complete heart block and rapid ventricular pacing.

– Cerebral embolism may occur during retrograde catheterization of the aortic valve and may result from the dislodgement of calcific valvular particles. Atheromatous plaque dislodgement from the aortic root or the ascending aorta, or formation of thrombi from catheters and guidewire may be other reasons for embolism. MRI has shown cerebral abnormalities consistent with clinically hidden embolic lesions in 15% to 22% of cases at 48 hours after retrograde aortic valve catheterization (5) with 1.7% to 3% (6) of clinically apparent neurological deficit, which are often reversible.

CONCLUSION

An optimal technique for crossing the aortic valve can make the procedure successful, quick and safe, turning it into a meaningless step toward balloon aortic valve predilatation and transcatheter valve implantation.

REFERENCES

1. Cribier A, Savin T, Saoudi N, et al. Percutaneous transluminal valvuloplasty of acquired aortic stenosis in elderly patients: An alterative to valve replacement? Lancet 1986; 1:63–67.
2. Letac B, Cribier A, Koning R, et al. Results of transluminal aortic valvuloplasty in 218 adults with valvular aortic stenosis. Am J Cardiol 1988; 62:598–605.
3. Agatiello C, Eltchaninoff H, Tron C, et al. Balloon aortic valvuloplasty in the adult. Immediate results and in-hospital complications in the latest series of 141 consecutive patients at the University Hospital of Rouen (2002–2005). Arch Mal Cœur Vaiss 2006; 99(3):195–200.
4. Feldman T, Caroll JD, Chiu YC. An improved catheter for crossing stenosed aortic valves. Catheter Cardiovasc Diagn 1989; 16:279–283.`
5. Omran H, Schmidt H, Hackenbroch M, et al. Silent and apparent cerebral embolism after retrograde catheterization of the aortic valve in valvular stenosis: A prospective, randomized study. Lancet 2003; 361:1241–1246.
6. Meine TJ, Harrison JK Should we cross the aortic valve: The risk of retrograde catheterization of the left ventricle in patients with aortic stenosis. Am Heart J 2004; 148 (1):41–42.

14 | Preimplantation Percutaneous Aortic Balloon Valvotomy (Retrograde Approach)

Alain Cribier and Hélène Eltchaninoff

Department of Cardiology, Hôpital Charles Nicolle, University of Rouen, Rouen, France

Introduced by our group in 1986 (1), and intensively investigated thereafter (2–7), percutaneous balloon aortic valvotomy (BAV) is currently recognized as a valuable palliative procedure in unstable or critically ill patients or those considered high surgical risk because of comorbid conditions or advanced age. Mechanisms of action include intraleaflet fractures within calcific deposits, leading to greater leaflet flexibility (Fig. 1), separation of fused commissures (uncommon in elderly patients), and stretch of the aortic annulus (5,8). This leads to a relatively modest increase in effective orifice area and decrease in transvalvular gradient with subsequent hemodynamic and functional improvement. Over the last two decades, the technique and the procedure have significantly improved, with new balloons catheters, new sheaths, and the use of rapid right ventricular pacing (RVP) allowing more stable and effective balloon dilatation, leading to better results and less morbidity, and explaining the current revival of this old method (5–7).

Over the last years, the development of transcatheter aortic valve implantation (TAVI) has contributed to the renaissance of BAV since the procedure plays a crucial role in preparing the native aortic valve for implantation. BAV has become an integral part of TAVI, whatever the bioprosthesis (balloon-expandable or self-expanding), or the approach (retrograde or transapical) used. The native calcified aortic valve must in all cases be predilated and made more flexible before being crossed by the devices. Thus, each operator must become familiar with the updated technique of balloon aortic valvotomy.

We describe here the equipment and the procedure currently used before retrograde implantation of the balloon expandable Edwards SAPIEN valve. The equipment used in the context of self-expanding CoreValve system is slightly different and is described elsewhere, but the principles remain similar.

EQUIPMENT

Arterial Introducers

The current balloon catheters used for BAV require the placement of a 14-F introducer in the femoral artery, either percutaneously or after surgical cut-down. The arterial sheath generally used is the Check-Flo introducer from Cook (Cook Europe, Bjaeverskov, Denmark). The set comprises three dilators of increasing size, which may be helpful in case of resistance to sheath progression (Fig. 2). The sheath can be placed into the femoral artery over a regular 0.035" guidewire at the beginning of the procedure, or over the extra-stiff wire previously placed inside the left ventricle if the aortic valve has already been crossed.

Contralateral Catheterization

Percutaneous sheaths are placed in the controlateral femoral artery (6 F) and femoral vein (6 or 7 F) (Fig. 3). A pigtail catheter is advanced through the arterial sheath to the aortic root to monitor the aortic pressure and perform angiographies. Through the venous sheath, a pacing lead is advanced to the right ventricle in preparation to rapid pacing.

Guidewires

The valvotomy balloon catheters must be advanced to the aortic valve over an extra-stiff guidewire that has been previously reshaped and placed inside the left ventricle, as described in chapter 10. This wire is the 260-cm long, 0.035" Amplatz Extra Stiff J Guidewire

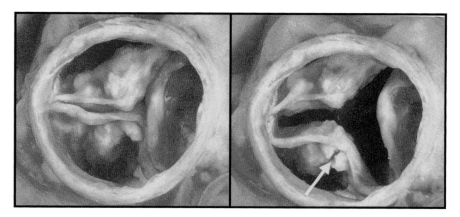

Figure 1 Effect of a 23-mm balloon inflation on a calcific aortic valve. After balloon valvotomy (*right panel*), the orifice is enlarged and one leaflet has been fractured (*arrow*).

(Cook, Bjaeverskov, Denmark), which offers an optimal support for valve predilatation as for implantation of the bioprosthesis.

Valvotomy Balloons
During the early phase of TAVI, by using the antegrade transseptal approach (9) as for the first cases performed retrograde from the femoral artery (10), the balloon catheters used for predilatation were the Z-Med, from NuMed (Cornwall, ON, Canada). These catheters, 120 cm

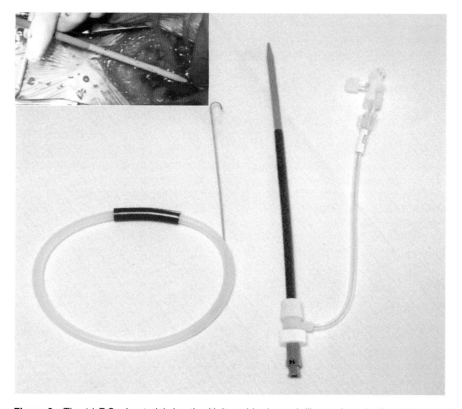

Figure 2 The 14-F Cook arterial sheath with its guidewire and dilators. Introduction of the sheath in the femoral artery after cut-down (*top panel*).

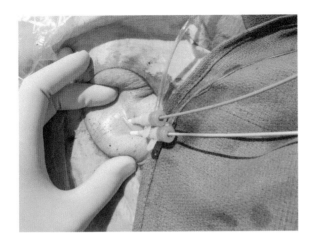

Figure 3 Controlateral catheterization: 6-F pigtail in 6-F sheath (right femoral artery); 6-F Soloist Intracardiac Electrode Catheter (Medtronic) in 7-F sheath (right femoral vein).

in length with a 9-F shaft size have a 4.0-cm long balloon, with various maximal diameters at inflation (20, 23, or 25 mm).

To date, Edwards Lifesciences (Irvine, CA, USA) provides a specific balloon catheter, the RetroFlex Balloon Catheter, recommended for valve predilatation, (Fig. 4). These catheters have a length of 130 cm and a 9-F shaft compatible with a 0.035" guidewire and require a 14-French introducer. The balloons are 30 mm in length with two diameters at full inflation, 20 and 23 mm. The rated burst pressure is 3 atm.

Selection of Balloon Size

The end point of aortic valve predilatation is not to obtain the "optimal result" usually expected after BAV (doubling the valve area) (2,7), but to sufficiently enlarge the valvular orifice and make the leaflets more flexible to facilitate retrograde crossing of the calcific valve with the bioprosthesis. Being less demanding on the result makes the predilatation procedure simpler and safer than regular BAV, which generally requires sequential balloon inflations with increasing sizes until the desired result is reached.

Predilatation is achieved by using single size balloon inflations. Balloon size is selected according to the expanded external diameter of the bioprosthesis planned to be implanted, which depends on the aortic annulus size. The diameter of the aortic annulus is measured from the transthoracic parasternal or transesophageal long-axis view. Two models of Edwards SAPIEN valve are currently available. The 23-mm valve size is considered appropriate for an annulus diameter of 18 to 21 mm whereas the 26 mm valve size is recommended for an annulus larger than 21 mm, up to 25 mm. The 20-mm balloon size is recommended before implantation of the 23-mm valve and the 23-mm size before implantation of the 26-mm valve.

This strategy can be modified in particular cases. When a 26-mm valve is planned in patients with massive valvular calcification or porcelain aorta, it may be preferred to use cautious sequential predilatation (20 mm followed by 23 mm balloon size) to decrease the risk of aortic

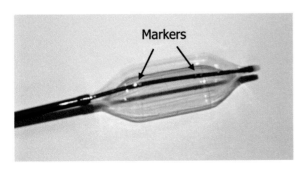

Markers

Figure 4 The RetroFlex balloon catheter from Edwards Lifesciences.

valve or annulus disruption. In many cases, when the annulus has been measured between 20 and 22 mm, the valve size may not be formally determined before the procedure. In this setting, it may be helpful to use a 23-mm balloon and perform an aortogram at the time of full balloon inflation to determine the optimal valve size, as described later.

Preparation of Valvotomy Balloon

Before predilation the balloon must be carefully purged of air to avoid the possibility of air embolization in the event of balloon rupture. De-airing the balloon is accomplished using the 15:85 contrast media/saline solution, which is used for valvotomy. This contrast dilution is adequate to visualize the balloon on fluoroscopy and reduces viscosity thus facilitating the inflation-deflation cycles. To facilitate the introduction of the deflated balloon inside the 14-F sheath and to prevent any injury to the balloon structure, it is recommended to purge the balloon in the aorta, either the descending or ascending aorta. Doing it in the ascending aorta has the potential advantage of preserving the low balloon profile while crossing the aortic arch and thus decreasing the risk of friction and plaque migration. The maneuver consists in fully inflating and deflating the balloon two or three times until residual air is removed, as assessed by fluoroscopy.

Hardware for Balloon Inflation

To inflate the balloon, either a specific device or a regular syringe can be used. In the set of transcatheter Edwards valve, a special inflation device is provided, which is used for valve delivery as well as for balloon valve predilatation. The Atrion QL inflation device (Fig. 5) (Atrion Medical Products, Inc., Arab, AL, USA) is a disposable system with a lock lever design that controls the piston, a manometer, and a connecting tube with a male rotating adapter. The manometer allows pressure measurement with a gauge marked in 1 atm increment. The syringe is completely filled with the contrast-media solution and the syringe and connecting tube purged of air. The connecting tube is then hand-tighten securely to the balloon inflation port. For the procedure of valvotomy, we would not recommend however to turn the palm grip on the piston clockwise slowly, but rather to push it rapidly with the palm until full inflation is obtained, as confirmed on fluoroscopy and by the high resistance felt. Balloon deflation is rapidly obtained by releasing the piston and pull back. The negative pressure is maintained by sliding the lock lever back to lock. Of note, the inflation pressure is not routinely monitored and the maximal pressure that can be delivered almost never reaches the bursting point. As a matter of fact, balloon ruptures are exceptional. In our institution, the technique has been simplified with the use of a simple 30 mL Luer-Lok syringe (BD Plastipak, Drogheda, Ireland), connected by a three-way stopcock to an extension tube, 25 cm long, 2.5 mm in diameter. The same technique is used for purging the system of air. The syringe is filled with 20 to 25 mL of contrast/saline solution. Pushing rapidly the piston with the palm is easier with this technique.

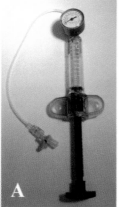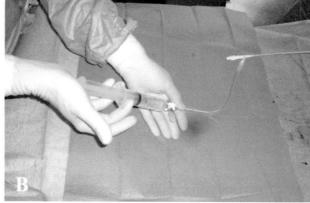

Figure 5   The Atrion QL balloon inflation device.

For deflation, the piston is easily pulled back whereas the negative pressure is obtained by locking the stopcock.

Pacing Lead, Pacemaker, and Pacing Rate

For many years, maintaining the balloon "locked" in the valve to deliver adequate dilating force has been a key issue for efficient BAV. In the course of the BAV experience, several tips and tricks have been proposed to prevent ejection of the balloon by the ventricle during inflation (9,11). However rapid ventricular pacing (RVP) has been a determinant for successful BAV and subsequently for transcatheter valve implantation. RVP-induced ventricular tachycardia accomplishes an optimal reduction of the cardiac output, creating a transient cardiac standstill. As a way to arrest the forceful contractions of the heart and stabilize the balloon in the optimal position, RVP was tried by us during BAV in 2001 and used on regular basis thereafter (6). This technique was then successfully extended to transcatheter valve implantation (9) and appeared to be crucial for accurate balloon expandable valve positioning.

Pacing Lead

The best pacing lead should offer a good suppleness/stiffness compromise and be easily and reliably placed at the mid-part of the right ventricle's posterior wall with low risk of dislodgement or ventricular perforation. After having tried a number of pacing catheters, our personal choice is currently the Soloist Intracardiac Electrode Catheter (Medtronic, Inc., Minneapolis, MN, USA) (Fig. 6). The lead has a 6F size and a length of 110 cm with a Josephson curve tip. In some patients with heart enlargement, it may be useful to straighten the curved tip by hand before use to facilitate the intraventricular placement. The worst pacing catheters for TAVI are the balloon tip catheter leads, often used by the anesthesiologists from the jugular vein approach. The risk of premature dislodgement of these pacing catheters is high during RVP and may result in premature discontinuation of pacing during valve implantation and subsequent valve embolization.

In case of difficulties in crossing the tricuspid valve and/or positioning and stabilizing the lead at the desired place in the right ventricle, it appears very helpful to place a 8-F Mullins sheath in the right atrium, direct its tip toward the tricuspid valve, and then advance the pacing lead into the right ventricle. The pacing catheter will be securely placed be stable during the whole procedure.

Pacemaker

In RVP, it is essential to use a pacemaker that allows a sharp start and discontinuation of rapid pacing at the expected rate. Among the number of pacemakers available, we have selected the Medtronic 5348 (Medtronic Inc., Minneapolis, MN, USA) (Fig. 7).

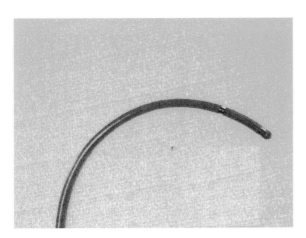

Figure 6 The Soloist Intracardiac Electrode Catheter (Medtronic).

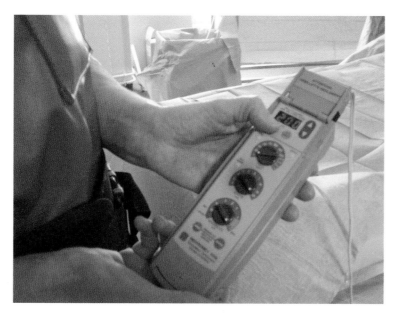

Figure 7 The Medtronic 5348 temporary pacemaker used for rapid pacing.

Rate of Rapid Pacing

Pacing is usually initiated at a rate of 200 bpm and the capture tested. Repeat pacing at decrement of 10 bpm is performed if capture is unreliable. In patients with normal left ejection fraction, the minimum pacing rate should not be lower than 180 bpm. In the absence of 1/1 capture setting atropine (1 mg IV) can be administered and the test repeated. Change in the position of the pacing lead inside the right ventricle should be attempted in case of failure. An appropriate pacing rate should lead to a stable reduction of systolic arterial pressure to below 60 mm Hg. Pacing must be repeated at a rate of 220 bpm if this goal is not reached. In patients with severely depressed left ventricular ejection fraction (<30%), lower pacing rate can however be used (i.e., 150–160 bpm).

TECHNIQUE OF BALLOON VALVOTOMY

Procedure (Video 1)

In our institution, the procedure of valvotomy is performed under local anesthesia and sedation (Midazolam 2 mg IV and Nebuphine 5 mg IV). Heparin, 50 U/kg IV is administered after cut-down of the femoral artery at the groin. The sheaths have been placed in the controlateral femoral artery and femoral vein. A pigtail catheter has been advanced to the aortic root and a supra-aortic angiogram obtained in a view showing the aortic valve perpendicular to the screen and assessing the degree of associated aortic regurgitation. This view is displayed on a screen to facilitate balloon positioning and later on positioning of the prosthesis. The 14-F sheath has been placed in the femoral artery, the aortic valve crossed, the transvalvular gradient measured and the extra-stiff wire positioned inside the left ventricle as described in chapter 10.

The pacing lead is advanced in the femoral vein to the right ventricle. Adequate threshold for pacing is confirmed and the appropriate pacing rate determined. The steps of balloon valvotomy are shown on (Fig. 8). The balloon catheter is advanced through the 14 French sheath over the extra-stiff guidewire and de-aired into the aorta [Fig. 8(A)]. Before crossing the valve with the balloon catheter, the aortic pressure should be stabilized at baseline level. If general anesthesia is used, induced hypotension usually requires norepinephrine infusion to maintain adequate blood pressure. The balloon is then advanced across the aortic valve, positioning it with the aortic calcification slightly above midway between the two markers [Fig. 8(B)]. The first operator then asks an assistant (generally a nurse or an anesthesiologist) to initiate pacing (Fig. 9). As soon as the reliable capture is confirmed, the balloon is rapidly fully

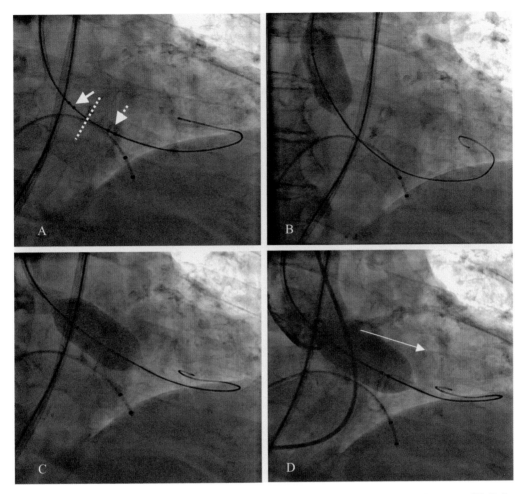

Figure 8   Phases of balloon valvotomy (23 mm balloon). (**A**) Balloon purged of air in the aorta. (**B**) Balloon placement across the valve (*arrows*: balloon markers; *dotted* line: valvular calcification line). (**C**) First balloon inflation. (**D**) Second balloon inflation with aortogram: in this patient with a 21-mm annulus diameter, the free space between balloon edges and aortic wall and the aortic regurgitation (*arrow*) confirm the need for a 26-mm valve.

inflated and deflated [Fig. 8(C)], pacing is turned off and the balloon is withdrawn from the valve, maintaining safe wire position in the left ventricle. Rapid balloon deflation and restoration of blood flow is important to minimize the duration of hypotension and hypoperfusion. It is mandatory to await recovery of aortic pressure to baseline before additional balloon inflation. A second balloon inflation can then be performed. In most cases, this additional inflation will be done with simultaneous aortogram [Fig. 8(D)]. After valvotomy, the balloon catheter is retrieved and the guidewire left in place for bioprosthesis implantation. In most cases, it is not required to assess the residual transvalvular gradient.

Aortogram During Balloon Inflation: Technique and Interest
Performing an aortogram during balloon inflation is recommended in many cases. It is obtain by injection at full balloon inflation of a small volume of nondiluted contrast media (about 10 mL), using the pigtail catheter placed at immediately above the balloon.

One of the interests is to assess the risk of left main or right coronary occlusion in the presence of huge calcific nodules located on the left or right coronary cusps. Pushed aside by the deployed bioprosthesis, the nodules may come into contact with the coronary ostia, compromising or blocking the coronary blood flow (Fig. 10). Injection of contrast media during

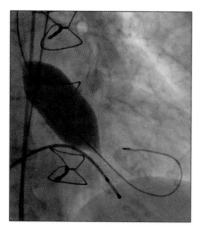
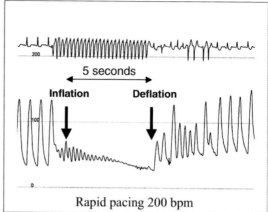

Figure 9   Effect of rapid pacing on blood pressure and phases on balloon inflation/deflation.

balloon inflation allows a good delineation of the calcific nodules and visualization of the coronary ostia. This can lead to cancellation of a TAVI or possibly protection of the coronary artery lumen with an angioplasty guidewire to be prepared for urgent angioplasty and stent implantation after valve deployment. Another indication is to confirm the adequate size of the bioprosthesis when the aortic annulus diameter has been measured from 20 to 22 mm. In this setting, a 23-mm balloon should be systematically used for valvotomy. Assessment of the free space between balloon edges and aortic wall, and the degree of paravalvular leak will easily confirm the optimal bioprosthesis size.

BALLOON VALVOTOMY FAILURES

Impossibility of Crossing the Valve with the Balloon

Crossing the native calcified valve with the balloon may prove impossible in rare cases with massively calcific aortic valves, more particularly when the guidewire is entrapped eccentrically within the valve cusps. To overcome the wire bias, it may be useful to slightly inflate the balloon and try to cross the valve during active deflation and simultaneous traction on the guidewire. The wire can also be pushed forward inside the left ventricle to modify the crossing position of its stiff part across the aortic orifice. Finally, it may be needed to first enlarge the aortic orifice with smaller size/lower profile balloons (15 or 18 mm) before using the larger size balloon.

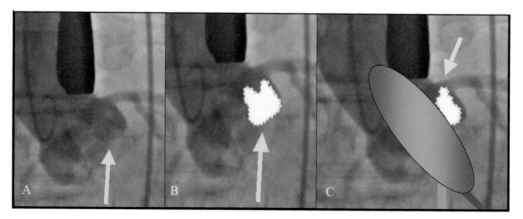

Figure 10   Schematic representation of the assessment of the risk of left main coronary occlusion by aortogram during balloon inflation. The huge calcific nodule seen on baseline aortogram [*arrows* on (**A**) and (**B**)] is pushed aside during balloon inflation and comes into contact with the left main.

Instability of the Balloon During Inflation

"Locking" the balloon across the aortic valve during maximal inflation is essential for effective valvotomy. In spite of RVP, the 30-mm long RetroFlex Balloon Catheter may often slide inside the left ventricle or be ejected into the aorta at first balloon inflation. In general, a slight change in initial balloon positioning will solve the problem at the second try. In exceptional cases, the balloon is consistently ejected in the aorta during inflation, whatever the balloon size, the initial positioning and the pacing rate. This may be associated with considerable left ventricular muscular hypertrophy or subvalvular septal hypertrophy that can be detected by echocardiography. In this setting TAVI may be cancelled even if we are aware of rare cases that could be undertaken successfully by using the transapical approach that allows a better control of the catheter shaft displacement during balloon inflation.

COMPLICATIONS

A number of serious adverse events have been reported with BAV. In the 1990s, total periprocedural complications ranged between 22.6% and 25% in the Mansfield Scientific (3) and NHLBI registries (4) with procedural deaths reaching 4.9% and 3%, respectively. With more experience and technological improvements, major complications have been reduced by about 50% as shown in the latest series (6,7,12).

The risk of complication is definitely much lower during preimplantation valvotomy than during regular BAV due to less aggressive valve dilatation with smaller size balloons. The complications specifically associated with predilatation valvotomy are not clearly reported in the literature, included in the "intention to treat" overall complications of transcatheter valve implantation. However, even infrequent, major and minor complications may occur during the procedure as shown from our personal experience of 75 cases of retrograde Edwards SAPIEN valve implantation, and from unpublished data from other groups.

(1) Sustained cardiovascular collapse after balloon inflation is the predominant issue and may be fatal. Individual cases have been reported in the multicenter registries of TAVI (unpublished data). This results from left ventricular depression from balloon occlusion of the outflow track, and is much more likely to be observed in patients with severely depressed myocardial contractility or associated severe coronary artery disease. It can also result from ventricular perforation, rupture of the aortic annulus, or massive aortic regurgitation. In all patients, but more particularly in those with unstable hemodynamics, balloon inflation/RVP-induced hypotension should be as short as possible. Balloon inflation should never be initiated in the presence of acute unstable hemodynamics or before restoring baseline systemic pressure with atropine, adequate fluid administration, and/or vasopressors administration.

Left ventricle perforation and tamponade is prevented by careful manipulation of guidewires and catheters inside the left ventricle and preshaping of the extra-stiff wire (see chapter 10). Massive aortic regurgitation may result of leaflet avulsion or tear, rupture or dissection of the aortic root. The undersized balloons required for predilatation decrease the risk of mechanical complication, but aortic dissection may occur, more particularly in patients with porcelain aorta (one case in our series).

(2) Permanent or transient cerebrovascular accidents (one and two cases respectively in our series) and other embolic events are associated with retrograde catheterization of the aortic valve and may occur during valve crossing with the wire and balloon valvotomy (13). Incidence of stroke was <2% in recent series of BAV (6,7). The causes and consequences have been described in chapter 10. Transient hypoperfusion induced by balloon inflation and RVP can have clinical consequences in patients with severe cerebrovascular or coronary atherosclerotic disease, which enforce the need for short periods of induced hypotension.

(3) Ventricular arrhythmias (extra systoles and nonsustained ventricular tachycardia) are frequently observed during manipulations of wires and catheters inside the left ventricle but can be easily prevented. Complete heart block may result from a pressure effect on the interventricular septum and conduction system with the balloon, more likely if underlying right bundle branch block is present. This can be rapidly overcome by the transient pacemaker in place for rapid pacing.

Rapid pacing is generally well tolerated and sustained ventricular tachycardia or ventricular fibrillation are rarely observed: 3% in our series like in Webb's experience (11), in all cases immediately responsive to electrical defibrillation. Occurrence of RVP-induced ventricular arrhythmias is favored by underlying severe coronary artery disease, depressed left ventricular function or hypokalemia.

CONCLUSION

Preimplantation percutaneous BAV is a mandatory procedure before TAVI in all cases. Failure in predilating the aortic valve would result in unsuccessful crossing of the native valve with the bioprosthesis. The technique has become simpler and safer and benefits of the large experience and technological improvements of primary BAV. Besides its role in preparing the native valve to receive the prosthesis, its combination with aortogram can help in determining the optimal valve size and assess the risk of coronary occlusion after implantation. The procedure also allows simulating the behavior of valve implantation and preparing the operators to the protocol of rapid ventricular burst pacing that is crucial for valve deployment.

ACKNOWLEDGMENT

The authors wish to thank Alan Zacharias, MD, for his help in reviewing the chapter.

REFERENCES

1. Cribier A, Savin T, Saoudi N, et al. Percutaneous transluminal valvuloplasty of acquired aortic stenosis in elderly patients: An alterative to valve replacement? Lancet 1986; 1:63–67.
2. Letac B, Cribier A, Koning R, et al. Results of transluminal aortic valvuloplasty in 218 adults with valvular aortic stenosis. Am J Cardiol 1988; 62:598–605.
3. Mc Kay RG. The Mansfield scientific aortic valvuloplasty registry: Overview of acute hemodynamic results and procedural complications. J Am Coll Cardiol 1991; 17:485–491.
4. NHLBI Balloon Valuloplasty Registry. Percutaneous balloon aortic valvuloplasty: Acute and 30-day follow-up results in 674 patients from the NHLBI Balloon Valvuloplasty Registry Circulation 1991; 84:2383–2397.
5. Hara H, Pedersen WR, Ladich E, et al: Percutaneous balloon aortic valvuloplasty revisited: Time for a renaissance? Circulation 2007; 115:334–338.
6. Sack S, Kahlert P, Khandanpur S, et al. Revival of an old method with new techniques: balloon valvuloplasty of the calcified aortic stenosis in the elderly. Clin Res Cardiol 2008; 97:288–297.
7. Agatiello C, Eltchaninoff H, Tron C, et al. Balloon aortic valvuloplasty in the adult. Immediate results and in-hospital complications in the latest series of 141 consecutive patients at the University Hospital of Rouen (2002–2005). Arch Mal Cœur Vaiss 2006; 99(3): 195–200.
8. Letac B, Gerber L, Koning R. Insight in the mechanism of balloon valvuloplasty of aortic stenosis. Am J Cardiol 1988; 62:1241–1247.
9. Cribier A, Eltchaninoff H, Tron C, et al. Early experience with percutaneous transcatheter implantation of heart valve prosthesis for the treatment of end-stage inoperable patients with calcific aortic stenosis. J Am Coll Cardiol 2004; 43:698–703.
10. Webb JG, Chandavimol M, Thompson R, et al. Percutaneous aortic valve implantation retrograde from the femoral artery Circulation 2006; 113:842–850.
11. Webb JG, Pasupati S, Achtem L, et al. Rapid pacing to facilitate transcatheter prosthetic heart valve implantation. Catheter Cardiovasc Interv 2006; 68:199–204.
12. Klein A, Lee K, Gara A et al. Long-term mortality, cause of death, and temporal trends in complications after Percutaneous aortic balloon valvuloplasty for calcific aortic stenosis. J Interv Cardiol 2006; 19: 269–275.
13. Omran H, Schmidt H, Hackenbroch M, et al. Silent and apparent cerebral embolism after retrograde catheterization of the aortic valve in valvular stenosis: a prospective, randomized study Lancet 2003; 361: 1241–1246.

15 | Advancing the Delivery System Across the Aorta and Valve (Edwards SAPIEN Valve)

Peter C. Block, Vasilis Babaliaros, and Zahid Junagadhwalla

Emory University Hospital, Gruentzig Cardiovascular Center, Atlanta, Georgia, U.S.A.

INTRODUCTION AND PROCEDURAL PLANNING

Historical Perspective

The first case of transcatheter heart valve (THV) implantation for aortic stenosis was performed by Cribier et al. in April 2002 (1). Because the first patient had severe peripheral vascular disease that precluded insertion of a 24-F sheath into the ileo-femoral arteries, the femoral vein was cannulated and the THV was implanted by an antegrade transseptal approach. The majority (82%) of patients in the initial feasibility study were implanted by this route with 85% success (2). The major limitation of this route was difficulty in maintaining hemodynamic stability in patients with small ventricles because of tethering of the anterior mitral leaflet by the delivery system (1–3). In addition, the early cases of retrograde implantation had less success (57%) because of the bulky introducer sheath and lack of steerability/pushability of the delivery catheter (2,4). For the THV procedure to progress, a better introducer sheath and delivery system were developed for the retrograde technique (5,6), and the antegrade technique was abandoned. This chapter describes the current retrograde implantation from preprocedural evaluation to cross the aortic valve with the THV.

Preprocedural Evaluation to Avoid Problems

Preprocedural planning is critical to maximize the chances for successful passage of the delivery catheter from the introducer sheath through the distal, transverse, and proximal aorta, and then across the stenotic aortic valve. Careful examination of the CT scan (chest, abdomen, and pelvis) as well as the aorto-iliac angiogram delineates the anatomy of the aorta and ileo-femoral vessels, and is critical to answer a series of questions for each patient: (i) Are the ileo-femoral vessels large and distensible enough for placement of a 22- or 24-F sheath? (ii) Will the delivery sheath reach well above the aortic bifurcation, and if not, is the bifurcation clear of atherosclerotic disease on the side contralateral to the sheath insertion to allow safe passage of the delivery catheter and valve? (iii) How much atherosclerotic plaque and calcification is present in the descending, transverse, and ascending aorta? (iv) How long is the transverse aorta, and thus how wide is the transverse arch? This translates into the amount of flexing that the Retroflex catheter will need to safely traverse the arch. (v) What is the angle of the valve annulus plane (horizontal or more vertical)? (vi) What is the best angle for retrograde crossing of the stenotic valve with the THV after balloon aortic valvuloplasty (BAV)? Also during the preprocedural evaluation, the echocardiogram (TTE and occasionally TEE) must be carefully reviewed to select the smallest THV that will adequately treat the patient and concomitantly improve deliverability. All of the potential barriers to implantation should be identified in advance as patient selection remains the most important variable for procedural success.

The evaluation of the iliac and femoral arteries deserves additional discussion as currently this is the major limitation to transfemoral implantation (7–9). Because atherosclerotic disease commonly affects these vessels so as to produce stenoses or foci of calcification, learning to read an abdominal/pelvis CT and the abdominal aortogram with run-off to the level of the femoral head is time well spent to avoid vascular complications. We have routinely used both imaging modalities to evaluate prospective candidates for THV implantation. A biplane aortic angiogram using oblique projections at 30 to 45 degrees, or an anterioposterior projection in one plane with a 30-degree angle in the second plane is best performed at the time of coronary angiography, which is normally done during screening. A pigtail catheter is placed with its tip

8 to 10 cm above the aortic bifurcation. We use a pigtail catheter with radio-opaque markers at 1-cm intervals (Cook Medical, Bloomington, IN) to assist in measuring vessel diameter. The image intensifiers for both angiographic planes should be as close to the patient as possible to minimize magnification, though if the pigtail is in the artery that is being measured, there is little error produced. However, if the marker pigtail catheter is in the contralateral artery (a usual strategy since minimizing arterial punctures of the artery that is to be used for THV placement avoids the chances of local dissection, hematoma, etc., which could complicate the cut-down at the time of the procedure), care must be taken to try and measure the 1-cm interval as close to the contralateral artery as possible. This usually means measuring the reference 1-cm distance near the aortic bifurcation. Quantitative angiographic techniques are then used to measure the minimum diameter of the ileo-femoral vessels.

The CT scan can confirm the lumen diameter measured at angiography, but more importantly, shows the degree and distribution of vessel calcification that can be equally or more important than lumen diameter. In our experience, heavier calcification occurs in the common iliac vessels and less in the external iliacs. Although heavy calcification in the common iliacs is usually of no significant consequence as the lumens are large and the vessels are straight, calcification of any extent in the external iliacs may be prohibitive for sheath placement because of tortuosity and smaller lumen size. The entry point into the common femoral artery should ideally be without calcification (even if this requires a "high" entry at the level of the inguinal ligament before the vessel dives into the pelvis), and the bifurcation of the external and internal iliac should ideally be without calcification to allow straightening without "trapping" the sheath during insertion or removal. If there is calcification in these areas, the common iliac should be scrutinized for feasibility of an iliac conduit (Dacron graft anastomosis end-to-side to the common iliac; conduit externalized through groin incision; sheath inserted via the conduit). Alternatively, the patient might be considered for transapical valve implantation (10–12).

In its current profile, the 23-mm Edwards SAPIEN valve can fit through a sheath with a 22-F inner diameter (a "22-F" sheath). It must be remembered, however, that the outer diameter of the "22-F" sheath is actually larger because of sheath wall thickness (25 F or 8.3 mm). The 26-mm Edwards SAPIEN valve fits through a "24-F" sheath that has an outer diameter of 28 F or 9.3 mm. In general, for the 23-mm Edwards SAPIEN device the iliofemoral arteries must have a minimal lumen diameter of 7.0 mm (assuming a paucity of calcification to allow the vessels to stretch), and for placement of the 26-mm THV, a minimal lumen diameter of 8 mm.

Intraprocedure Evaluation

Before crossing the aortic valve for the first time we perform multiple injections of contrast through a pigtail catheter placed just above the aortic valve or in one or more of the aortic sinuses. We change projections by moving the X-ray tube/image intensifier so that the base of each aortic sinus is projected in a straight line (Fig. 1, Video 1(A), 1(B)). This allows imaging of the aortic annulus in a superimposed straight line (often a 0° annular plane (AP) projection or a shallow LAO projection with mild cranial angulation will "line up" the AP). This maneuver is critical to avoid deploying the THV too caudal or cephalad because of a fore-shortened radiographic view of the aortic valve. In addition, since the position of the THV predeployment is rarely coaxial with the aortic root (and thus rarely perpendicular to the AP), identification of the AP greatly helps in understanding how the THV will expand/orient within the aortic valve once inflation of the balloon occurs. The angle of the image intensifier is best chosen before BAV as hemodynamic instability during the procedure may preclude doing this later.

The initial crossing of the aortic valve with a straight guidewire [usually placed through an AL1 (Amplatz) catheter] also gives the operator important information. The level of the stenotic valve orifice and the subsequent position of the guidewire and the AL1 catheter must be noted. For example, if the wire crosses into the commissure between the right coronary cusp and the noncoronary cusps (a common scenario), it may initially be difficult to cross the aortic valve even with the valvuloplasty catheter. Though the BAV balloon catheter can usually be advanced across the valve regardless of its crossing position, later passage of the THV across the aortic valve may be impossible if the guidewire remains deep in the commissure, and it is potentially dangerous if too much forward pressure is applied. Tearing of the sinus of Valsalva or proximal aortic disruption or dissection may occur. Placing a 30 to 40-degree bend in the

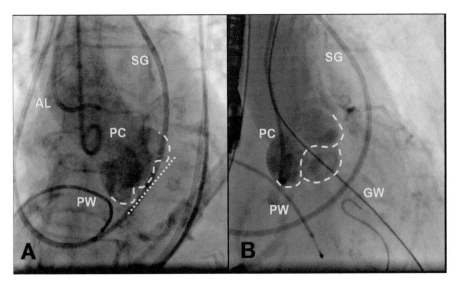

Figure 1 Lining up the annular plane (AP) of the aortic valve. (**A**) An AP or slight LAO projection with cranial angulation will image the aortic cusps (*dotted curvy lines*) on a tangential plane (*dotted straight line*). This lines up the annulus of the aortic valve. (**B**) Example of a malaligned aortic valve with the three cusps (*dotted lines*) out of plane. A foreshortened view of the aortic valve can result in malposition of the THV. *Abbreviations*: AL, Amplatz catheter; SG, Swan–Ganz catheter; PW, temporary pacing wire; PC, pigtail catheter; GW, guidewire.

extra-stiff guidewire approximately 15 to 20 cm above the transition point of the soft tip may help place the transannular position of the guidewire toward the center of the aortic valve orifice and further out of the commissure.

ADVANCING THE DELIVERY SYSTEM ACROSS THE AORTA

Placement of the Introducer Sheath
Ultimately the introducer sheath should have its tip above the distal aortic bifurcation and should be oriented so that the THV can exit the sheath safely. Because we perform the majority of our sheath insertions via cut-down to the femoral artery with a counter-incision in the skin (this insures that the sheath is in the plane of the common femoral artery prior to cannulation), the distance of the cannulation site and counter-incision must be carefully chosen in tall patients. Insertion of serial dilators (including dilators that are equal in size to the outer diameter of introducer sheath) increases the chances of successful insertion of the 22-or 24-F sheaths. The use of excessive force to pass the dilators or sheath into the aorta should be avoided as this can cause fatal vascular complications during insertion or during removal (separation or dissection of ileo-femoral vessels).

Traversing and Exiting the Sheath
Once the sheath has been successfully placed with its tip in the distal aorta, the delivery system (Retroflex catheter and THV mounted on a balloon catheter) should move smoothly through it without resistance. If resistance to advancing the device is felt by the operator, the source must be immediately evaluated under fluoroscopy. If the delivery system enters the sheath for a few millimeters and cannot be advanced beyond the arteriotomy site, it is likely that the sheath has too severe a bend between the skin incision and arteriotomy. The struts of the THV cannot traverse a sharp bend. We have experienced a case where the stent struts caught the inside of the sheath and penetrated the sheath wall, thereby prohibiting forward movement of the delivery system (Fig. 2, Video 2). Once the problem was identified, the sheath was removed over the extra-stiff wire already in place, a new sheath was placed, the angle of entry at the arteriotomy lessened, and the device then was advanced without difficulty.

Since the sheath is positioned with a dilator in place it is unlikely that a vascular stenosis will compress the sheath, but it is possible that vessel rebound can locally constrict it slightly.

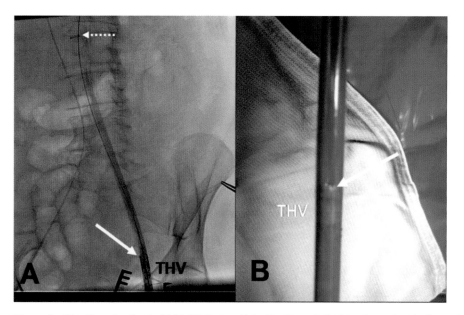

Figure 2 Sheath perforation by THV. (**A**) Contrast injection through the introducer sheath shows the THV with a strut that has exited the sheath wall (*solid arrow*) preventing further advancement of the delivery system (*dotted arrow*. proximal end of the sheath). (**B**) Sheath was removed from patient and perforation by the stent struts (*arrow*) is evident. THV is seen faintly through the sheath wall.

In that case the device will not advance easily. This can be overcome by retracting the sheath approximately 2 to 3 cm while at the same time gently advancing the delivery system to the area of stenosis. The combination of the delivery system and the sheath can then be advanced together through the offending area.

In elderly patients the common iliac arteries may bifurcate from the aorta at a wide angle and then loop back toward the femoral head, producing a double bend. The extra-stiff guidewire helps straighten these vessels in many cases. However if there is still an area of angulation, once the dilator is removed from the sheath the sheath may kink at that spot. The kink cannot be seen fluoroscopically, but obviously the device and delivery catheter cannot traverse the kink. This problem is mostly encountered at or near the aortic bifurcation. Attempting to straighten out the kink by forward pressure of the deliver catheter will not work. To remedy this, the previously described maneuver is usually successful. The sheath is withdrawn for a few centimeters, and the delivery system is advanced until resistance is felt. The sheath and delivery system are then advanced together. It should be emphasized, however that the tip of the introducer sheath should not be brought back to the iliac vessels. The protective effect of the sheath surrounding the device as it is advanced is essential to avoid iliac dissection, which is more likely to occur if the device is advanced "naked." Ultimately the introducer sheath could be replaced with a new sheath (Edwards Lifesciences) or a stiffer sheath (Cook Medical, Bloomington, Indiana) if manipulating the sheath/delivery system does not work.

Finally, as the device exits the sheath tip, care must be taken to avoid aortic injury. Atherosclerotic plaque is common at or above the bifurcation. As the device, which is easily seen under fluoroscopy, exits the sheath the operator can feel a "release" as the constricted device/delivery system moves cephalad. Observation under fluoroscopy at this point is essential. The device may exit the sheath at an angle and not coaxial to the descending aorta since the guidewire is biased against the aortic wall opposite the iliac artery, which is used for the sheath. This often occurs if the aortic bifurcation is widely angulated, and the device may "catch" on plaque in the distal aorta. This is both felt by the operator and seen on fluoroscopy—the device does not continue to move smoothly cephalad. Forward pressure will cause damage to the descending aorta. However simply retracting the delivery system a few millimeters and advancing again usually allows clearance of the opposite aortic wall. Pulling back the guidewire a few millimeters can help in this maneuver, but remember that the distal tip of the guidewire must remain well positioned in the left ventricle. If neither of these two maneuvers allows the delivery system to proceed cephalad smoothly, the introducer sheath, and delivery system should all be withdrawn a few centimeters. This re-orients the guidewire slightly as it lies in the descending aorta, and almost always then allows safe passage of the delivery system in a cephalad direction. Flexing of the Retroflex catheter has also been used to move the device into a more coaxial position in the descending aorta. If the sheath has been withdrawn during these maneuvers, remember that forward movement of the introducer sheath to return it to its initial position should not be done. The "mouth" of the sheath may cause an aortic tear as it moves forward. The final position of the sheath should be secured by suturing the distal end to the skin, preventing future movement of the sheath during manipulation of the THV through the aorta and valve.

Crossing the Transverse Aorta

After exiting the introducer sheath, the delivery system usually moves cephalad through the thoracic aorta smoothly. If resistance is encountered it signifies impingement on aortic plaque [Fig. 3(A), Video 3(A)]. Simply withdrawing the delivery system a few millimeters and then advancing again usually solves this problem. Once the distal portion of the transverse arch is reached by the tip of the delivery system it is important to change the imaging plane to a left anterior oblique projection [Fig. 3(B), Video 3(B)]. This avoids foreshortening in fluoroscopic imaging of the transverse arch and shows how much flexion of the Retroflex catheter is needed to bring the THV to a more horizontal position as the transverse arch is crossed. We usually begin flexing the Retroflex catheter just as the delivery system enters the distal transverse arch, thereby anticipating the bias of the wire and catheters against the greater curvature of the arch. Slight rotation of the Retroflex catheter may be needed to help "clear" any plaque in the transverse arch. It is important to remember that the Retroflex catheter is not designed to be rotated more than a few degrees in either direction. Rotation of the Retroflex catheter of course also moves the tip of the delivery catheter either anteriorly or posteriorly, which may make later crossing of the aortic valve more difficult. Also, greater amounts of rotation may produce torsion and kinking of the Retroflex catheter. Kinking the Retroflex catheter causes

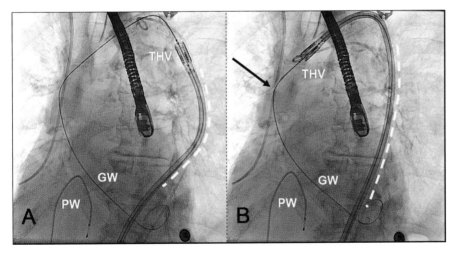

Figure 3 Advancing the delivery system across the aorta. (**A**) The delivery system has encountered a plaque in the aortic valve. Pushing the delivery system only causes the Retroflex catheter to buckle (*white dotted line*). Pulling the catheter back with mild flexing can re-direct the catheter into the lumen of the aortic arch. (**B**) The aortic arch is best visualized in the LAO projection. The delivery system is advanced forward with active flexing of the Retroflex catheter to prevent bias of the THV into the outer curvature of the aorta. Notice the bowing of the delivery system is now absent (*dotted line*) and a secondary bend in the guide wire (arrow) should facilitate passage of the THV across the native aortic valve. *Abbreviations*: GW, guidewire; PW, pacing wire.

dysfunction of the flexing mechanism. If this occurs, placement of the delivery catheter and the valve in the proper position may be far more difficult or impossible.

ADVANCING THE DELIVERY SYSTEM THROUGH THE ASCENDING AORTA AND ACROSS THE AORTIC VALVE

Once the delivery system enters the ascending aorta, the X-ray tube and image intensifier should be moved back to the position in which the aortic annulus is superimposed in one plane (see earlier). As the delivery system is advanced into the ascending aorta, the guidewire almost always is biased against the greater curvature of the aorta. This usually produces a transvalvular position of the guidewire in the commissure between the right coronary cusp and the noncoronary cusp. Without taking any flex off, the delivery system can then be advanced to the aortic valve and an initial attempt at crossing can be performed. If successful, further exact placement of the THV is then done. However, it is often not possible to advance the delivery system across the native valve orifice in this position because bias within the commissure causes the balloon catheter and THV to catch in the base of the commissure [Fig. 4(A), Video 4(A)]. Further advancement attempts are usually fruitless and may result in native valve damage or aortic root disruption. In this situation, the delivery system should be pulled back over the wire guide to a position about 2 cm above the native valve. Attempts must then be made to minimize the bias of the wire guide toward the greater curvature of the aorta and into the commissure. If the wire has been previously shaped with a bend approximately 15 to 20 cm up the ascending aorta, either advancing the guidewire or retracting it might change the "crossing" position and allow the delivery system to cross the native valve. Other attempts to change the guidewire crossing configuration include a number of options:

a. "Unflexing" the Retroflex catheter: The Retroflex catheter can be "unflexed" varying amounts. We have had some success with this maneuver but in general this simply biases the wire further against the greater curvature.
b. Telescoping the THV/balloon valvuloplasty catheter: The Retroflex catheter can be withdrawn 6 or 8 cm, so its tip is at the top of the ascending aorta, leaving the delivery catheter just above the native valve. This maneuver may make the delivery catheter more flexible. Advancing the delivery catheter alone at that point may allow it to better follow the wire guide in its passage through the native valve. If a different position of the delivery catheter

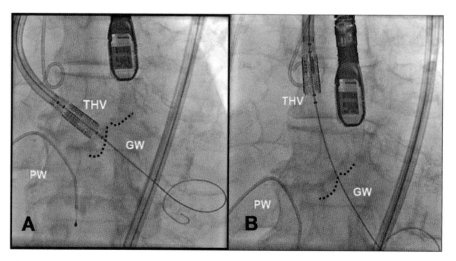

Figure 4   Crossing the native aortic valve with the THV. (**A**) Initial attempts to cross the native aortic valve were unsuccessful as the THV is biased into the outer curvature of the aorta, and the wire is biased into the commissure (*dotted line*, outline of right and left aortic cusps). Forward pressure causes the delivery system to bow (**B**) After an initial failure to cross, the delivery system is withdrawn into the ascending aorta, un-flexed and then re-flexed with mild clockwise torque to return the guidewire into the center of the valve orifice. The system can then be re-advanced with a favorable result as the THV crosses the native valve. (dotted line, outline of right and left aortic cusps). *Abbreviations*: PW, pacing wire; GW, guide wire.

tip and the THV are noted, but the THV/balloon catheter will not advance, the Retroflex catheter can then be carefully advanced over the balloon catheter as it is again flexed until it comes in contact with the THV. This allows more force to be transmitted to the THV for crossing.

c. Re-aligning the guide wire: We have had the best success in re-aligning the guidewire more centrally in the aortic orifice by withdrawing the unflexed delivery system from the ascending aorta to the proximal transverse aorta. The Retroflex catheter is then maximally re-flexed with moderate clockwise rotation (45–90 degrees). As the delivery system is again advanced with maintenance of clockwise rotation (moderate rotation of the Retroflex catheter moves the THV anteriorly and can be performed safely without kinking the catheter), the wire guide moves toward the inner curvature of the aorta with the result that the position of the wire guide as it crosses the aortic valve is considerably more central. Holding the wire in place the operator then carefully can advance the delivery system over the wire guide to the native valve orifice [Fig. 4(B), Video 4(B)]. Crossing is then easier and achieved by gentle forward pressure.

Other techniques can also be considered, though their use is unusual.

i. If wire bias is repetitively within the commissure between the right coronary cusp and noncoronary commissure even after attempting all above-mentioned maneuvers, the balloon catheter can be advanced with its tip through the native valve. The extra-stiff wire could then be replaced with another wire—either with a more marked bend proximally (Fig. 5) in it or replaced with a softer wire (allows more flexing toward the inner curvature of the aorta), which might allow better passage of the THV through the native valve orifice. Loss of wire position may be permanent if the balloon catheter tip is "pushed out" of its position across the aortic valve when re-advancing a new wire. It might be possible to re-cross the stenotic native valve with the guidewire but the potential difficulty of that maneuver is daunting.

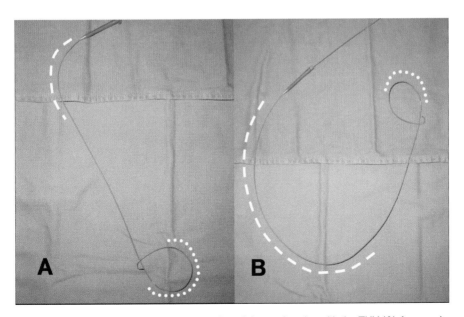

Figure 5   Wire techniques to facilitate crossing of the aortic valve with the THV (**A**) A secondary curve (*dashed lines*) can be made 15 to 20 cm distal to the primary pigtail curve (*dotted lines*) to bias the THV/delivery system away from the outer curvature of the aorta and away from the commissure of the right coronary cusp and noncoronary cusps. The guidewire can be shaped prior to implantation of the THV or re-shaped after failed attempt at crossing. (**B**) A long, gradual secondary bend (*dashed lines*) can be made 15 cm distal to the primary pigtail curve (*dotted lines*) to bias the THV/delivery system away from the outer curvature of the aorta and away from the commissure of the right coronary cusp and non-coronary cusps. This secondary bend can facilitate flexing of the Retroflex catheter.

ii. A second guidewire could be placed across the native valve, using the pigtail catheter already in position in the aortic root or replacing it with an AL1 catheter and re-crossing in the classic manner. The second guidewire also biases in the commissure next to the first. A small valvuloplasty balloon catheter can then be advanced and inflated within the native valve, essentially blocking the commissure and deflecting the delivery system toward the center of the native valve.

iii. A low-volume inflation of the balloon catheter distal to the crimped THV can be performed. The tip of the catheter balloon inflates first, before the valve is expanded and before the balloon portion proximal to the crimped THV begins to inflate. A small inflation of the distal balloon with a few cc's of contrast makes the tip more globular and moves the shaft and crimped THV out of the commissure. Advancement of the delivery system through the stenotic valve may then be possible.

iv. Re-valvuloplasty of the native valve with a larger balloon from the contralateral access site.

v.   Transseptal puncture with snaring of the delivery system (wire and/or balloon catheter) from the left ventricle via the left atrium.

Second-Generation Catheters

The second-generation delivery systems greatly facilitate the passage of THV through the introducer sheath, the aorta, and across the aortic valve compared to the first-generation systems. The first-generation delivery systems have the balloon catheter and THV uncovered. Though the THV is crimped tightly over the balloon center, the ends of the balloon, especially the forward portion, have a folded surface that can produce some friction. More importantly, the THV always has a slightly larger diameter than the folded balloon in front and behind it. Thus, especially in passage through the native aortic valve, it is the shoulder of the crimped THV in the center of the delivery balloon that "catches" on plaque or in the commissure of the native valve. The new-generation devices have a nose cone that tapers at the front end and is integrated into the forward portion of the delivery balloon on the back end (Fig. 6). The portion of the nose cone that integrates with the forward half of the balloon has the same outer diameter of the crimped THV. Passage through the introducer sheath is smoother, and traversing the native

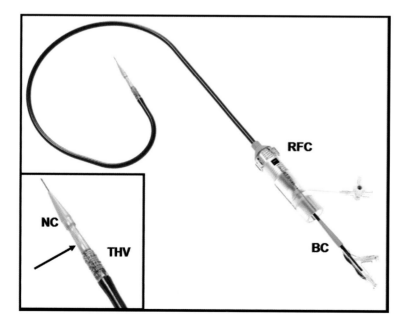

Figure 6 Next-generation Retroflex catheter. The new Retroflex catheter combines a nose cone (picture insert, NC) that is integrated with the forward part of the balloon (*arrow*) creating a smoother transition from balloon to THV and facilitating crossing of the native valve. The RFC covers the back part of balloon during crossing and is then sleeved before deployment. *Abbreviations*: BC, balloon catheter; RFC, Retroflex catheter.

aortic valve does not require force. Once the nose cone and THV pass through the native valve orifice, the Retroflex catheter is then withdrawn until the distal portion of the delivery balloon is free and exact placement and deployment of the THV is then performed. In addition, the second-generation devices have a lower profile, as low as 18 F for the smaller 23 mm THV. This reduction in size increases the number of potential patients for THV implantation, and also greatly facilitates the procedure.

CONCLUSIONS

THV implantation can be performed successfully if patients are carefully selected. However, even in the best selected patients, vessel tortuosity, atherosclerotic plaque, wire bias, or the stenotic aortic valve itself can produce unforeseen problems in guiding the THV to its proper position within the aortic annulus. Attention to detail minimizes most surprises, and fortunately, most of these problems can be solved after they arise. A guiding principle that cannot be overemphasized is that if any resistance to forward movement of the sheath or delivery system is noted, re-evaluation is critical rather than trying to force through a problem. The "tricks" and "tips" already listed should greatly aid in solving issues that may occur during THV procedures.

REFERENCES

1. Cribier A, Eltchaninoff H, Bash A, et al. Percutaneous transcatheter implantation of an aortic valve prosthesis for calcific aortic stenosis: First human case description. Circulation 2002; 106:3006–3008.
2. Cribier A, Eltchaninoff H, Tron C, et al. Treatment of calcific aortic stenosis with the percutaneous heart valve: Mid-term follow-up from the initial feasibility studies: the French experience. J Am Coll Cardiol 2006; 47:1214–1223.
3. Cribier A, Eltchaninoff H, Tron C, et al. Early experience with percutaneous transcatheter implantation of heart valve prosthesis for the treatment of end-stage inoperable patients with calcific aortic stenosis. J Am Coll Cardiol 2004; 43:698–703.
4. Hanzel GS, Harrity PJ, Schreiber TL, et al. Retrograde percutaneous aortic valve implantation for critical aortic stenosis. Catheter Cardiovasc Interv 2005; 64:322–326.
5. Webb JG, Chandavimol M, Thompson CR, et al. Percutaneous aortic valve implantation retrograde from the femoral artery. Circulation 2006; 113:842–850.
6. Webb JG, Pasupati S, Humphries K, et al. Percutaneous transarterial aortic valve replacement in selected high-risk patients with aortic stenosis. Circulation 2007; 116:755–763.
7. Feldman T, Leon MB. Prospects for percutaneous valve therapies. Circulation 2007; 116:2866–2877.
8. Babaliaros V, Block P. State of the art percutaneous intervention for the treatment of valvular heart disease: A review of the current technologies and ongoing research in the field of percutaneous valve replacement and repair. Cardiology 2007; 107:87–96.
9. Babaliaros V, Cribier A, Agatiello C. Surgery insight: Current advances in percutaneous heart valve replacement and repair. Nat Clin Pract Cardiovasc Med 2006; 3:256–264.
10. Ye J, Cheung A, Lichtenstein SV, et al. Transapical transcatheter aortic valve implantation: 1-year outcome in 26 patients. J Thorac Cardiovasc Surg 2009; 137:167–173.
11. Ye J, Cheung A, Lichtenstein SV, et al. Six-month outcome of transapical transcatheter aortic valve implantation in the initial seven patients. Eur J Cardiothorac Surg 2007; 31:16–21.
12. Walther T, Simon P, Dewey T, et al. Transapical minimally invasive aortic valve implantation: multi-center experience. Circulation 2007; 116:I240–I245.

16 | Advancing the Delivery System Across the Aorta and Valve (CoreValve)

Eberhard Grube, Ulrich Gerckens, Georg Latsios, and Lutz Buellesfeld

Department of Cardiology and Angiology, HELIOS Heart Center Siegburg, Siegburg, Germany

This chapter assumes that the interventionist, during the procedure of transfemoral aortic valve implantation, is at that point where a wire is placed in the left ventricle retrogradely across the stenotic aortic valve. By using the transfemoral retrograde approach, the wire passes the common femoral artery, external and common iliac artery, the abdominal aorta, and thoracic aorta. At each location, vascular abnormalities such as calcifications, stenoses, aneurysms or thrombi, as well as elongations and kinkings can be present. All of these problems should be and can be overcome not only by careful patient selection but also by various—more or less—ingenious tricks. We will try to cover this road step by step, and illustrate some of the problems and solutions.

The standard technique for implantation of the CoreValve ReValving system uses an Amplatz Super Stiff ST1 (ST, short tip) guidewire (Boston Scientific) (0.035 in. or 0.89 cm) 260 cm in length, PTFE-covered, which possesses the special characteristic of having only 1 cm of flexible floppy atraumatic tip. Prior to insertion, this tip has to be bent manually to a pigtail-like configuration. We have learned in the past that this specific configuration is mandatory to provide an atraumatic support during the procedure. The tip is ideally placed in the apical part of the left ventricle (Video 1). The manipulation of the wire against the left ventricular apex allows repositioning of the valve in a manner similar to that of ostial stenting, that is, pushing the wire causes the prosthesis to come back and vice versa.

Before detailed description of the insertion maneuver, we would like to comment briefly on the handling of the sheath. We prefer to keep the 18-F sheath in the common femoral artery as short as possible to minimize complications. For this reason, the introduction takes place just before balloon predilation. This time point is best as it is a compromise of keeping the sheath in place as short as possible, but being able to insert the prosthesis after predilation without delay due to a sheath exchange. This can be of critical importance in case of hemodynamic instability after predilation because of significant regurgitation. It could be disastrous if this situation occurs but the operator is unable to insert an 18-F sheath to implant the valve prosthesis to stabilize the situation. So, only predilate a transcatheter aortic valve implantation (TAVI) case with an 18-F sheath in place.

In our laboratory we routinely use either the Ultimum EV 18-F sheath (St Jude Medical, Minnetonka, Minnesota) or the Check-Flo Performer 18-F Introducer (Cook Inc, Bloomington, Indiana). Both have a diameter of 6.00 to 6.17 mm and a length of 30 cm. The tip of the sheath dilator should be bent slightly, which helps to direct the sheath during introduction. Over the stiff wire, the sheath is slowly introduced in the common femoral artery. At all times, constant wire tension should be applied and the wire tip position should be controlled under fluoroscopy. This helps to avoid accidental perforation of the ventricular wall with the wire or accidental pulling of the wire out of the ventricle into the aorta.

ADVANCEMENT OF THE 18-F COREVALVE DELIVERY SYSTEM FROM THE SHEATH TO THE AORTIC ARCH

Meticulous screening of patients before the procedure is mandatory to identify patients with adequate access. This is one of the fundamentals for a successful procedure. Once a suitable access site is identified, the wire is placed in the ventricle, the 18-F sheath is inserted, and the valve is properly predilated, the prosthesis is advanced into the sheath in a standard over-the-wire technique.

During entry of the delivery system into the sheath, some resistance is usual at the sheath's hemostatic valve. A second resistance is usually observed when the distal housing of the prosthesis exits the sheath (Video 1). Now, various problems can arise, caused by either a possibly calcified stenosis at the level of the iliac artery or by a more or less severe kinking of the vessels.

In case of *kinking*, the vessel can be usually straightened using a stiff guidewire. If the regular "super stiff" wire is not stiff enough, a buddy wire or wires such as a Meier extra back-up wire can be used.

In case of aortoabdominal kinking, this wire can be placed from the contralateral side as well (Videos 2 and 3).

The *diameter* of the entire arterial bed, from the level of the bifurcation of the abdominal aorta all the way through the common iliac, the external iliac, and the common femoral arteries should be—by protocol—equal to or larger than 7 mm. Borderline values equal or greater than 6 mm are also accepted, so long as the vessel is not severely calcified. In the event of periprocedural detection of significant lesions in the access vessels, two options are available:

1. Change of access site—If the initially intended access turns out to be unfavorable, the contralateral femoral side can be used. If both femoral arteries are unsuitable, a transsubclavian or transapical approach can be used. Both options are discussed in greater detail in other chapters of this book.
2. Percutaneous transluminal angioplasty of the stenosis—Stenoses of the femoral or iliac arteries that preclude the advancement of the CoreValve system might be effectively treated with angioplasty, regaining a lumen area that allows insertion of the prosthesis. This can be done either simultaneously with the TAVI procedure or in two sequential sessions.

The latter approach has some advantages, such as split of the total volume of contrast agent used in two separate time settings, and better fixation of a stent after a certain healing period. In this way there is no risk of stent dislodgement or disruption by meticulous interaction between the CoreValve delivery system and stent struts. According to common knowledge and our experience, 4 weeks are time enough for a TAVI procedure to be carried out safely and effectively after a stent is implanted peripherally in a diseased artery. It is obvious that the diameter of the stent should fulfill the already discussed anatomic criteria, that is, more or equal to 6 to 7 mm.

Pathologies of the abdominal aorta other than severe kinkings, that is, aneurysms with or without thrombus, usually do not cause significant problems during the TAVI procedure.

ADVANCEMENT OF THE 18-F COREVALVE DELIVERY SYSTEM THROUGH THE AORTIC ARCH AND THROUGH THE CALCIFIED VALVE

The process of advancing the CoreValve prosthesis, which is securely fixed inside the delivery system, all the way through the aortic arch and through the calcified, stenosed aortic valve usually does not cause any problems. However, the more bulky a device the more problematic are these two steps. The aortic arch turns itself in a 180-degree fashion with multiple secondary three-dimensional curves as well, and can be severely calcified, which poses an additional risk for liberating embolic debris. Therefore, particularly these steps can be related to stroke events that are reported in the literature.

During the evolution phase of the CoreValve system, and namely the profile reduction from 25 F (introduced in 2004) to 21 F (introduced in 2005) and today to 18 F (introduced in 2006) and the improvement in the capability and experience of the physicians that perform this procedure, the percentage of patients suffering a stroke has drastically decreased from 17% in the 21-F study (1) to 1.4% in the ongoing evaluation of the 18-F device (personal communication).

In the early first-in-man trials using the 25-F first-generation device, the procedure required a surgical cut-down in the iliac artery. To pass around the aortic arch with that bulky device, an additionally inserted snare was used to bend the distal tip of the catheter (Video 4). The simultaneous pushing of the delivery catheter and pulling of the snare, which was anchored at the tip of the prosthesis, enabled the advancement of the CoreValve delivery catheter in almost all occasions.

Nowadays, the lower profile facilitates tremendously the way around the arch as well as the insertion into the diseased native valve with the latest generation CoreValve prosthesis so that a snare is usually no longer needed (Video 5). However, in the rare event of passage problems, use of a snare inserted via the femoral artery might help overcome these problems.

When the prosthesis reaches the aortic valve, the Amplatz Super Stiff ST1 wire needs to be checked once again, so that it is completely straightened and tensed, and also that its manually curved tip rest comfortably against the left ventricular apex with its stiff part (Video 6). If the wire has lost the ideal apical position during balloon valvuloplasty or any other time point before advancement of the prosthesis, wire repositioning with a pigtail catheter should be considered.

The advancement of the CoreValve prosthesis across the native valve usually does not pose any special difficulties either. In case the delivery catheter does not cross the native aortic valve, repeat balloon aortic valvuloplasty might be helpful to optimize native valve opening.

So finally, the prosthesis crosses the native valve. Its final position before its deployment sequence is just across the valve, with its lower part just below the noncoronary sinus. The latter is delineated by a normal 5-F pigtail catheter. Most of the times the CoreValve prosthesis tends to be forwarded to a deeper than optimal position, and should be corrected, positioned, and subsequently deployed, as it will be described in the following chapter.

The whole procedure of advancing the 18-F CoreValve delivery system takes usually less than 30 seconds, so it is a rather rapid procedure inside the whole implantation process—a helpful fact in case of hemodynamic problems after balloon predilation.

REFERENCE
1. Grube E, Schuler G, Buellesfeld L, et al. Percutaneous aortic valve replacement for severe aortic stenosis in high-risk patients using the second- and current third-generation self-expanding CoreValve prosthesis: Device success and 30-day clinical outcome. J Am Coll Cardiol 2007; 50(1):69–76.

17 | Implantation of the CoreValve ReValving System

Peter de Jaegere, Nicolo Piazza, A. Tzikas, Carl Schultz, Robert Jan van Geuns, and Patrick W. Serruys

Department of Interventional Cardiology, Erasmus University Medical Center, Thoraxcenter, Rotterdam, The Netherlands

INTRODUCTION

The correct positioning and implantation of the CoreValve ReValving system (CRS) in aortic position in patients with valvular aortic stenosis implies a profound understanding of the recipient anatomy, the geometry of the prosthesis, and the various imaging techniques that are used for guidance, control, and evaluation and the prosthesis itself.

In chapter 1 and the paper by Piazza et al., the complex anatomy of the aortic root has been translated into helpful information for the clinician (1). At variance with surgical valve replacement, catheter-based (aortic) valve implantation is performed using various imaging techniques such as X-ray and transesophageal echocardiography and, thus, lacks the real-time three-dimensional (3D) sight of the valve and surrounding structures as seen during surgical valve replacement. Therefore, correct positioning and implantation of the valve implies the correct use and interpretation of the resultant images. The integration of the anatomic information and information derived from the two-dimensional (2D) imaging techniques allows—so to speak—a mental 3D view of the aortic root, which is illustrated in Figure 1.

The details of the CRS are described in chapter 7. Analogous to the role of imaging, a thorough understanding of the CRS prosthesis is mandatory for successful valve implantation, which is the subject of this chapter. For that matter, the following will be addressed:

- The CRS prosthesis—details that one must know and understand before embarking on implantation.
- The base of the aortic root—how to use X-ray angiography to accurately depict the base of the aortic root.
- Sizing—which inflow size CRS for which patient.
- Positioning and deployment, and pitfalls in deployment (how to avoid and how to solve).

THE COREVALVE REVALVING SYSTEM

As discussed in chapter 7, the CRS consists of a self-expanding Nitinol frame to which is sewn a porcine pericardium valve in a trifoliate configuration [Fig. 2(A) and 2(B)]. The multilevel design incorporates three different areas of radial force and function. *The base* of the frame is 12 mm high and provides high-radial force. It functions to anchor the prosthesis within the patient's annulus. The base is covered with a skirt composed of a single layer of porcine pericardium that functions to create a seal to prevent paravalvular aortic regurgitation after implantation. It is important to understand that in this area there is no valvular function. *The middle segment* of the frame is constrained to avoid jailing of the coronary arteries after implantation. This segment hosts the zone of coaptation of the leaflets, which stretches from the central point where the three leaflets meet (central coaptation) up to the commissures that are located on the frame at a higher level. As such, the valve is implanted intra-annularly, but functions supra-annularly. This segment has high hoop strength (resistance to deformation) to maintain size and shape to guarantee normal leaflet geometry and function within design limits. *The upper part or outflow portion* of the frame has low radial force, implants itself in the ascending aorta, and orients the prosthesis across the aortic root in the direction of blood flow. The lower part of this segment hosts the top of the commissures of the leaflets.

In addition to the gross anatomic breakdown of the CRS, it is the detailed structure of the CRS that is used for guiding the positioning and deployment in the aortic root.

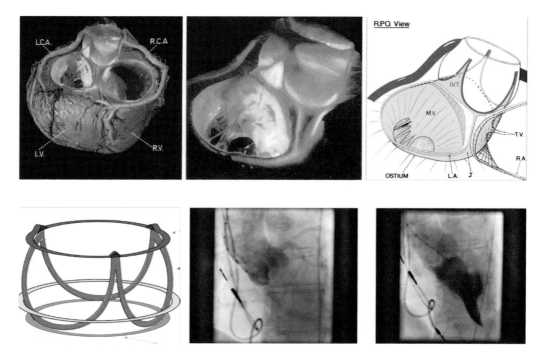

Figure 1 Ex vivo 3D view of the aortic root in relation to the mitral apparatus (upper row) and in vivo 2D angiographic view (lower row).

Upper row: gross 3D overview of the aortic root seen from slightly posterior and the right. The intimate relationship between a large part of the base of the aortic root and the mitral apparatus is clearly seen (magnification in middle picture) and illustrated by the drawing on the right. In addition, the Intervalvular Trigone (IVT) is clearly seen. Bottom row: the aortic root can be seen or reduced to three rings of which the lower green ring corresponds with the true base of the aortic root (transition left ventricular outflow tract and the most basal attachment of the aortic leaflets). The upper blue ring corresponds to the sino-tubular junction. These rings can be seen on contrast angiography if properly performed (see text for explanantion).

Abbreviations: LCA: left coronary artery, RCA: right coronary artery, LV: left ventricle, RV: right ventricle, MV: mitral valve, TV: tricuspid valve, LA: left atrium, RA: right atrium. Pictures: courtesy to W.A. McALpine. Heart and Coronary arteries. Springer-Verlag Berlin Heidelberg, New York 1975.

The frame consists of a series of cells, which have a diamond configuration when fully deployed A full cell is 8 mm high and consists of three joints (each joint is 4 mm apart) [Fig. 2(B)]. Since Nitinol is radiopaque, these cells are clearly visible on X-ray fluoroscopy in their collapsed state and while being deployed. Since the joints have a higher Nitinol density, they are more easily discerned from the thin struts of the frame. The combination of this information and the appropriate settings of the X-ray gantry are the basis of a controlled and correct valve positioning and deployment that is described below.

BASE OF THE AORTIC ROOT

Notwithstanding the potential value of new software that may improve the guidance of catheter-based valve replacement therapies, it is our premise that conventional X-ray will remain the most widely used technique for guidance and control of these procedures. The reasons are: ubiquitous availability, ease of use and its high spatial (0.12 mm), and temporal resolution. Obviously, it only provides a 2D shadowgram of the aortic root that is a distant surrogate of the direct and real-time surgical 3D view. Yet, the base of the aortic root can easily been demonstrated and interpreted by contrast angiography provided the X-ray gantry is positioned in such a way that the three sinuses of the aortic root are visualized on one single line, one next to the other as shown in Figure 3 [Video 3(A), 3(B), 3(C)]. In almost all patients, a slight LAO in combination with some caudal or cranial rotation of the X-ray image intensifier will offer this view. Rarely a slight RAO with some caudal or cranial rotation or a straight anterior–posterior view is needed. Although multislice computed tomography (MSCT) is the most elegant technique to define

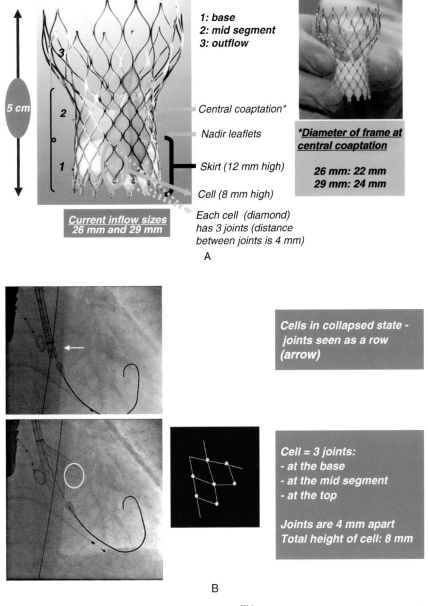

1: base
2: mid segment
3: outflow

5 cm

Central coaptation*

Nadir leaflets

Skirt (12 mm high)

Cell (8 mm high)

Current inflow sizes
26 mm and 29 mm

Each cell (diamond)
has 3 joints (distance
between joints is 4 mm)

*Diameter of frame at
central coaptation

26 mm: 22 mm
29 mm: 24 mm

A

Cells in collapsed state -
joints seen as a row
(arrow)

Cell = 3 joints:
- at the base
- at the mid segment
- at the top

Joints are 4 mm apart
Total height of cell: 8 mm

B

Figure 2 (**A**) The CoreValve Revalving System[TM]. (**B**) In vivo visualisation of the CoreValve Revalving System[TM].

the valve plane and obtain the X-ray gantry settings (see chaps. 3, 12, and 25), an experienced operator can easily find the correct plane with contrast angiography (2,3).

SIZING

At present, the CRS valve is currently available in two sizes based on the diameter of the base or inflow of the frame: 26 and 29 mm [Fig. 2(A)]. According to the instructions provided by the manufacturer, a 26-mm inflow CRS is intended for a patient annulus of 20 to 23 mm and a 29-mm inflow CRS is intended for a patient annulus of 24 of 27 mm (Appendix).

This proposal is subject of debate given the absence of validated scientific evidence and in view of the fact that the base of the aortic root (annulus) is oval rather than circular (1–4). Yet,

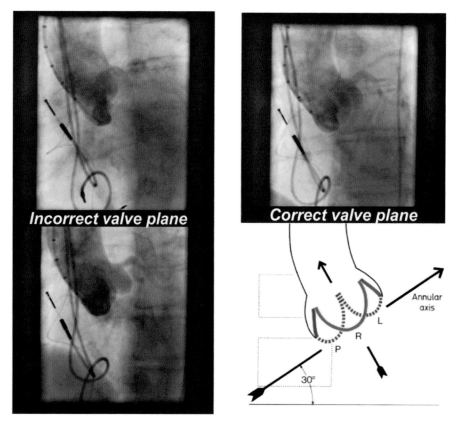

Figure 3 Visualisation of the aortic root during valve implantation. (**A & B**) inappropriate visualisation of the aortic root. (**C & D**) correct visualisation of the aortic root: the three aortic sinuses are seen on one line.

correct prosthesis–host match is imperative to avoid procedural complications such as valve embolization or paravalvular regurgitation in case of undersizing, and acute or long-term valve dysfunction due to leaflet distortion and/or local tissue injury in case of oversizing. (2,5–7)

With respect to the measurement of the base of the aortic root, we use MSCT as it is a 3D imaging modality that allows the definition and precise measurement (spatial resolution 0.5 mm) of the true base of the aortic root (the three most caudal attachment points to the 3D crown shaped attachment line of the leaflets (Fig. 4). This is not possible with 2D imaging such as transthoracic echocardiography (TTE) and trans-oesophageal (TOE) echocardiography given their limitation to provide detailed information of the surrounding structures needed to define the nadir of the aortic root and, thus, the lowest level of the hinge points of the leaflets, their limited spatial resolution to define the hinge points of the aortic leaflet as well as the unknown angle between the incoming ultrasound beam and the base of the root leading to incorrect measurement of the true dimensions of the aortic root.

At the Thoraxcenter, we started using the matrix proposed by the manufacturer for the selection of valve size (Appendix). We gradually switched to an integrated assessment of the dimensions of the base of the aortic root on the basis of (*i*) clinical information (gender, length, and body weight), (*ii*) TTE, and (*iii*) the visual appreciation of the dimensions of the aortic root by means of contrast angiography (performed with the X-ray gantry settings already described). During the course of time, the latter became the most dominant factor in the decision of valve size. Later, as we became more acquainted with MSCT, it became the most important source of information on the basis of which we choose the valve size in our practice. Table 1 illustrates our modus operandi; it depicts the smallest (D1) and largest dimension (D2) of the annulus by MSCT and the CRS size that was used based upon the integration of clinical information, aortic root angiography and information of TTE and MSCT.

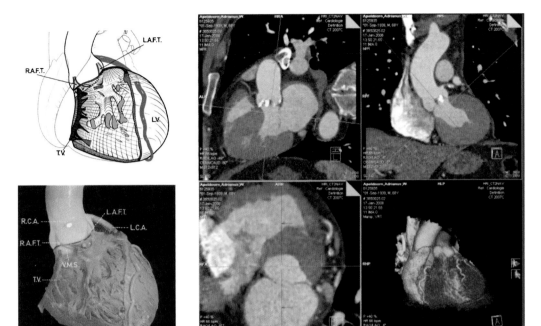

Figure 4   Definition of the base of the aortic root ("aortic annulus") Explanation: see text.
Abbreviations: RAFT & LAFT: right and left anterior fribrous trigone, LCA: left coronary artery, RCA: right coronary artery, LV: left ventricle, TV: tricuspid valve, VMS: ventricular membranous septum.

As mentioned earlier, a scientific basis for valve size selection is currently absent. In addition, the selection of the valve size is complicated by the availability of two prosthesis sizes for a wide range of dimensions of the root, and the fact that the frame is circular whereas the left ventricular outflow tract and base of the aortic root, where the prosthesis is anchored, is usually oval.

POSITIONING AND DEPLOYMENT

The CRS must be positioned and implanted in such a way that the base or inflow portion of the frame—that is covered by the pericardial skirt with a height of 12 mm—is located in the LVOT base of the aortic root. The ventricular end of the CRS should be preferably 6 mm but no deeper than 8 mm (1 diamond) below the base of the aortic root (Fig. 5). An implantation beyond 12 mm is not compatible with the concept of the design and will likely be associated with significant paravalvular aortic regurgitation (Fig. 6). We advocate a depth of 6 mm, since we observed that none of our patients in whom the valve was implanted within 6 mm below the base of the aortic root developed a left bundle branch block directly related to valve implantation. (8)

Table 1   Assessment of Annulus Dimensions (D1 and D2) by MSCT Before CRS Implantation

	D1 (mm) *N* = 12 patients	D2 (mm) *N* = 21 patients
26-mm inflow CRS	19.0 (17.6–22.4)	23.5 (20.5–26.8)
29-mm inflow CRS	22.8 (19.6–30.2)	27.5 (22.9–33.7)

Twelve patients received a 26-mm inflow CRS and 21 patients received a 29-mm inflow CRS. According to the manufacturer's matrix on valve selection, the matrix was not respected (retrospective analysis) in 7 out of the 12 patients in whom a 26-mm inflow CRS was implanted and in 10 out of the 21 patients in whom a 29-mm inflow was implanted.

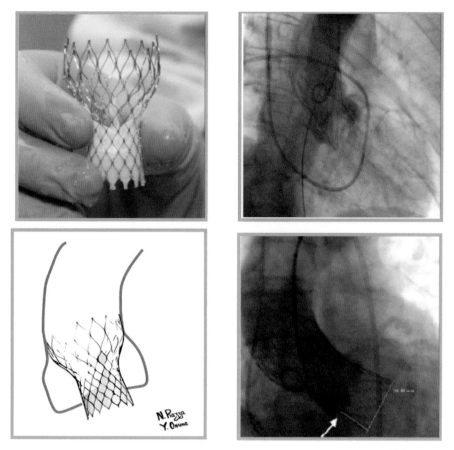

Figure 5   Positioning and depth of implantation of the CoreValve Revalving System™.

Exact visualization of the base of the aortic root is mandatory for correct positioning and subsequent deployment of the CRS. As discussed, the X-ray gantry is positioned in such a way that all three sinuses are depicted one next to each other on a single line, somewhat off-center on the monitor so that the left ventricle, LVOT, and ascending aorta are under continuous visual control (Fig. 7). It allows the constant control of the position of the wire in the ventricle and the entire deployment of the frame from the base of the aortic root up to the ascending aorta.

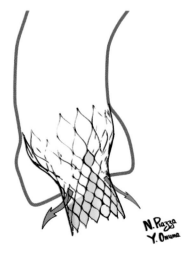

Figure 6   Aortic regurgitation due to a incorrect (too deep) implantation. The top pericardial skirt is below the base of the aortic root. As a result there is aortic regurgitation due to operator related misplacement of the valve.

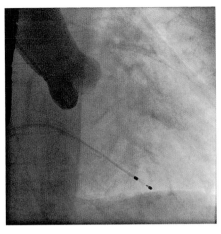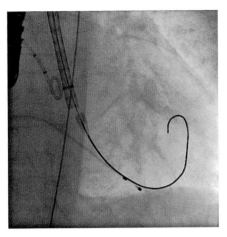

Figure 7 First phase of CoreValve Revalving System^TM implantation. Correct visualisation of the base of the aortic root (three aortic sinuses on one line – picture left), entering of prosthesis in left ventricular outflow tract and initiation of the withdrawal of the protective sheet (picture right).

A pigtail that sits firmly in the nadir of the noncoronary sinus is used as a reference target for the positioning and deployment of the valve [Fig. 8, Video 8(A), 8(B), 8(C), 8(D), 8(E)]. The nadir of the noncoronary sinus is used as a reference point because it is usually the lowest of the three coronary sinuses on contrast angiography with the X-ray gantry positioned in the way just described. It allows correct valve implantation, even in the absence of calcium. In case bulky calcified leaflets preclude the pigtail reaching the nadir of the leaflets, one may use these calcifications as a reference.

   With this X-ray gantry setting and control of the anatomy, the CRS that is crimped on a 18-F delivery catheter and covered with a protective sheath is entered into the LVOT. The CRS is entered into the LVOT a few millimeters below the plane of the base of the aortic root. In its collapsed state, one cannot discern the diamonds of the frame but one can use the radiopaque characteristics of the joints. In the collapsed state, they appear individually perpendicular to the axis of the frame and separated by 4 mm [Fig. 2(B)]. In case the position of the frame in relation to the base of the aortic root is unclear, a contrast angiogram (we typically use 15 cc at a flow of 15 cc/sec) will confirm its position. An experienced operator may choose to only enter the cone of the delivery catheter in the LVOT (Fig. 9, Video 9) because the CRS has the tendency move forward into the LVOT when the protective sheath is slowly being withdrawn.

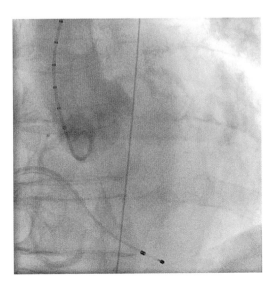

Figure 8 Pigtail in the nadir of the non-coronary sinus. Correct positioning of a pigtail in the nadir of the non-coronary sinus will help the operator to correctly position and implantation of the CoreValve Revalving System^TM.

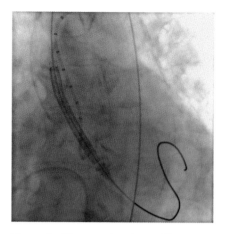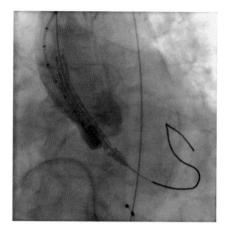

Figure 9 The control of the position of the CoreValve Revalving System™ in the left ventricular outflow tract before valve implantation. The pigtail that is positioned in the nadir of the non-coronary sinus helps the operator the check the position (picture left). Contrast angiography (picture right) confirms the position.

The deployment of the valve consists of a coordinated action of the two operators; while the first operator controls the positioning of the prosthesis, the second executes a gentle and controlled clockwise rotation of the microknob that results in the gradual withdrawal of the protective sheath (Fig. 10). The process of valve implantation is performed in a stepwise manner.

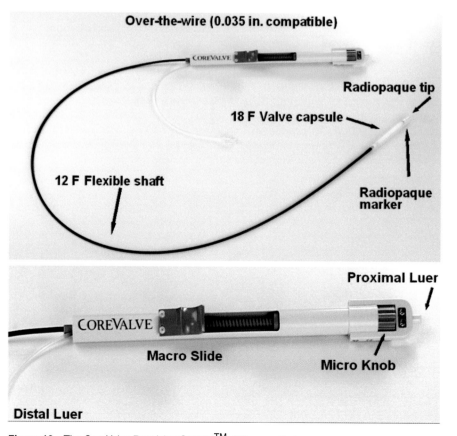

Figure 10 The CoreValve Revalving System™ delivery catheter.

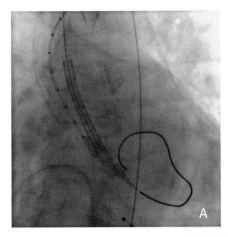
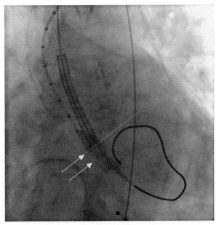

Upper arrow: pigtail in nadir of noncoronary sinus
Lower arrow: distal end CRS prosthesis
Dotted line: aortic valve plane

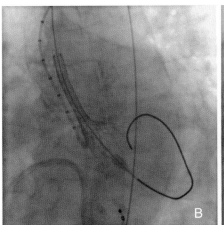
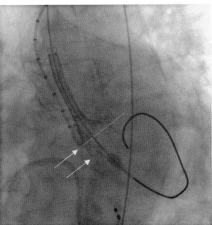

Figure 11 (**A**) The control of the depth of implantation during valve implantation during the initiation of the withdrawal of the protective sheet. (**B**) The control of the depth of implantation during valve implantation during the flaring of the frame upon further release.

In the very first phase of the withdrawal of the protective sheath, there is no flaring of the frame. One can observe the separation of the radiopaque marker of the protective sheath from the cone of the delivery catheter. The frame of the CRS is still collapsed [Fig. 11(A), Video 11(A1), 11(A2)]. Upon further withdrawal of the protective sheath, the frame will begin to flare [Figure 11(B), Video 11(B1), 11(B2)].

During this phase of deployment, there is abundant time to control the position of the frame. For that matter, both operators verify the relation of the ventricular end of the frame at relative to the pigtail as an anatomic reference since it is located in the nadir of the noncoronary sinus. One should not be misled or consider the opposite side, that is, the part of the aortic root that is in juxtaposition with the mitral valve apparatus. In case the frame enters the left ventricle, the first operator may gently pull on the delivery to bring the CRS in its desired position. [Video 11(A1)] Some advocate a gentle push on the wire that is located in the LV by the second operator. In case this is done, both operators must be in complete synchrony with one another. One should also realize that pushing the wire may cause ventricular wall injury and possibly AV conduction disturbances or more dramatically, LV perforation. This

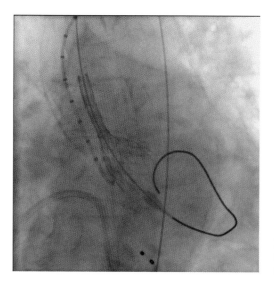

Figure 12 The use of the position of the pigtail in the nadir of the non-coronary sinus to control the position of the valve during implantation.

latter complication may occur more frequently in small, hypertrophied heart. In case of doubt of the CRS position, contrast angiography must be performed.

In the initial phase of the flaring, there is no drop in blood pressure since there is no obstruction of flow across the "native" aortic valve. At this moment, one may discern the diamonds of the inflow part of the frame. Inspection of the relation between the lower most diamonds and the pigtail in the nadir of the noncoronary sinus, allows the first operator to correct the position of the frame.

Blood pressure will go down when the frame reaches the opposite side of the aortic root because the "native" aortic valve is excluded from the circulation and the bioprosthetic leaflets cannot move freely yet. We call this the parachute phase [Fig. 12, Video 11(C1)]. The deployment has to be continued [Video 11(C2), 11(D1), 11(D2)] to allow pressure recovery while avoiding the CRS being propelled into the ascending aorta, which may occur in patients with hypertrophic left ventricle and a pronounced systolic function [Fig. 13, Video 13(A) and 13(B)]. Deployment is continued in the way described with special emphasis on the control of the position of the frame and the nadir of the noncoronary sinus. Once the blood pressure has stabilized, it is the moment to double check the position of the valve. In case the valve is still somewhat too low in the aortic root, the first operator may exert traction on the delivery catheter. This should be

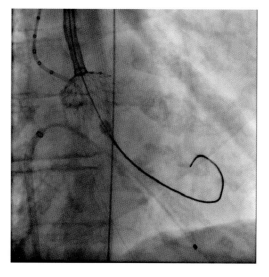

Figure 13 Embolisation of The CoreValve Revalving System^{TM} into the ascending aorta.

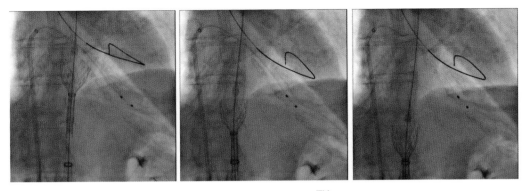

Figure 14   Complete retrieval of The CoreValve Revalving System^{TM} from the circulatory system.

done carefully without a brisk pull on the delivery catheter since it may result in expelling the valve into the ascending aorta. If this occurs, one has to remove the valve, delivery catheter, and sheath en bloc out of the body and restart the implantation all over again (Fig. 14, Video 14). If the valve is implanted too deep one may try to pull the prosthesis into its correct position with a goose neck snare. Obviously, this is a technique to be avoided given its inherent risk of embolism of calcified tissue from the ascending aorta, vessel wall injury, or valve dislodgement, by ensuring correct valve position during expansion of the frame as discussed above. If the degree of aortic regurgitation is grade 3 or more or not well tolerated, a second CRS should be implanted in the first CRS (valve-in-valve) (9) [Fig. 15, Video 15(A1), 15(A2) and Video 15(B1), 15(B2), 15(B3), 15(B4), 15(B5), 15(B6)].

In case of a correct position, the pigtail is removed from the noncoronary sinus, and the deployment is completed. The deployment is completed when the two hooks of the frame are released from the delivery catheter. This should be checked in at least two views. In case of doubt, one should not pull on the delivery catheter but continue the inspection. One may carefully advance the delivery catheter and check whether the hooks move in conjunction with the forward movement of the frame. Complete release is sometimes achieved by further pushing the delivery catheter towards the base of the aortic root forcing the release of the hook or by a gentle clock- and counter-clockwise rotation of the delivery catheter [(Fig. 16, Video 16(A1), 16(A2), 16(A3), 16(A4)]. Once the hooks are completely detached from the delivery catheter, the soft part of the stiff wire that is located in the left ventricle is pulled to the level of the cone of the delivery catheter [Fig. 16, Video 16(B)]. This allows the cone to move away from the interventricular septum into the direction of the inlet of the frame. In this position, the cone can safely be removed out of the left ventricle. In case the cone is removed while it is in contact with the interventricular septum, it may become entangled with the ventricular end of the frame and result in dislocation of the valve.

Advancing the macroslide then recaptures the cone of the delivery catheter. It is recommended to check the recapture in two projections to ensure coaxial alignment and a safe withdrawal through the 18-F sheath.

The final step consists of a contrast angiogram with the pigtail just above the CRS leaflets and sufficient contrast volume (e.g., 20 cc) and rate of injection (e.g., 20 cc/sec at 1200 -psi) to verify: (1) valve position, (2) presence and degree of aortic regurgitation, and (3) visualization of coronary arteries.

Checking the distance between the nadir of the non- and left coronary sinus and the base of the radiopaque frame can readily assess the depth of implantation (Fig. 5). It goes without saying that this angiogram is made with the X-ray gantry positioned in the way described earlier (visualization of all three sinuses on one single horizontal line).

In general there is some degree of aortic regurgitation (grade 1 or 2) after CRS implantation. In case of aortic regurgitation grade 3 or more or in case the aortic regurgitation is not well tolerated, one has to first define its cause by contrast angiography of the aortic root and transesophageal echo-Doppler. In case of correct position of the valve, one should exclude incomplete expansion or apposition of the frame due to, for instance, bulky calcified native

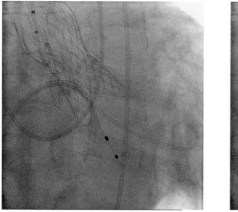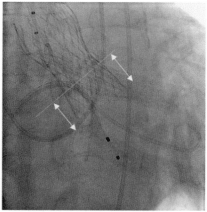

Dotted line: level of the base of the aortic root
Visual assessment of the diamonds of the frame
allows appreciation of the depth of implantation

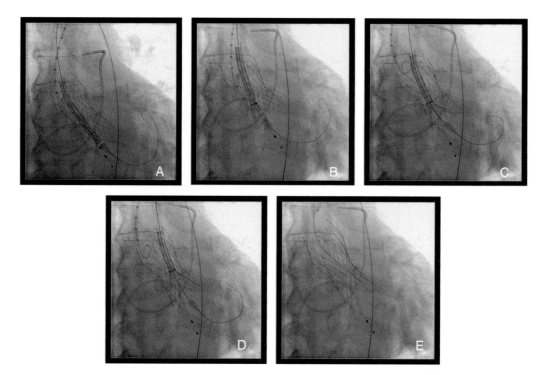

Figure 15 (**A**) Assessing the depth of implantation of The CoreValve Revalving System™. (**B**) Valve-in-valve procedure to correct aortic regurgitation because of a too deep implantation of the first valve.

leaflets. In such a case, additional in-valve balloon dilatation must be performed. Balloon size is selected on a combination of the dimensions of the annulus (preferably by MSCT before implantation) and the size of the CRS that was implanted [Fig. 17, Video 17(A), 17(B), 17(C)]. In case the CRS is implanted too deep (>12 mm below the base of the aortic root) one is committed to a valve-in-valve procedure already described.

It is important to verify the appearance of the coronary arteries to rule out unexpected coronary occlusion. In our experience, the coronaries can easily be checked by indirect visualization via the aortic root angiography (Fig. 18, Video 18). In case of doubt, selective coronary

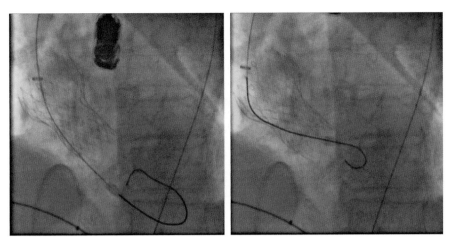

Figure 16 Removal of the cone out of the left ventricular outflow tract. To safely remove the cone out of the left ventricular outflow tract, the soft part of the stiff wire over which was used to delver the valve, is retracted up to the cone. This allows the safe withdrawal of the cone since the cone has moved to a more aligned position in relation to the frame and is more central position in the outflow tract.

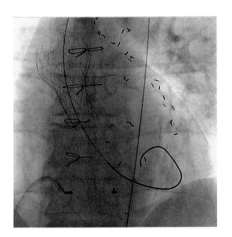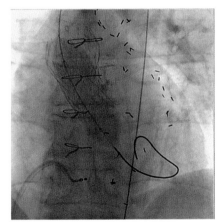

Figure 17 Balloon dilatation post valve implantation.

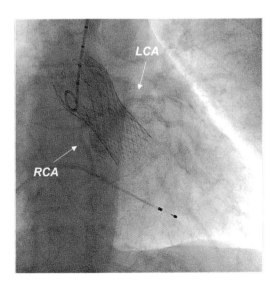

Figure 18 Indirect visualisation of the coronary arteries after the implantation of the CoreValve Revalving System^{TM}.

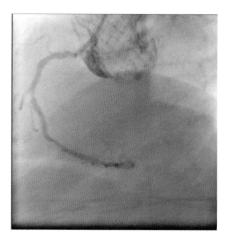 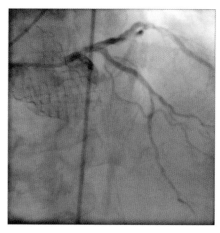

Figure 19 Selective contrast angiography of the right and left coronary artery after the implantation of The CoreValve Revalving System™.

angiography should be performed followed by appropriate further management in case of blockage or occlusion [Fig. 19, Video 19(A) and 19(B)].

REFERENCES

1. Piazza N, de Jaegere P, Schultz C, et al. Anatomy of the aortic valvar complex and its implications for transcatheter implantation of the aortic valve. Circ Cardiovasc Interv 2008; 1:74–81.
2. Schultz CJ, Weustink A, Piazza N, et al. The geometry and degree of apposition of the CoreValve Revalving system (CRS®) with multislice computer tomography after implantation in patients with aortic stenosis. J Am Coll Cardiol. 2009; 54:911–918.
3. Tops LF, Wood DA, Delgado V, et al. Noninvasive evaluation of the aortic root with multislice computed tomography: Implications for transcatheter aortic valve replacement. JACC Cardiovasc Imaging 2008; 1:321–330.
4. Doddamani S, Gruskho MJ, Makaryus AN, et al. Demonstration of left ventricular outflow tract eccentricity by 64-slice multi-detector CT. Int J Cardiovasc Imaging 2009; 25:175–181.
5. Thubrikar M, Piepgrass WC, Deck JD, et al. Stresses of natural versus prosthetic aortic valve leaflets in vivo. Ann Thorac Surg 1980; 30:230–239.
6. Thubrikar M, Piepgrass WC, Shaner TW, et al. The design of the normal aortic valve. Am J Physiol. 1981; 241:H795–H801.
7. Zegdi R, Ciobotaru V, Noghin M, et al. Is it reasonable to treat all calcified stenotic aortic valves with a valved stent? Results from a human anatomic study in adults. J Am Coll Cardiol 2008; 51:579–584.
8. Piazza N, Onuma Y, Jesserun E, et al. Early and Persistent Intraventricular Conduction Abnormalities and Requirements for Pacemaking After Percutaneous Replacement of the Aortic Valve. JACC Cardiovasc Interv 2008; 1:310–316.
9. Piazza N, Otten A, Schultz C, et al. Results of implantation of two self-expanding aortic bioprosthetic valves during the same procedure—Insights into the valve-in-valve implantation. Catheter Cardiovasc Interv 2009; 73:530–539.

APPENDIX

Elements below reflect Indications for Use according to the CE Mark

Diagnostic Findings	Non-Invasive			Angiography			Selection Criteria	
	Echo	CT/MRI	LV	Ao Root	CAG	Vascular	Recommended	Not Recommended
Atrialor Ventricular Thrombus	X						Not Present	Present
Sub Aortic Stenosis	X	X	X				Not Present	Present
LV Ejection Fraction	X		X				>20%	<20% without contractile reserve
Mitral Regurgitation	X						≤Grade 2	>Grade 2 Organic Reason
Vascular Access Diameter		X				X	≥6 mm Diameter	<6 mm Diameter
Aortic and Vascular Disease		X				X	None to Moderate	Sever Vascular Disease
Indications for 26 mm CoreValve Device								
Annulus Diameter	X	X					20-23 mm	<20 mm or >23 mm
Ascending Aorta Diameter		X		X			≤40 mm	>40 mm
Indications for 29 mm CoreValve Device								
Annulus Diameter	X	X					24-27 mm	<24 mm or >27 mm
Ascending Aorta Diameter		X		X			<43 mm	>43 mm

General medical guidance for use CoreValve*

Diagnostic Findings	Non-Invasive			Angiography			Selection Criteria	
	Echo	CT/MRI	LV	Ao Root	CAG	Vascular	Recommended	Moderate-High Risk
LV Hypertrophy	X	X					Normal to Moderate 0.6 - 1.6 cm	Severe ≥ 1.7 cm
Coronary Artery Disease		X			X		None, Mid or Distal >70%	Proximal Lesions >70%
Aortic Arch Angulation		X				X	Large Radial Turn	Sharp Turn
Aortic Root Angulation		X				X	<30 degrees	30-45 degrees
Aortic and Vascular Disease		X				X	No or Light Vascular Dosease	Moderate Vascular Disease
Vascular Access Diameter		X				X	>6 mm	Calcified and elongated >7 mm
Anatomic Considerations for 26 mm CoreValve Device								
Sinus of Valsalve Width	X	X		X			≥27 mm	<27 mm
Sinus of Valsalva Height	X	X		X			≥15 mm	<15 mm
Anatomic Considerations for 29 mm CoreValve Device								
Sinus of Valsalva Width	X	X		X			≥29 mm	<29 mm
Sinus of Valsalva Height	X	X		X			≥15 mm	<15 mm

*-General medical guidance reflects the experience to date with the product, but final judgment remains with the implanting physicians(s).

Consult with a certified proctor to determine if your patient is Moderate-High Risk

INTERNATIONAL
CAUTION: The CoreValve System is not currently available in the USA for clinical trials for sale.
CoreValve is a registered trademark of Medtronic CV Luxembourg S.a.r.l.

18 | Implantation of the Edwards SAPIEN Valve

Fabian Nietlispach and John G. Webb
St. Paul's Hospital, University of British Columbia, Vancouver, British Columbia, Canada

This discussion will focus on procedural elements specific to deployment of the Edwards SAPIEN valve (Edwards Lifesciences, Inc., Irvine, California). Device sizing, positioning, and deployment will be reviewed (see Video 1 for a complete overview of an Edwards SAPIEN implantation procedure). As patient selection and other elements of the procedure have been discussed elsewhere (see chap. 5), these will not be reviewed in detail here.

THE EDWARDS SAPIEN VALVE

An understanding of certain characteristics of the valve and delivery system are fundamental to optimal implantation. The current Edwards SAPIEN valve is constructed of a balloon-expandable stainless-steel frame, bovine pericardial leaflets, and a synthetic PET fabric-sealing cuff [Fig. 1(A)] (1). The valve is currently available in two sizes, with expanded external diameters of 23 or 26 mm and lengths of 14.28 and 16.07 mm, respectively. The next-generation SAPIEN XT valve substitutes a cobalt chromium alloy frame with thinner struts and a more open cell structure to allow tighter crimping [Fig. 1(B)]. When expanded the 23- and 26-mm SAPIEN XT valves have lengths of 14.34 and 17.02 mm, respectively (2).

VALVE DELIVERY SYSTEM

Initially the valve was delivered on a standard valvuloplasty balloon. The limitations of this system required transvenous, transseptal valve delivery. Subsequently, the development of the deflectable RetroFlex catheter facilitated development of a reproducible transarterial procedure (1,3,4). The more recent RetroFlex III catheter incorporates a fixed nosecone for atraumatic passage through the aorta and native valve (Fig. 2). A lower profile RetroFlex 4 delivery system specifically designed to take advantage of the low-profile SAPIEN XT valve is anticipated.

SIZING

Ideally the implanted prosthesis with its fabric seal is completely apposed to the native annular tissue, so as to prevent paravalvular regurgitation. An undersized or underexpanded prosthesis may not provide adequate sealing. Moreover undersizing increases the likelihood of embolization and patient–prosthesis mismatch.

A strategy of routine oversizing appears desirable to minimize paravalvular regurgitation, device embolization, and maximize valve orifice area. However there are limitations to oversizing. First, a larger prosthesis requires a larger diameter catheter system. Consequently, where arterial access is borderline, a smaller valve and delivery system may be desirable to reduce the risk of arterial injury. Second, inability to fully expand an oversized valve in a rigid, calcified annulus may result in suboptimal leaflet coaptation and reduced durability. Most importantly, overdilation of the aortic annulus increases the risk of dissection or rupture of the aortic root. Although rare, the risk may be a greater in patients with extensive calcification.

The current strategy is to oversize when possible by 10% to 20%. An annulus diameter of 18 to 22 mm would be appropriate for a 23-mm valve while an annulus of 21 to 25 mm would be appropriate for a 26-mm valve. These represent general guidelines rather than strict criteria, however, greater degrees of under- or oversizing may be associated with increasing risk of paravalvular regurgitation or aortic root injury.

MEASUREMENT OF THE ANNULUS

Accurate estimation of the annulus diameter is important for selection of the appropriate prosthesis diameter and appropriate patients. Transthoracic echocardiography (TTE) is the routine initial screening imaging modality. However, transesophageal echocardiography (TEE)

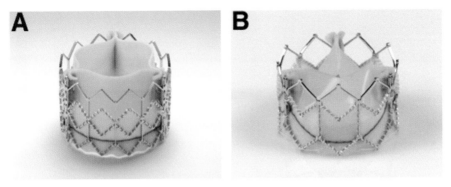

Figure 1 (**A**) Edwards SAPIEN valve. (**B**) Edwards SAPIEN XT valve.

estimates in the long-axis midesophageal view at approximately 120 degrees appear to be more accurate. The annulus is measured in this view as the distance between the basal insertion of the noncoronary and the right coronary leaflets (Fig. 3). Typically, TEE results in an annulus measurement 1 to 2 mm larger than a transthoracic study, although occasionally the discrepancy can be larger (5).

There are several common problems with echocardiographic annular measurements: (*i*) standard measurements of the left ventricular outflow tract should not substitute for annular measurements. (*ii*) Aortic leaflet attachments extend in a crown-like fashion into the larger diameter aortic root. Measurements not obtained at the most basal attachment of the valves may overestimate annular diameter. (*iii*) Suboptimal imaging and blooming may reduce apparent annulus diameter. In addition, there are inherent problems with echocardiographic assessment in that (*i*) the distance from the basal insertion of the noncoronary cusp to the right coronary cusp does not represent a true aortic diameter and (*ii*) long axis echocardiographic measurements evaluate only one axis of an annulus that is more often oval than truly circular.

Aortographic measurements of the aortic annulus have been utilized. However, aortography visualizes the aortic root above the valve, not the area below the leaflets where the prosthesis will be seated. More useful is fluoroscopy or aortography during valvuloplasty. Comparison of the valvuloplasty balloon to the aortic root may occasionally be of help.

Multislice computed tomography (MSCT) offers the advantage of improved two-dimensional visualization of the plane of the annulus (6–8). The annulus is seen to be not so much circular as slightly oval with diameters that vary in long and short axis by 1 to 3 mm. Coronal diameters tend to exceed sagittal diameters. Coronal diameters, which in a very general way correspond with echocardiographic long-axis views, tend to be slightly larger than those reported by TEE. Although MSCT may assume a greater role in the future, currently measurements are not well standardized and clinical correlation is lacking.

Despite the limitations noted above, extensive experience supports echocardiographic estimation of annular diameter as the current clinical standard. TTE is currently used for screening and may be adequate for many patients. Annular diameters measured with TEE are on average 1 to 2 mm larger but differences may be larger and TEE is a much more reliable assessment (5). TEE is particularly desirable in patients where prosthesis sizing is borderline when assessed by TTE.

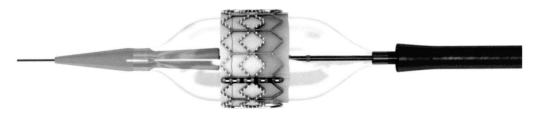

Figure 2 RetroFlex III catheter.

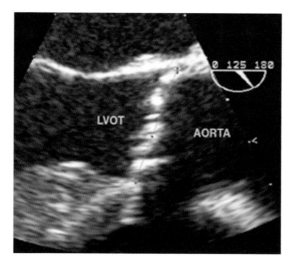

Figure 3 TEE measurement of annular diameter: a parasternal long-axis view is chosen. In a zoomed view, the distance between the basal insertion of the noncoronary and the right coronary leaflets is measured.

IDEAL POSITIONING

The SAPIEN valve is designed to sit within the native valve (9). Ideally, the frame extends superiorly just to the tips of the native leaflets. Any portion of the frame extending above the leaflets serves no specific function as the diameter of the supravalvular aorta exceeds the diameter of the valve frame. Although it is unlikely that the sealing skirt of a valve placed in a functional position could obstruct a coronary ostium, it is rarely possible for a valve strut to overlay and obstruct a coronary ostium. On the other hand, a frame that does not extend to the tips of the leaflets may allow residual native valvular stenosis and may lead to insufficient anchorage of the valve stent.

Ideally the frame extends into the ventricle just enough to provide anchoring and sealing against the subvalvular annulus. Any portion extending further into the outflow tract runs the risk of contact with the mobile portion of the anterior mitral valve leaflet (with the risk of mitral regurgitation) or the interventricular septum (with the risk of heart block). Moreover, a valve positioned too low may leave the sealing skirt unopposed to the subvalvular tissue, resulting in paravalvular regurgitation.

POSITIONING PRIOR TO DEPLOYMENT

Imaging is key to optimal positioning and planning should begin prior to actual positioning of the valve. Since the distribution of calcium varies, it is prudent to spend the time to distinguish whether this is present in the leaflet tips, base or annulus prior to positioning. Accurate valve positioning requires that the plane of the valve is accurately defined. Typically the aortic valve is directed cranially, to the left and slightly anteriorly. Consequently RAO (right anterior oblique) views tend to require caudal angulation and LAO (left anterior oblique) views require cranial angulation to achieve perpendicularity to the valve plane (Figs. 4 and 5). A baseline aortogram is performed. With a pigtail placed directly on the valve, a power injection of 20 mL of contrast over 2 seconds is adequate. Generally an AP–caudal or LAO–cranial view is selected with the valve magnified and centered in the field of view. Aortography is repeated with slight changes in angulation as required, until all three cusps seen in profile in the same horizontal plane. Ideally, identical angulation and magnification will be used at the time of valve positioning.

Introduction and passage of the prosthesis through the native valve are discussed in chapter 12. Once the prosthesis has been delivered into the ventricle, a number of steps must follow in rapid sequence as the catheter system is partly obstructive within the valve orifice. First, the RetroFlex catheter must be withdrawn to reduce obstruction. A pigtail previously placed in the ascending aorta is advanced so as to directly contact the native valve and act as a readily visible landmark. Then the prosthesis is positioned, taking advantage of visible calcification and the pigtail as landmarks. Minor adjustments are made and evaluated by repeated small 5-mL hand injections through the pigtail catheter. If available, TEE or intracardiac echo (ICE) are used to confirm optimal positioning.

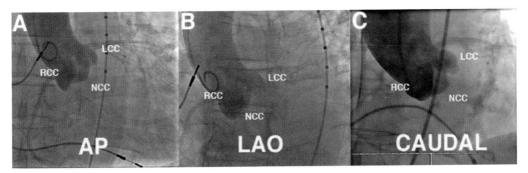

Figure 4 Effect of fluoroscopic angulation on visualization of the valve plane. When all three cusps are similarly visualized, this suggests perpendicularity. *Abbreviations*: RCC, right coronary cusp; LCC, left coronary cusp; NCC, noncoronary cusp.

IDEAL POSITION PRIOR TO DEPLOYMENT

As the deployment balloon and stent valve expand, they move due to a combination of factors. Transaortic flow tends to eject the obstructive balloon. The expanding balloon may contact the outflow tract and move unexpectedly. The expanding prosthesis may move with the native valve leaflets as they are forced outwards and upwards. The net result is typically movement of the prosthesis during deployment in the direction of the aorta, typically this ranges from 1 to 3 mm. Movement may occasionally occur in the opposite direction, toward the ventricle. This occurs when the stent is initially positioned below the native leaflets such that the stent slides down inside them rather than gripping the leaflets and rising with them.

As movement is typically in the direction of the aorta, our practice is to initially position the outflow of the stent just at the tips of the native leaflets while at the same leaving about two-thirds of the stent below the visible plane of leaflet attachment. Achieving both of these goals may not be possible when the stent is short in relation to the diameter of the annulus, where the stent is not coaxial within the annulus, or if the leaflets extend to a peak well above the plane of the valve. Compromise may be necessary.

TEE visualization is a helpful adjunct during positioning (5). Often its contribution is greater in the absence of extensive calcification, just when fluoroscopic imaging becomes less reliable. The value of TEE is highly dependent on the experience of the echocardiographer

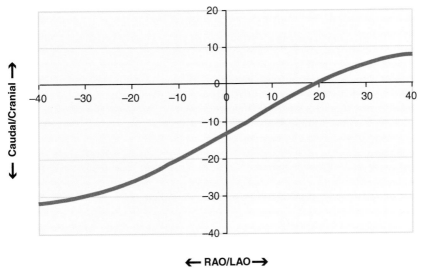

Figure 5 Graph showing a typical line of perpendicularity. In this case AP–caudal or LAO–cranial view might commonly be chosen for visualization of the valve plane during positioning.

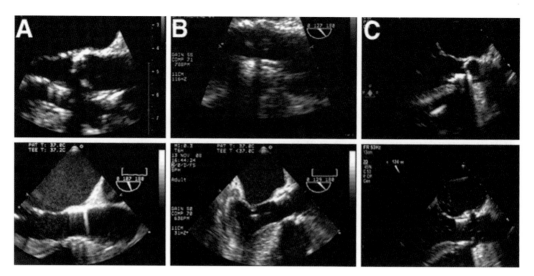

Figure 6   TEE positioning: Columns depicting pre- and postimplantation images. (**A**) Proper valve position. (**B**) Valve position too high (aortic). (**C**) Valve position too low (ventricular).

and the ready accessibility of the images to the operator during positioning. Ideally, echocardiographic images are displayed immediately adjacent to the fluoroscopic images for quick correlation. The three-chamber long-axis view at approximately 120° is typically used during positioning. With training the operator can usually distinguish the ventricular end of the stent with its slightly thicker fabric cuff. The aortic end of the stent may be more difficult to distinguish because of shadowing from the native valve. The ventricular end of the stent should be at the hinge point of the anterior mitral leaflet while the aortic end should just extend to the tips of the leaflet [Fig. 6(A)].

DEPLOYMENT
Rapid ventricular pacing is routinely used at the time of valve deployment to reduce transvalvular flow and cardiac motion (10). A transvenous right ventricular pacemaker is placed and a threshold of less than 1 mA is assured, following which the output is increased to 10 mA to assure reliable capture. Unreliable capture may lead to unexpected movement of the prosthesis during deployment [Fig. 7(A)]. Typically pacing is initiated at ~200/min . If 1:1 capture is not achieved, pacing is terminated (Fig. 7(B) and (C)). After a brief period of recovery the pacing rate is incrementally reduced by 20 beats/min. Typically 1:1 capture is achieved at rates between 160 and 220 beats/min associated with a reduction in systolic pressure to below 60 mm Hg and a marked reduction in pulse pressure (Fig. 8).

It is important to ensure clear communication. We typically follow a protocol where the physician requests "pacer ready," "pacer on," and "pacer off." The pacer operator repeats and immediately implements each request. It is important that pacing be initiated promptly when requested, as the stent may move if there is delay. Once 1:1 capture is assured, a few seconds are

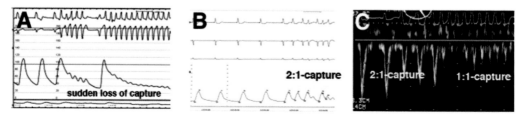

Figure 7   (**A**). Loss of capture during rapid pacing. (**B**) Ineffective rapid pacing due to 2:1 capture. (**C**) Pulsed wave Doppler signal of the left ventricular outflow tract during burst pacing with initial 2:1 capture, followed by effective burst pacing with 1:1 capture.

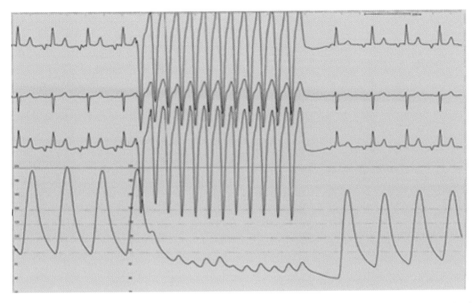

Figure 8 Rapid pacing with an effective drop in blood pressure below 60 mm Hg and marked reduction in pulse pressure amplitude.

allowed to pass to allow pulse pressure to fall, at which time the balloon is rapidly inflated with dilute 10% contrast. When the inflation device is emptied of contrast, the balloon is deflated after 3 seconds of full inflation. Only when the balloon is deflated does the physician request that pacing be stopped. Termination of pacing with the balloon inflated can result in ejection of the occlusive balloon and dislodgement of the stent.

Once the balloon is deflated it is immediately withdrawn into the ascending aorta so as to allow normal valve function. The guidewire is left in place. Adequate positioning is assessed [Figs. 6(A) and 9(A)]. TEE provides rapid assessment of paravalvular regurgitation. If the positioning is adequate and the paravalvular regurgitation not severe, the guidewire is withdrawn. Any valvular regurgitation tends to resolve with removal of the guidewire. Aortography may be performed for final assessment if desired.

It is important to minimize the ischemic stress associated with burst pacing in the setting of aortic stenosis (11,12). Bursts are kept as short as possible (typically under 15 seconds), time is allowed for hemodynamic recovery between pacing episodes, pacing in the presence of hypotension is avoided and vasoconstrictors are used as necessary to maintain coronary perfusion pressure (e.g., 100–200 mg bolues of phenylephrine). Of course, if the prosthesis is positioned and ready for deployment it may be desirable to proceed even in the presence of hypotension.

PARAVALVULAR REGURGITATION

The frequency of paravalvular regurgitation varies with the aggressiveness with which it is looked for. TEE is the most sensitive method and shows some paravalvular regurgitation in most patients. Typically this is trivial or mild, most often adjacent to the anterior mitral leaflet [Fig. 10(A)]. Even if moderate this appears to be well tolerated and without apparent clinical relevance. More severe degrees of paravalvular regurgitation are uncommon, but do occur. The first clue may be a low diastolic pressure or, if very severe, severe systolic hypotension. Aortography may be misleading due to the presence of valvular regurgitation while a guidewire lies across the valve. TEE is very helpful in understanding the severity and etiology of paravalvular regurgitation [Fig. 10(A) and (B)].

If the prosthesis is positioned much too aortic or ventricular implantation of a second overlapping prosthesis may rarely be considered (Fig. 11). More often redilation to assure full expansion of the valve is the initial approach. The deployment balloon is typically used.

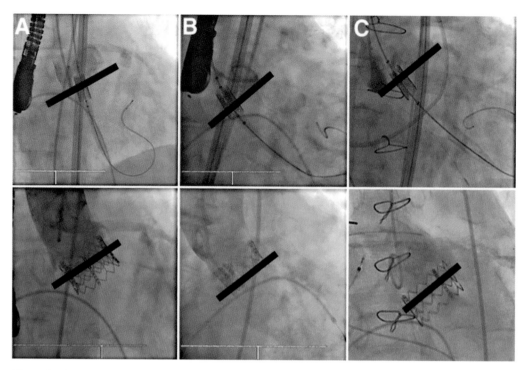

Figure 9 Aortograms postdeployment: Columns depicting pre- and postdeployment position. (**A**) Valve just right. (**B**) Valve too high (aortic). (**C**) Valve too low (ventricular).

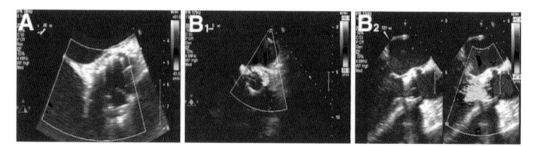

Figure 10 TEE showing trivial (**A**) and severe (**B**) paravalvular leaks. B_1: short axis, B_2: three-chamber long axis.

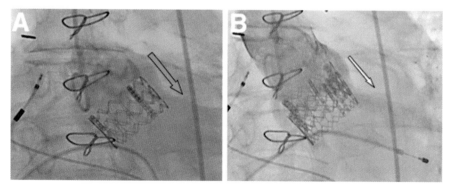

Figure 11 (**A**) Valve implantation too low (ventricular) with severe paravalvular regurgitation. (**B**) Implantation of a second overlapping, but more aortic, valve dramatically reduced regurgitation.

There is no value in the use of a larger balloon as the fabric-sealing cuff will not dilate beyond the nominal diameter. In most cases, redilation will result in a reduction in regurgitation. Although valve injury and dislodgement are potential concerns these have not been observed.

SUPRANNULAR POSITIONING
This is the most common positioning error [Figs. 6(B) and 9(B)]. As long as the stent is fixed in place the major concern is failure of adequate apposition of the fabric cuff in the annulus, resulting in paravalvular regurgitation. Redilation can be considered; however, if regurgitation is severe, the only effective option may be to implant a second valve within the first but positioned slightly lower, so as to extend the fabric seal into the outflow tract. This can be highly effective.

EMBOLIZATION
Embolization may occur at the time of implantation if the prosthesis is deployed too aortic such that neither the subvalvular annulus nor the native leaflets provide adequate fixation. Late embolization has not been observed. The frequency of embolization has fallen dramatically with improved understanding of positioning and deployment (13).

The embolized valve tends to float in the ascending aorta. Only if the guidewire is pulled back does the valve flip over and become obstructive. Prompt implantation of an aortic stent may be necessary to hold the obstructive leaflets open. As long as coaxial position of the guidewire is obtained the valve is not obstructive and management can be more leisurely and considered. A valvuloplasty balloon is advanced over the guidewire and inflated to low pressure within the prosthesis after which both are withdrawn as a unit to a point in the transverse or descending aorta, where the prosthesis can be overdilated and fixed in place. As long as the fabric cuff does not overly a sidebranch and aortic atheroembolism does not occur from this maneuver, the long-term consequences appear relatively benign.

CORONARY OBSTRUCTION
This is a rare complication, occurring in ~1% of patients (1). A sudden drop in blood pressure and acute heart failure immediately after stent deployment may be due to acute obstruction of the left main coronary. This typically occurs when the native left leaflet is sandwiched between the stent and the left coronary ostium [Fig. 12(A)]. In approximately half of the population, the length of the left coronary cusp exceeds the distance from the annulus to the ostium of the left coronary artery (6). Percutaneous coronary intervention with stenting of the left main through the valve-stent struts has been successful [Fig. 12(B) and 12(C)]. Alternatively, open-heart bypass surgery might be an option. So far, no data on chronic obstruction of coronary ostia are reported.

SUBANNULAR POSITIONING
With current implantation techniques subannular positioning is uncommon. The first clue to this is typically fluoroscopic visualization of the stent descending as it slides under the native leaflets, rather than riding up with them. If the native leaflets extend far above the valve there

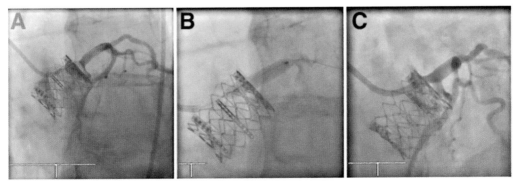

Figure 12 (**A**) Coronary obstruction by the native leaflet sandwiched between the aortic wall and the valve stent. (**B**) Stenting of the left coronary ostium through the stent-struts. (**C**) Final result after stenting.

may be residual stenosis. If the fabric-sealing skirt does not appose the outflow tract, there may be paravalvular regurgitation. Modest degrees of either may be tolerated, but on occasion hemodynamic instability may occur. Immediate implantation of a second valve within the first but positioned slightly higher may be a very effective option (Fig. 11). If, however, the stent is so ventricular as to interfere with the mitral valve or ventricular function, surgical removal may be the only option.

SUMMARY

Implantation of the Edwards SAPIEN valve can be a relatively reliable procedure with excellent clinical outcomes. Critical assessment and planning, optimal imaging, an experienced team and attention to detail are the elements of success.

REFERENCES

1. Webb JG, Pasupati S, Humphries K, et al. Percutaneous transarterial aortic valve replacement in selected high-risk patients with aortic stenosis. Circulation 2007; 116:755–763.
2. Webb JG, Altwegg L, Masson JB, et al. A new transcatheter aortic valve and percutaneous valve delivery system. J Am Coll Cardiol 2009; 53(20):1855–1858.
3. Webb JG, Chandavimol M, Thompson CR, et al. Percutaneous aortic valve implantation retrograde from the femoral artery. Circulation 2006; 113:842–850.
4. Eltchaninoff H, Zajarias A, Tron C, et al. Transcatheter aortic valve implantation: Technical aspects, results and indications. Arch Cardiovasc Dis 2008; 101:126–132.
5. Moss RR, Ivens E, Pasupati S, et al. Role of echocardiography in percutaneous aortic valve implantation. JACC Cardiovasc Imaging 2008; 1:15.
6. Tops LF, Wood DA, Delgado V, et al. Noninvasive evaluation of the aortic root with multislice computed tomography implications for transcatheter aortic valve replacement. JACC Cardiovasc Imaging 2008; 1:321–330.
7. Wood DA, Tops LF, Mayo JR, et al. Role of multislice computed tomography in transcatheter aortic valve replacement. Al J Cardiol 2009; 103(9):1295–1301.
8. Leipsic J, Wood D, Manders D, et al. The evolving role of MDCT in transcatheter aortic valve replacement: A radiologist's perspective. AJR Am J Roentgenol 2009; 193(3):W214–W219.
9. Piazza N, Jaegere P, Schultz C, et al. Anatomy of the aortic valvar complex and its implications for transcatheter implantation of the aortic valve. Circ Cardiovasc Intervent 2008; 1:74–81.
10. Webb JG, Pasupati S, Achtem L, et al. Rapid pacing to facilitate transcatheter prosthetic heart valve implantation. Catheter Cardiovasc Interv 2006; 68:199–204.
11. Ree RM, Bowering JB, Schwarz SK. Case series: Anesthesia for retrograde percutaneous aortic valve replacement—Experience with the first 40 patients. Can J Anaesth 2008; 55:761–768.
12. Walther T, Dewey T, Borger MA, et al. Transapical aortic valve implantation: Step by step. Ann Thorac Surg 2009; 87:276–283.
13. Al Ali AM, Altwegg L, Horlick EM, et al. Prevention and management of transcatheter balloon-expandable aortic valve malposition. Catheter Cardiovasc Interv 2008; 72:573–578.

19 | Transapical Aortic Valve Implantation—Procedural Steps

Thomas Walther and Jörg Kempfert

Universität Leipzig, Herzzentrum, Klinik für Herzchirurgie, Leipzig, Germany

Todd Dewey

Heartcenter, Medical City, Dallas, Texas, U.S.A.

INTRODUCTION

Conventional aortic valve replacement surgery is a standard and safe procedure for many patients with symptomatic aortic stenosis. However, in elderly patients suffering from relevant comorbidities, the operative risk may be increased. Some of these patients are deferred treatment due to a perceived high risk. New minimally invasive transcatheter techniques aim at reducing the risk of conventional aortic valve replacement while attempting to keep up with the excellent outcomes of conventional surgery.

Transapical (TA) aortic valve implantation (AVI) is—besides the transfemoral (TF) approach—one of these new transcatheter techniques to treat such patients with symptomatic aortic stenosis who have an increased risk profile. The goal is to treat patients by using a minimally invasive, off-pump approach. The left ventricular apex is reached through a left anterolateral mini-thoracotomy for direct antegrade AVI. Feasibility of TA-AVI has been proven by recent clinical studies (1–3). At present TA-AVI has been performed at more than 50 different centers in several countries. As of February 2009, the total number of patients treated by means of minimally invasive TA-AVI is above 500. The Edwards SAPIEN (Edwards Lifesciences, Inc., Irvine, California) transcatheter heart valve has been granted CE approval for transapical implantation using the Ascendra delivery system (Edwards Lifesciences, Inc., Irvine, California). Another device, the Ventor Embracer (Medtronic Inc., St. Paul, Minnesota) technology, is currently undergoing an initial feasibility study for transapical implantation. Due to the current availability of only preliminary results for the Ventor-Medtronic valve, this article will focus exclusively on the Edwards SAPIEN prosthesis.

PATIENT SCREENING

Patients with symptomatic, severe aortic stenosis (AS), and high surgical risk should be considered candidates for transcatheter AVI and specifically TA-AVI at present (4,5). High surgical risk can be defined as a logistic EuroScore calculated risk of mortality $\geq$ 15%, STS score risk of mortality $\geq$ 10% or presence of other comorbidities rendering conventional aortic valve surgery difficult, such as a porcelain aorta, previous cardiac surgery with presence of patent grafts or severe adhesions, previous radiation therapy, liver cirrhosis, need to avoid sternotomy due to patient immobilization, or marked patient frailty. Risk assessment should be performed individually for each patient with the recognition that risk scoring systems are helpful, but not completely comprehensive. The logistic EuroScore is known to overestimate the individual's risk, therefore a strategy of dividing the logistic EuroScore by three, even though not yet scientifically tested, may render a good estimate for potential outcome.

Patients who are referred with symptomatic aortic stenosis should be evaluated first whether they are fit enough to undergo any type of procedure or whether they are moribund, which may lead to a conclusion that no invasive therapy (besides medical management) should be performed.

Patients scheduled for TA-AVI should undergo similar screening as all other patients scheduled for conventional cardiac surgery. This includes standard preoperative testing, particularly echocardiography to exclude other significant lesions requiring intervention. Concomitant mitral regurgitation is frequently present in elderly patients with severe AS, but should

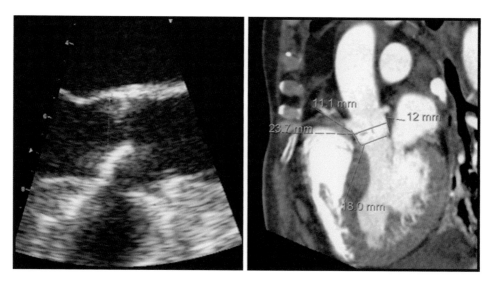

Figure 1   Measurement of the aortic annulus by using TEE and of aortic root geometry by using CT.

not be considered as a contraindication to AVI unless it is severe or unless there is structural disease of the mitral valve leaflets. Carotid ultrasound should be performed to exclude significant carotid stenosis and cardiac catheterization to rule out significant coronary artery disease (CAD). In the presence of relevant CAD, a conventional surgical approach with combined coronary artery bypass grafting and aortic valve replacement should be reconsidered; alternatively preoperative coronary stent placement followed by TA-AVI or combined MIDCAB plus TA-AVI, depending on the individual situation, are suitable options.

Delineation of the aortic root geometry is essential before performing TA-AVI. Transesophageal echocardiography (TEE) is the most reliable tool to measure the diameter of the aortic root (mid-esophageal long-axis view) as well as to evaluate the amount and pattern of calcification of the native aortic valve cusps (short axis). The diameter of the aortic annulus is measured, including all cusp calcifications, at mid-systole from the insertion of the right coronary cusp at the junction between interventricular septum, aortic annulus, and aortic root and the insertion of the noncoronary cusp just opposite at the junction between the anterior mitral leaflet, aortic annulus, and aortic root (Fig. 1). Three repetitive measurements with midline imaging of the aortic root should be performed. Three-dimensional TEE may be helpful to be able to measure in the exact plane to avoid undersizing of the annulus. Valve size selection is based on TEE measurements and an oversizing of approximately 10% should be performed to obtain sufficient pressure to anchor the transcatheter valve inside the aortic annulus. To obtain sufficient oversizing, patients with an aortic annulus diameter ≤ 21 mm usually are scheduled to receive a 23-mm prosthesis and patients with an aortic annulus diameter between 22 and 24 mm are scheduled to receive a 26-mm prosthesis. A larger 29 mm valve is currently under development and will allow patients with an annular diameter of up to 27 mm to be treated in the near future. Some oversizing is essential to avoid severe paravalvular leakage. However, in presence of a rigid aortic root aggressive oversizing should be avoided.

Aortic root dimensions may also be measured during initial cardiac catheterization, but this method is not as sensitive as TEE. Computerized tomography (CT) is another method of determining the width of the aortic annulus and has the added ability of measuring the distance from the aortic annulus to the coronary ostia (Fig. 1).

Although the right coronary orifice is usually higher than the left and therefore not at risk of obstruction, the inferior aspect of the left coronary orifice should be 10 to 12 mm from the aortic annulus especially if heavy eccentric calcification is present in the left cusp. If such a situation is present, consideration can be given to placement of a guidewire in the left coronary artery prior to valve deployment.

HYBRID OR SETUP

TA-AVI should ideally be performed in a hybrid operative theatre. This includes full opera-tive capabilities including the availability of cardiopulmonary bypass (usually on stand-by) if required and with laminar air flow for an optimal hygienic standard. In addition optimal imaging by means of a high-quality fixed fluoroscopic system equivalent to that of a cardiac catheterization laboratory with a large image intensifier and immediate replay capability is required. If such a room is not available, it is advisable to convert a large cardiac catheterization room into an operative setting than vice versa, since AVI is being performed without direct vision and thus optimal imaging quality is the most crucial factor for success. Optimally, the imaging arm should come from the right side of the patient to allow maximal access to the left side for the surgical team. Placement of monitors on both sides of the patient including a slave monitor on the right side allows for optimal visualization for the whole team. Expertise in TEE is helpful both for determination of valve positioning and evaluation of postdeploy-ment ventricular function and possible paravalvular leaks. Besides anesthetist, cardiologist, and cardiac surgeon further team members should include those with expertise in catheteriza-tion equipment, a surgical scrub team, and a perfusionist. Future advanced imaging modalities will revolve around three-dimensional visualization, including online three-dimensional TEE, and online Dyna-CT to improve the periprocedural visualization of the aortic root anatomy and dimensions.

OPERATIVE PROCEDURE STEP BY STEP

The TA approach takes advantage of the close proximity of the fifth or sixth intercostal space and the apex of the left ventricle. By using an anterolateral mini-thoracotomy the apex can be approached directly. Pursestring sutures are used to secure the apex during antegrade placement of wires and a delivery sheath. There is no real limitation for sheath diameter and ventricular function is well preserved after the TA approach (2). Current outcomes are favorable in high-risk, elderly patients (3). TA-AVI includes several procedural steps as indicated in Table 1.

Table 1   Transapical (TA) Aortic Valve Implantation (AVI): Procedural Steps

		Figure
a.	Measurement of the aortic annulus by using routine transesophageal echo (and eventually additional CT scan) to perform valve size selection.	1
b.	Placement of femoral arterial sheath, aortic root pigtail catheter, and femoral venous wire as a safety net.	2
c.	Anterolateral mini-thoracotomy in the sixth/fifth intercostal space to obtain access to the left ventricular apex, pericardiotomy, and stay sutures.	2
d.	Placement of two pledget reinforced apical pursestring sutures (Prolene 2–0) and an epicardial pacing wire.	3
e.	Preparation of the application catheter and crimping of the valve under sterile conditions, all steps performed in parallel to the surgical steps.	4
f.	Apical puncture followed by antegrade placement of a soft and later on superstiff guidewire across the stenotic aortic valve and the aortic arch into the descending aorta.	5
g.	Balloon valvuloplasty of the native aortic valve during a brief episode of rapid ventricular pacing.	6
h.	Insertion of the 26-F introducer sheath and positioning of the crimped valve inside the aortic annulus.	7,8
i.	Valve implantation during another short episode of rapid ventricular pacing.	9
k.	Functional control of the implanted aortic valve prosthesis using transesophageal echo and aortic root angiography.	10
l.	Routine closure of the access site.	
m.	Early extubation of the patient in PACU unit.	

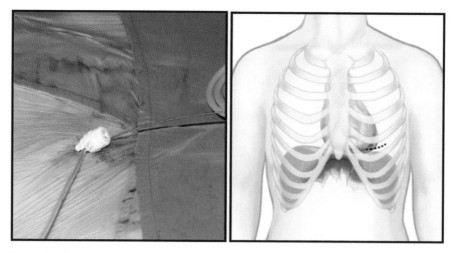

Figure 2   Femoral guidewires (safety net) and lateral minithoracotomy.

The patient is positioned supine with slightly elevated left chest. Femoral vascular access are placed using a femoral venous wire and an arterial sheath; this allows for fast cannulation and connection to cardiopulmonary bypass if required (safety net) (Fig. 2). A pigtail catheter is placed from the femoral arterial sheath into the aortic root for angiography during the procedure. Heparin is given at a dose of approximately 100 IU/kg aiming at an activated clotting time of 300 seconds.

An anterolateral mini-thoracotomy is performed in the midclavicular line fifth or possibly sixth intercostal space aiming at a straight approach to the apex (Fig. 2). Usually the direction is toward the right shoulder of the patient.

After a longitudinal pericardiotomy and stay sutures the apex is exposed, regular ventilation can be maintained and there is no need for double lumen intubation. An epicardial pacing wire is placed and tested. Two apical pursestring sutures [Prolene 2–0, large (MH) needle with 5 interrupted Teflon pledgets] are placed lateral to the LAD with sufficiently deep bites (approximately 3–5 mm, not penetrating completely) into the myocardium (Fig. 3). The fatty tissue immediately at the apex is avoided and the sutures are placed slightly more anterior.

In parallel to these surgical steps the application catheter system is prepared, the valve rinsed (three times for one minute) and then crimped upon the application catheter (Fig. 4).

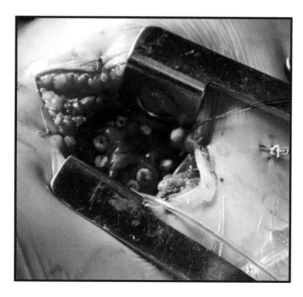

Figure 3   Left ventricular apical pursestring sutures (Prolene 2–0) with Teflon reinforcement.

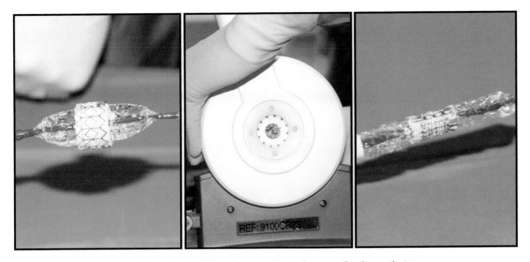

Figure 4   Crimping of the Edwards SAPIEN valve upon the balloon application catheter.

Care is taken for positioning the valve in the correct antegrade orientation upon the catheter. Crimping is performed inside the operative theatre under sterile conditions. Training of one of the team members, for example, the pump technician, is helpful.

Following these preparatory steps the fluoroscopic system is positioned perpendicular to the annulus, usually this is achieved at angulations between AP and LAO ~10° and cranial ~10° position. Further adjustment can be performed once the crimped valve is at the annular level and after angiography. All further steps are performed in close cooperation with the anesthetist. Prior to valvuloplasty completely stable baseline hemodynamics are critical to ensure hemodynamic stability through the rest of the procedure including the two episodes of rapid ventricular pacing. Volume loading and low-dose inotropes (usually norepinephrine) may be required to keep the mean blood pressure above 80 mm Hg.

The apex is punctured and a soft guidewire inserted antegrade across the stenotic aortic valve, followed by a soft tip 14 F (30-cm long) sheath. A superstiff guidewire (Amplatz superstiff, 260 cm) is then positioned into the descending aorta with the help of a right Judkins catheter (Fig. 5). This minimizes any manipulation in the aortic arch that might embolize atheromatous debris. Valvuloplasty is performed using a 20 mm balloon that is filled with 1:4 diluted contrast

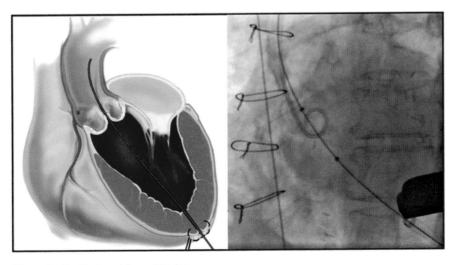

Figure 5   Positioning of the guidewire.

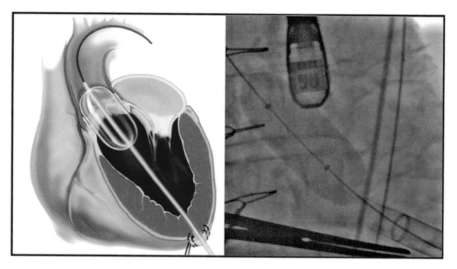

Figure 6   Balloon valvuloplasty of the stenosed aortic valve.

during a brief episode of rapid ventricular pacing (RVP) between 170/min and 220/min (Fig. 6) (Video 1). RVP is used for temporary cessation of left ventricular ejection. The balloon catheter is immediately retrieved together with the 14-F sheath and the 26-F transapical delivery sheath is inserted bluntly (5–6 cm on the external indicators) over the stiff wire and then its introducer retrieved. The crimped valve is inserted over the wire after checking for proper antegrade orientation, connected to the sheath with the loader before de-airing the system. The valve is introduced into the annulus and the pusher retrieved.

Valve positioning is performed under angiographic guidance aiming at implanting one-third (maximum one-half) of the stent above and the other two-thirds (minimum one-half) below the level of the aortic annulus (Fig. 7) (Video 2). Once in good position, online fluoroscopic imaging should be performed until valve implantation. Slight axial movement should be counter-acted. An extra episode of RVP may be required to confirm optimal positioning. Valve orientation should be in line (coaxial) with the long axis of the ascending aorta and just perpendicular to the aortic annulus, optimally in the middle of the aortic annulus or more laterally. Adjustments with the wire may correct for an oblique position of the valve: Pushing the wire slightly inward

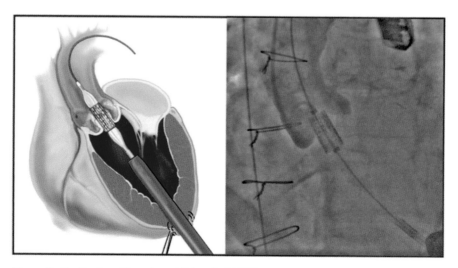

Figure 7   Positioning of the crimped Edwards SAPIEN prosthesis in the aortic annulus, approximately one-third above and two-thirds below.

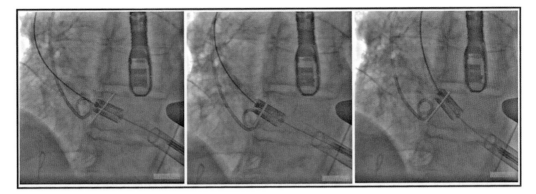

Figure 8 Perpendicular orientation of the crimped valve inside the aortic annulus (*middle*), and oblique orientations (*left* and *right*), depending on the tension on the wire. For further explanation see text.

(thereby producing slack) leads to a more rightward position in the annulus while pulling back on the wire (thereby tightening it) leads to a more leftward position of the valve in the aortic annulus (Fig. 8). In addition, inward and outward motions can be performed relatively easily.

Repeat RVP is used for valve implantation (Fig. 9) (Video 3). To confirm exact valve position immediately prior to balloon inflation, valve implantation should be performed as follows: a stable hemodynamic situation should be obtained, optimally aiming at a mean arterial pressure of 80 mm Hg. Then rapid pacing is initiated. As soon as there is no ventricular output contrast injection is performed to visualize the aortic root and to confirm the position of the crimped valve in a subcoronary position inside the aortic annulus. The valve can then be implanted either by a controlled slightly stepwise balloon inflation or a more rapid inflation technique to immediately fix the position of the valve in the annulus. After balloon deflation, rapid pacing is discontinued. This episode should usually take only 10 to 15 seconds and can be tolerated well by most patients. After deflation the balloon is retrieved and regular cardiac function usually recovers. Valve function is assessed using TEE and root angiography (Fig. 10) (Video 4). The wire is retrieved in case of good valve function, the sheath removed and the apex closed using the pursestring sutures. Repeat dilatation can be useful in individual situations but should be avoided in others as indicated in Table 2.

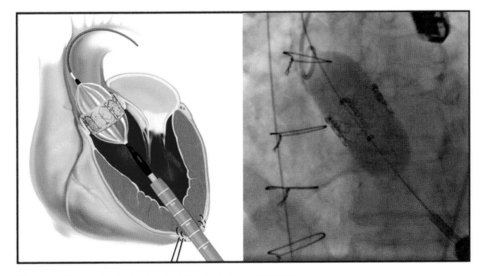

Figure 9 Transapical valve implantation by balloon dilatation.

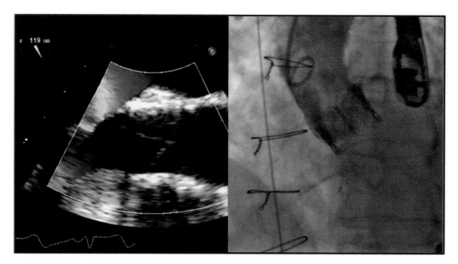

Figure 10   Angiographic and echocardiographic control after valve implantation showing patent coronary arteries and good aortic valve function.

At the end of the procedure Protamine is administered and the pericardium is slightly closed. A pleural chest drain is inserted, the incision controlled for bleeding, local anesthetic injected, and the chest wall closed in a routine fashion. The patient can undergo early extubation in the postanesthetic care unit and is transferred to intermediate care afterwards.

POSTOPERATIVE CARE

Postoperative care is important for all patients. The older the patient and the more complex the comorbidities, the more intense postoperative care needs to be. We usually attempt very early extubation. Close monitoring of hemodynamic function is mandatory. Renal function requires special attention because the patients receive contrast agent during the procedures. Aortic valve implantation using an oversizing technique while leaving the native calcified aortic valve cusps in situ may be responsible for the occurrence of late AV block in some patients. Therefore close monitoring for 5 days together with holter ECG has to be recommended. Besides these aspects patients receiving TA-AVI will require the same type of care as other patients after conventional aortic valve replacement.

COMPLICATIONS, SOLUTIONS, AND BAIL OUT

TA-AVI is a minimally invasive off-pump procedure that usually proceeds in a straightforward fashion. However, unpredictable events with serious hemodynamic consequences can occur at any time.

Hemodynamic compromise may occur after balloon dilatation or after valve insertion, which may require immediate conversion from the off-pump to an on-pump technique. Cannulation for CPB can usually be safely accomplished using the existing femoral access. Further

Table 2   Indications for Postdilatation After Transcatheter AVI of a Balloon Inflatable Device and Circumstances to Rather Avoid Postdilatation

Consider postdilatation	Rather avoid postdilatation
Paravalvular leak	Central leak
Regular coronaries	Calcium close to coronaries
Stable hemodynamics	Unstable hemodynamics
	Porcelain aorta

diagnostic (valve and coronary function) and therapeutic interventions (repeat valve dilatation, percutaneous transluminal angioplasty (PTCA), etc.) can then be performed.

Details on the optimal straight alignment between the apical sheath, the superstiff guidewire and the aorta have been previously mentioned. Repositioning may be required in case of an oblique angle or if the wire is accidentally caught in the mitral valve apparatus. TEE is helpful for diagnosing this latter problem.

Paravalvular leak usually is minimal when using moderate oversizing of the implanted valves. It has been infrequently necessary to perform postdilatation of the valve prosthesis because of a paravalvular leak.

Coronary obstruction is fortunately a rare complication of this procedure. Additional coronary artery bypass grafting or PTCA plus stent implantation are useful therapeutic options, depending on the severity of obstruction and the individual situation.

Severe valve dysfunction is uncommon but can occur either due to intrinsic prosthetic valve leaflet dysfunction or due to low placement of the stented valve, resulting in overhang of the native leaflet tissue and subsequent insufficient back pressure to close all of the leaflets during diastole. This problem may be solved by implanting a second valve (partially) inside the first one ("valve-in-valve" implantation). Valve embolization retrograde into the ventricle requires conversion to a conventional surgical technique.

Excessive bleeding from the apex is rare after the transapical approach. If it occurs, additional Teflon-reinforced sutures should be used. Arterial blood pressure should be lowered during pursestring closure, and can be accomplished pharmacologically or with repeat RVP.

Tear or rupture of the aortic root has been infrequently observed and requires conversion to a conventional aortic valve replacement with repair of the tear or a complete root replacement operation.

Excessive motion of the balloon during inflation may occur due to several factors: axial motion of the heart (usually in patients with a good ejection fraction), a small sinotubular junction leading to valvular "downshift," or a prosthetic mitral valve leading to an "upshift." These movements of the balloon should be carefully watched for during balloon valvuloplasty.

OVERVIEW OF RESULTS

Current results are highly dependent on patient selection, technical equipment, and center experience. Patient selection is the most important aspect, especially when comparing the outcomes of TF versus TA-AVI. However, no randomized clinical trial is available at present. Patient selection strategies may vary. Some centers apply a "TF-first" strategy; this will definitely lead to worse outcomes in the TA cohorts, which can be explained by higher patient complexities in presence of peripheral vascular disease.

Current results indicate that 30-day survival above 90% can be anticipated in high-risk elderly patients with a logistic EuroScore above 20% with TA-AVI.

The obvious strengths of the TA approach are the avoidance of the femoral arteries as well as a very low stroke risk due to minimal manipulations in the aortic arch. Therefore this approach should be chosen in all patients with questionable or borderline femoral access vessels and in those with severe calcifications of the aorta. As peripheral vascular disease is a major risk factor in elderly patients this has to be kept in mind whenever comparing transapical to TF results at any later stage.

Current results of transcatheter aortic valve implantations, by using the retrograde TF or the antegrade transapical (TA) approach are summarized in Table 3. We all have to keep in mind that these techniques are relatively new and that further developments such as further improved imaging and setup, improved team interactions, optimized bail-out procedures, and further technical developments will occur. This will certainly lead to improved outcomes in the future. A prospectively randomized trial, however, is required before applying these promising techniques to younger patients (6).

In summary TA-AVI is a truly minimally invasive procedure that can be performed using a standardized approach (14). TA-AVI allows for precise beating heart off-pump and thus minimally invasive aortic valve implantation in high-risk patients at present.

Table 3 Overview of Literature Results

Author	Year	Access	Device	Patients (n)	Logistic EuroSCORE [%]	30-day Mortality (%)	Stroke (%)	Study design, (reference)
Cribier	2006	TF	CE	27	~ 27%	22.2	3.7	SC (7)
Grube	2006	TF	CV	25	11	20	12	SC (8)
Lichtenstein	2006	TA	CE	7	35	14	none	SC, com-passionate use (1)
Grube	2007	TF	CV	86	21.5	12	10	MC (9)
Webb	2007	TF	ES	50	28	12	4	SC, selected patients (10)
Walther	2007	TA	ES	30	27	10	none	SC, all comers (2)
Walther	2007	TA	ES	59	27	13.6	3.4	MC (3)
Walther	2008	TA	ES	50	28	8	none	SC, all comers (11)
Svensson	2008	TA	ES	40	35.5	17.5	none	MC, US feasibility (12)
Piazza	2008	TF	CV	646	23	8	0.6	MC, Registry data (13)

Abbreviations: TF, transfemoral; TA, transapical; CE, Cribier–Edwards; CV, CoreValve; ES, Edwards SAPIEN; SC, single center; MC, multicenter.

REFERENCES

1. Lichtenstein SV, Cheung A, Ye J, et al. Transapical transcatheter aortic valve implantation in humans: Initial clinical experience Circulation 2006; 114:591–596.
2. Walther T, Falk V, Borger MA, et al. Minimally invasive transapical beating heart aortic valve implantation – proof of concept. Eur J Cardiothorac Surg 2007; 31:9–15.
3. Walther T, Simon P, Dewey T, et al. Transapical minimally invasive aortic valve implantation: Multicenter experience. Circulation 2007; 116(suppl I):I240–I245.
4. Bonow RO, Carabello BA, Chatterjee K. ACC/AHA 2006 Guidelines for the management of patients with valvular heart disease: Executive summary. Circulation 2006; 114:450–527.
5. Vahanian A, Alfieri O, Al-Attar N, et al. Transcatheter valve implantation for patients with aortic stenosis: A position statement from the European Association of Cardio-Thoracic Surgery (EACTS) and the European Society of Cardiology (ESC), in collaboration with the European Association of Percutaneous Cardiovascular Interventions (EAPCI). Eur Heart J 2008; 29:1463–1470.
6. Walther T, Chu MWA, Mohr FW. Transcatheter aortic valve implantation: Time to expand? Curr Opin Cardiol 2008; 23:111–116.
7. Cribier A, Eltchaninoff H, Tron C, et al. Treatment of calcific aortic stenosis with the percutaneous heart valve: Mid-term follow-up from the initial feasibility studies: the French experience. J Am Coll Cardiol 2006; 47:1214–1223.
8. Grube E, Laborde JC, Gerckens U, et al. Percutaneous implantation of the CoreValve self-expanding valve prosthesis in high risk patients with aortic valve disease. The Siegburg first-in-man study Circulation 2006; 114:1616–1624.
9. Grube E, Schuler G, Buellesfeld L, et al. Percutaneous aortic valve replacement for severe aortic stenosis in high risk patients using the second- and current third- generation self-expanding CoreValve prosthesis. Device success and 30-day clinical outcome. J Am Coll Cardiol 2007; 50:69–76.
10. Webb JG, Pasupati S, Humphries K, et al. Percutaneous transarterial aortic valve replacement in selected high-risk patients with aortic stenosis. Circulation 2007; 116:755–763.
11. Walther T, Falk V, Kempfert J, et al. Transapical minimally invasive aortic valve implantation—the initial 50 patients. Eur J Cardiothorac Surg 2008; 33:983–988.
12. Svensson LG, Dewey T, Kapadia S, et al. United States feasibility study of transcatheter insertion of a stented aortic valve by the left ventricular apex. Ann Thorac Surg 2008; 86(1):46–54; discussion 54–55.
13. Piazza N, Grube E, Gerckens U, et al. Procedural and 30-day outcomes following transcatheter aortic valve implantation using the third generation (18 F) CoreValve ReValving system: Results from the multicentre, expanded evaluation registry 1-year following CE mark approval. EuroIntervention 2008; 4:242–249.
14. Walther T, Dewey T, Borger MA, et al. Transapical aortic valve implantation (TA-AVI): Step by step. Ann Thorac Surg 2009; 87:276–283.

20 | Complications at the Time of Transcatheter Aortic Valve Implantation

Jean-Claude Laborde
Cardiology Department, Glenfield Hospital, Leicester, U.K.

Sabine Bleiziffer and Rüdiger Lange
Clinic for Cardiovascular Surgery, German Heart Center Munich, Munich, Germany

INTRODUCTION

Complications at the time of transcatheter aortic valve implantation (TAVI) can be classified as cardiac or noncardiac complications. Furthermore, some of these complications may be or may not be particular to TAVI such as valve malposition, paravalvular aortic regurgitation, and coronary obstruction in some cases or vascular access complications, cardiac perforation/tamponade, respectively. Proper patient selection is essential to maintain a heightened awareness for possible complications that may occur during particular steps of the procedure. Operators must have an in-depth knowledge of the implantation technique and be familiar with techniques and materials required for bail-out procedures. In addition, each hospital should identify a heart team (specifically, an interventional cardiologist and cardiac surgeon)—this is crucial for a successful outcome and management of potential complications that may arise during implantation of the CoreValve ReValving system.

CARDIAC COMPLICATIONS

Valve Malposition

Deployment of the CoreValve prosthesis is performed in a controlled and step-wise manner. Having said that, valve positioning remains one of the most challenging steps of the procedure—even after all necessary precautions have been considered, valve malposition may still occur. Only in rare and extreme instances does malposition actually jeopardize the hemodynamic status of the patient.

Correct evaluation for the degree of malposition is best evaluated using either transesophageal echocardiogrpahy or contrast angiography. A minimum of 20 mL of contrast media should be used to best appreciate the position of the prosthesis relative to the "aortic valve annulus" (i.e., at the level of the basal attachment line of the native aortic valve leaflets).

Normally, the CoreValve prosthesis should be positioned approximately 4 to 8 mm below the aortic valve annulus.

A "too low" implantation is defined as the distal edge of the valve frame (commonly referred to as the "inflow" aspect) positioned more than 12 mm below the annulus, into the left ventricular outflow tract (LVOT). This can be estimated with quantitative angiographic techniques using a graduated pigtail for calibration or by noting the number of joints or cells that lie below the aortic valve annulus.

A "too high" implantation is defined as the inflow aspect positioned above the annulus level.

Low Implantation

Except in cases of severe left ventricular hypertrophy, a low implantation is generally associated with moderate (grade II) to severe (grades III–IV) degrees of aortic regurgitation (AR) on contrast aortography. Transesophageal echocardiography can confirm the nature of the regurgitation (i.e., paravalvular vs. central).

The anecdotal and extremely rare association between moderate to severe mitral regurgitation observed by postimplant transesophageal echocardiography and a relatively "low" implant is likely related to shifts in hemodynamic parameters (e.g., left ventricular afterload) as opposed to anatomical considerations such as impingement of the anterior mitral valve leaflet by the inflow portion of the CoreValve prosthesis.

In the case of too-low positioning associated with significant aortic regurgitation and hemodynamic instability, the first objective would be to (a) manually reposition the valve by using a "goose-neck" catheter. If unsuccessful, the second option to consider is (b) implantation of a second valve inside the first one (i.e., valve-in-valve technique) but positioned slightly higher.

Primary Recommendation: the "Lasso" Technique
Description of the Lasso technique
The choice of projection on fluoroscopy is crucial and is dictated by the valve frame that should be aligned as perfectly as possible. In other words, the distal edges of the inflow portion of the valve should be aligned in one plane. This will provide a reliable reference line when repositioning the valve.

Advance and position a 0.035 guidewire inside the noncoronary sinus with the use of a 5-F multipurpose catheter to serve as a landmark for the annulus particularly in cases of poorly or noncalcified aortic valves. Advance a regular 20 to 35 mm goose-neck catheter alone or through a 7-F guiding catheter to engage one of the "loops" of the implanted valve. At this stage it is critical to understand that the success of this maneuver is dependent upon applying torsion to the frame ("unscrewing the valve") rather than applying direct axial force (which frequently results in ejection of the valve into the ascending aorta). It is for this reason that the simultaneous use of two goose-neck catheters is strongly discouraged.

Note: Success of this maneuver is largely dependent on the relative position of the frame loops within the patient's anatomy. Ideal position of the loops is in the anterior and posterior location on the AP projection (Fig. 1). The worst position is when one loop lies on the external curve of the ascending aorta (almost unreachable with the goose-neck catheter.) The other loop is easy to engage with the goose-neck catheter but it is impossible to apply anything other than axial force to the valve frame (Fig. 2).

Upon loop engagement, apply gentle and slowly increasing torsion/traction to the goose-neck catheter under constant fluoroscopic guidance. At this intermediate stage, it is not rare to reach a level of traction where one feels the heartbeat throughout the entire length of the catheter.

Next, apply quick, short, and intermittent torsion/traction movements to the goose-neck catheter and gradually increase force until mobilization of the valve in a more satisfactory position is achieved. Depending of the degree of visualization of the anatomy under fluoroscopy,

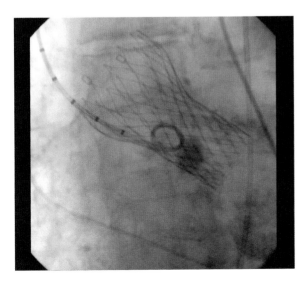

Figure 1 A left anterior oblique projection demonstrating the loading hooks of CoreValve in the anterior-posterior orientation. Goose neck snaring of loading hooks feasible.

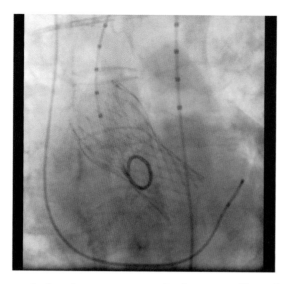

Figure 2 A left anterior oblique projection demonstrating the loading hooks of the CoreValve along the short and greater curvature of the ascending aorta. Goose neck snaring of the loading hooks more difficult than example in figure 1; especially the loading hook along the greater curvature which is likely impossible to grasp with the goose neck snare.

control angiograms may need to be repeatedly performed at different stages of the process to confirm the mobilization of the valve. After confirmation with hemodynamic analysis, angiogram and TEE, the goose-neck catheter is carefully detached and retrieved (Case 1).

Valve-in-Valve Technique (as an Alternative)
If the previously described technique of repositioning the valve is unsuccessful or is deemed too dangerous due to an unfavorable position of the loops, the correction of the severe AR can still be obtained using a second CoreValve implanted inside the first one in a slightly higher position.

Description of the Technique of "Valve-in-Valve"
As with the previous technique, the correct projection is crucial and is dictated by the frame of the valve that should be aligned as perfectly as possible. Advance the second valve into the previously implanted valve and calculate the position for implantation with regards to the patient's anatomy. Measure the overlap distance of the two valves to better understand the position of the second valve that will be implanted.

Improving the Accuracy of Implantation
While focusing on the distal (inflow) aspect, release the second valve until it is one-third deployed. Then focus on the proximal (outflow) aspect of the second valve and determine the optimal distance between the frame loops of the first and the second valve. Note: It is important not to focus anymore on the distal aspect (inflow) of the valves, because the "criss-cross" appearance of the struts will make it difficult to differentiate the individual valve frames.

Once optimal distance between the outflow tips is determined, deploy the remainder of the valve while strictly maintaining the prescribed distance between the two frames. Note: Frame loops from individual frames may serve as the most convenient marker.

After complete release of the second valve, it is likely that there will be no significant AR observed, and as a result, no need for BAV postimplantation. When AR (grade ≥ 2) is observed, generally when tortuous anatomies challenge the implantation of the second valve, incomplete expansion and axialization of the second valve's frame should be questioned and assessed using control TEE or rotational fluoroscopy. If so, BAV postimplantation should be considered (Case 2).

High Implantation
With the possibility of full valve retrieval up to four-fifths of the deployment process, such a situation should rarely occur except in cases of technical mistakes during the last steps of the procedure as the following:

a. Failure to notice incomplete disengagement of both frame loops from the delivery catheter before withdrawing the catheter.

b. Failure to manage the distal tip of the delivery catheter (i.e., nose cone) through the prosthesis after successful valve deployment resulting in tip displacement of the valve frame.
c. Postimplant dilatation without the use of rapid pacing or rapid pacing terminated to early relative to balloon inflation resulting in ejection of the balloon-valve unit into the ascending aorta.

Unfortunately, a high implantation does not offer the same attractive options for correction as a low implantation.

However, it is important to first clearly define the criteria for acceptable parameters despite a too high implantation. To a certain extent, the sealing effect of the native calcified aortic valve around the frame (similar to a chimney above the annulus) can make a too high implantation perfectly compatible with a good result with none to mild or moderate AR (Case 3).

The control angiogram and the hemodynamic analysis provide the criteria for an acceptable result:

1. AR grade ≤ 2
2. No ventricular–aortic gradient
3. No coronary occlusion

The last criteria, being the most important to analyze, may require additional aortograms in different projections or/and eventually selective catheterization of the coronary ostia to ensure coronary flow.

This also highlights the importance of evaluating a "high implantation" option in the prescreening analysis of a patient for TAVI, specifically with regard to a CoreValve implantation.

In cases where valve implantation is definitively too high and incompatible with an acceptable result, the valve can be repositioned into the ascending aorta. (Note: Despite the fact that valve retrieval from ascending to descending aorta has been accomplished with the use of two goose-neck catheters resulting ultimately in possible full valve retrieval through the 18-F introducer sheath, such a maneuver is strongly discouraged due to the high probability of atherosclerotic plaque dislodgement or aortic dissection.) The primary goal is to ensure a safe area for the implantation of a second valve. As a result, repositioning of the first implanted valve high in the ascending aorta must be accomplished to avoid jeopardizing the functioning of the second valve by the following:

a. Severely restricting second valve expansion.
b. Potentially compromising coronary arterial flow by creation of a long skirt as a potential consequence of two valves placed in continuation.

Because the CoreValve prosthesis measures approximately 50 to 53 mm in height depending on valve size, a safe distance of >50 mm above the annulus level is therefore optimal.

Note: The Lasso technique for frame loop engagement for higher repositioning of the valve has been previously described. In small anatomies, this technique may not be feasible due to lack of space in the ascending aorta that can nullify any axial force exerted through the frame loop. In such a case, the goose-neck catheter can be advanced through the struts of the frame toward the inflow aspect, and "hooking" at that point. This allows for effective retrieval of the valve when pulling on the goose-neck catheter (Case 4).

Next, and again for additional safety, the first valve should be secured in the correct position high in the ascending aorta with the use of the goose-neck catheter when a second valve is advanced through the first valve. This is critical to avoid mobilization of the first valve at the time of crossing. As a result, if a safe distance of >50 mm between the two valves has been obtained, the result of the second implantation should not bear any risk of coronary ischemia or mid- to long-term malfunction of the implanted valve as previously described when this technique is not applied.

In rare cases where the valve cannot be retrieved with the Lasso technique, open surgical removal of the fully deployed prosthesis is required. If coronary flow is compromised by the tissue frame of the valve, cardiocirculatory bypass should be instituted prior to opening the chest, to ensure adequate perfusion pressure in case of myocardial ischemia. For this, the femoral vessels are cannulated in Seldinger technique. In all other cases the chest is opened through a partial or full sternotomy and cardiopulmonary bypass with moderate hypothermia at 32°C is instituted by cannulating the aorta and the right atrium in standard fashion. The aorta is clamped, cardioplegia instituted and the vessel incised transversely. Note that the stent frame of the prosthesis may be directly underneath the incision, so that in cases of a fairly large aorta, a longitudinal, "hockey stick" incision may also be considered. The supra-annually positioned prosthesis can usually easily be retracted without applying any force. Retraction of the valve is even facilitated by rinsing the valve frame with ice-cold water. Special care must be taken if prior maneuvers with the Lasso technique have led to multiple piercing of the stent frame into the adventitia. To avoid further injury to the aortic wall in these cases it may be necessary to cut the outflow aspect of the stent frame with wire-cutting pliers. But even when utmost caution is applied, ascending aortic replacement may in rare cases be required, especially in patients with small aortic anatomy and a thin walled aorta. After removal of the malpositioned valve standard aortic valve replacement is performed.

In patients with a "porcelain" aorta, open retrieval of the valve may be an unsurmountable challenge, because the aorta cannot be clamped. The only safe option to manage these cases is the anastomosis of a Dacron prosthesis to the proximal aortic arch during a short period of hypothermic cardiocirculatory arrest at 24°C. The Dacron prosthesis can then be clamped and the proximal part of the aorta including the valve is replaced. However, this approach bares an extremely high risk for major brain injury or multiorgan failure in the very old and considerably sick patients, so that the decision has to be carefully balanced.

The rare requirement of an open surgical retrieval of a malpositioned valve prosthesis underlines the exigence of a multidisciplinary implantation team of cardiologists, cardiac surgeons, and anesthesiologists. Furthermore, it underlines the common claim of the societies of the respective medical specialties that a "hybrid OR" is the ideal place for these procedures to allow for immediate intervention.

Paravalvular Regurgitation

Excluded from the discussion here is the management of paravalvular regurgitation in association with a too low implantation of the valve, and centrovalvular regurgitation, which represents a different situation, since it may result from technical mistakes at the time of loading of the valve or from inadequate postimplantation BAV. We will discuss only the management of grade ≥ 2 AR following correct implantation of the valve.

Albeit not a true complication, AR grade ≥ 2 on control angiogram or TEE is not rare (>20% of overall cases). This can occur for the following reasons:

a. Low implantation of the valve
b. Underexpansion of the frame in severely calcified aortic valve.
c. Underevaluation of annulus measurement

Before all, it is important to remember the following:
Due to the self-expandable nature of the frame (Nitinol), there is continual frame expansion after implantation and consequently a remodeling of the annulus and the native valve may take place. As a result, in numerous occasions where prolonged time has elapsed between the first control angiogram immediately following valve implantation and a later control aortogram taken at the end of the procedure, a distinct decrease in the degree of AR is observed, which validates the concept of remodeling of the anatomy after implantation of the CoreValve prosthesis.

Severity of the AR on aortogram should be evaluated carefully following minimum basic rules that include

a. a minimum of 20 mL of contrast media injection,
b. RAO projection, and
c. position of the pigtail catheter slightly above the functioning portion of the implanted valve for the angiogram to minimize the risk of underevaluation of the AR.

But, despite adherence to those rules, different parameters can influence the degree of AR as blood pressure, heart rate, left ventricular dysfunction bearing the risk of underestimating the severity of the regurgitation at the time of implantation and having to face, later at follow-up, under different hemodynamic conditions a more severe AR. Also, the experience with TAVI does not differ from BAV in aortic valve disease where grade III AR could be well tolerated in presence of left ventricular hypertrophy and grade II AR not tolerated in presence of a poor left ventricular function. Therefore, it is recommended to add to the evaluation of the severity of AR provided by TEE and aortogram, a hemodynamic analysis to evaluate the tolerance of AR.

As a result, one should always measure left ventricular and aortic pressures before and after valve implantation to better define the strategy when facing AR grade ≥ 2 post CoreValve implantation. Simple criteria can be proposed to establish the potentially bad hemodynamic tolerance of AR grade ≥ 2 after valve implantation that should lead to discuss BAV:

a. ≥ 10 mm Hg elevation of the left ventricular end-diastolic pressure above the value prior to the implantation, or an absolute value above 25 mm Hg.
b. ≥ 10 mm Hg decrease of the diastolic pressure below the value prior to the implantation for a similar systolic pressure or an absolute diastolic pressure value below 50 mm Hg.
c. No "dicrotic notch" on the aortic pressure tracing.
d. Tachycardia.

The decision to perform BAV after CoreValve implantation should always be evaluated carefully in regard to the potential consequences of BAV, such as dislodgement of the valve and structural damage to the valve tissue, which may not become evident before mid- or even long-term follow-up. Although to date, nothing is known about the effect of BAV on long-term durability of the valve, a conservative approach is mandatory.

Pericardial Effusion/Pericardial Tamponade

The causes of pericardial effusion are multifactorial. It is important to note that an effusion can occur promptly during valve implantation, but also delayed. The source of bleeding can be the right or left ventricle (LV), or the aortic root. Injury of the right ventricle may result from perforation of the transient pacemaker wire. Injury of the LV may result from perforation of the stiff guidewire (Amplatz Superstiff ST1), or of the catheters (Amplatz, Judkins right) after valve passage. Aortic root rupture may occur after balloon valvuloplasty or after valve implantation, especially in elderly women with fragile tissue where bulky calcifications can perforate the aortic root.

Some preventive strategies can help to avoid those injuries. The aortic valve passage and insertion of potentially traumatizing catheters (Amplatz/Judkins) into the LV should be performed via regular guidewires and favor the use of 5 F rather than 6-F catheters. The sole use of guidewires with a soft tip (Amplatz Superstiff) is paramount for valvuloplasty balloon and delivery catheter guidance. The guidewire should additionally be curved manually prior to insertion into the LV. A correct position of the guide wire within the LV is crucial. The tip should be nonattached to the ventricular wall, and the curve of the wire should line the septum and apex within the cavity of the LV. In case of a nonoptimal guidewire position, it is strongly recommended to reposition the wire only through a pigtail catheter. Extreme care should be given when severe circumferential left ventricular hypertrophy with small ventricular cavity, at risk for such complication. As a rule, the advancement and deployment of the preshaped extra-stiff guidewire into the left ventricular cavity should always be realized in a RAO projection to optimize visualization of the left ventricular cavity by using a pigtail catheter. To prevent aortic root rupture, meticulous annulus measurements should be performed by computed tomography, transthoracic echocardiography, and transesophageal echocardiography to avoid oversizing of the balloon or prosthesis.

In the following, an algorithm is described for the management of pericardial effusion. As standard of care, all patients should undergo echocardiographic control for the identification of pericardial effusion at the end of the implantation procedure. Small effusions <10 mm without hemodynamic impairment are monitored echocardiographically at close intervals. Patients with rapidly increasing effusions and with effusions with hemodynamic impairment (CVP increase, blood pressure decrease, tachycardia) undergo pericardial puncture (Case 5). If no improvement of the symptoms is achieved, an emergent surgical sternotomy is performed.

Herein, we describe the technique for pericardial puncture, which can be performed in the ICU or in the OR. A 16 to 18 gauge cannula is inserted 2 cm caudally and leftward of the xiphoid process toward the left shoulder. At a distance of 5- to 8 cm the effusion can usually be aspirated. After insertion of a guidewire, the cannula is removed, and the punctuation site is dilated with a 6 to 8 F sheath. Finally, a pigtail catheter is inserted into the pericardium and the effusion is aspirated. Pericardial puncture should be performed under echocardiographic monitoring to verify correct placement of the catheter in the pericardium. The pigtail catheter is left in place for at least 24 hours.

Low Cardiac Output—Cardiogenic Shock

Intraprocedural circulatory depression may occur in up to 20% of the patients during implantation. Predisposing factors are impaired left ventricular function, severe left ventricular hypertrophy, or severe pulmonary hypertension. Cardiac depression with low cardiac output may occur during periods of rapid pacing and may be the consequence of inadequate coronary perfusion due to low intra-aortic pressure. Coronary perfusion may also be impaired when the remaining aortic valve orifice is partially or completely occluded during the placement of the catheter-mounted valve. Another reason for cardiac depression may be the sudden onset of severe bradycardia or third-degree AV block following balloon dilatation of the aortic valve or deployment of the valve prostheses. Furthermore, obstruction of coronary ostia or severe aortic regurgitation after balloon dilatation or after the deployment of the valve prosthesis may also cause severe cardiac depression.

The most important measure to avoid cardiac depression during implantation is to wait for the restoration of a stable arterial blood pressure after an episode of rapid ventricular pacing before instituting another period of stimulation or before proceeding with the implantation. In this respect a close communication between the anesthesiologists and the implantation team is absolutely mandatory. In cases of bradycardia or sudden onset of third-degree AV block ventricular pacing may quickly improve the circulatory condition. In other cases, if mild hypertension does not resolve spontaneously it may easily be treated with bolus injections of catecholamines or a continuous infusion of low dose dopamine or dobutamine. In cases of a more severe blood pressure drop therapy should be instituted according to the systemic vascular resistance after the cardiac output measurement. If the resistance is normal, a continuous infusion of 5 to 10 μg/kg/min may restore adequate circulation, or if the resistance is low, 0.05 to 0.1 μg/kg/min of Norepinephrine. In cases of persisting low cardiac output a combination of Milrinone or Levosimendan together with epinephrine is recommended. Intraprocedural ventricular fibrillation (VF) is treated by electrical conversion followed by cardiopulmonary resuscitation. In those cases, usually bolus doses of epinephrine are applied to restore adequate cardiac output. If those measures do not help to restore the circulation, emergency institution of extracorporeal circulation is the only safe rescue therapy. The heart lung machine is connected to the circulation by cannulating the femoral artery and vein. In some centres wires are already placed in those two vessels as a safety measure prior to the implantation. In the few cases where we had to install normothermic extracorporeal circulation, the heart recovered amazingly quickly and every patient could be weaned from bypass in 20 to 30 minutes. In those cases the implantation of the valve should be continued during extracorporeal circulation, so that the patient is weaned with the valve prostheses already in place.

When the blood pressure drops after the beginning of the deployment of the valve, the procedure should be carried on promptly and cautiously, until the valve leaflets are deployed. After that, control of positioning and paravalvular leakage can be performed safely using TEE or fluoroscopy, even if the valve is not yet fully deployed, thus leaving the possibility to reposition the valve manually, if needed.

Coronary Obstruction

Coronary obstruction during implantation is a rare entity, occurring in about 2% of the patients. The reasons for this potentially catastrophic event include (a) displacement of calcium deposits or large native aortic valve leaflets in front of the coronary ostia during valve deployment; (b) embolization of calcium debris into one of the coronary arteries; (c) aortic dissection with continuity of the rupture into the intima of one of the coronary ostia with resultant obstruction; (d) a valve prosthesis that is implanted too high may also impair coronary flow. The first reason described may be more frequent in the setting of a low-lying coronary artery. In addition, coronary air embolism can lead to myocardial ischemia.

The first clinical sign of coronary obstruction is usually ST segment elevation in the EKG recording, or rhythm disturbances such as sudden third-degree AV block or VF. In those cases usually severe cardiac depression ensues and the patient may go into cardiogenic shock. In doubt of coronary obstruction, a bolus angiogram of the aortic root may reveal which coronary is concerned. After that, selective intubation of the coronary ensues, followed by balloon dilatation or stenting of the coronary ostium. If the valve is implanted too high and coronary flow is impaired by the skirt of the valve, the prostheses must be immediately retracted into the ascending aorta to relieve the obstruction. In the majority of these cases of coronary obstruction, emergency cardiopulmonary bypass will have to be instituted. If interventional measures fail to reconstitute coronary flow, emergent coronary artery bypass grafting or open removal of a malpositioned valve prosthesis is required.

Conduction Abnormalities

Considering the anatomic proximity of the conduction system to the aortic valve, it is not surprising that conduction abnormalities such as AV block or bundle branch block are known complication of TAVI even in the absence of surgical excision of valve or annulus tissue. The requirement for permanent pacing has been described to be necessary in up to 20% of the patients. The occurrence of new-onset left bundle branch block (LBBB) during the procedure may occur in up to 40% of patients.

Possible explanations include transient periprocedural inflammation, edema, and mechanical stress due to balloon or stent trauma or myocardial necrosis in the basal interventricular septum due to ischemia. In addition, this population of elderly patients, all with underlying organic heart disease frequently exhibit pre-existing conduction abnormalities, which are known to be associated with aortic stenosis.

There are no definitely known risk factors for the occurrence of peri- and post-procedural complete heart block, but the occurrence of intraprocedural complete heart block, even when it is transient, and the presence of right bundle branch block seem to be predisposing factors. In addition, relatively low positioning of the valve within the left ventricular outflow tract and efforts to oversize the implanted prosthesis to securely fix it within the aortic annulus and thus minimize paravalvular regurgitation might play a role.

Prior to the implantation procedure, conduction abnormalities should be thoroughly documented by a 12-lead ECG to diagnose preexisting AV block or left and right bundle branch block. Intra- and postprocedural monitoring with a 3-lead rhythm strip has to be done continuously up to five days after the procedure, because there have been case reports describing the late occurrence of complete heart block after TAVI. Other preexisting episodes of bradycardia such as sinus node disease or symptomatic bradyarrhythmia may have been undetected in some patients before the procedure and are unrelated to TAVI. If there is an indication for a pacemaker implantation postoperatively, it is important to distinguish between a new-onset high-grade AV block, which may be related to TAVI and other preexisting bradycardias unrelated to TAVI.

A new-onset LBBB is not an indication for the implantation of a permanent pacemaker. The clinical implications of new-onset LBBB are currently unknown but its occurrence after surgical aortic valve replacement is associated with 1-year mortality. The avoidance of a too deep implantation of the prosthesis might help to prevent the occurrence of high-grade AV block. Adequate sizing of the balloon and valve are mandatory to avoid serious complications such as valve migration or severe paravalvular leak. As with the use of relatively larger valve sizes the risk of damage to the conduction system due to balloon and frame trauma might be higher, the balance between the anticipated complications has to be considered carefully. Whether immediate pacemaker implantation without further hesitation even in cases of intermittent AV block might be called a somewhat liberal indication, is the subject of ongoing debate. In our opinion, in this population of elderly patients, all with underlying organic heart disease, we opt for patients' safety.

Rhythm Disturbances

Patients scheduled for TAVI are considered to be a high-risk population with multiple comorbidities such as left ventricular dysfunction and concomitant valve disease in up to one-fifth of patients, coronary artery disease in one-half, and atrial fibrillation in one-third.

Atrial Fibrillation

Atrial fibrillation (AF) is known to increase the risk of stroke, a fact that makes it difficult to distinguish between TAVI-related cerebrovascular accident (CVA) and thromboembolic stroke due to AF. Keeping the higher stroke risk in mind, specific attention should be paid to the anticoagulation management with Coumadin and the recommended antiplatelet therapy. So far, there are no data concerning the optimal combination or duration of antiplatelet therapy and anticoagulation after the implantation of a catheter-based aortic bioprosthesis especially in a population with a high risk of major bleeding events. When there is an indication for Coumadin therapy after TAVI, we start Coumadin after being sure that no bleeding complications have occurred (that are, for example, pericardial tamponade, bleeding at the vascular access site, etc.), having given the antiplatelet loading dose before the intervention as appropriate. We only use Aspirin in combination with Coumadin in patients with an indication for anticoagulation therapy, because we consider the risk of Coumadin therapy combined with a dual antiplatelet therapy to be too high.

Ventricular Tachycardia and Ventricular Fibrillation

Considering the incidence of left ventricular dysfunction in these patients and significant coronary artery disease, spontaneous and sustained ventricular tachycardia (VT) and VF occur rather seldom during TAVI procedures (1–2%). Short self-limited VT is common, especially when manipulating the guidewire loop within the LV. Sustained VT or even VF can follow the iatrogenic VT induced by rapid ventricular pacing, in particular, in patients with preoperatively compromised left ventricular function. Of course, VT or VF can always be indicative of severe coronary ischemia during the intervention.

Patients with a previous implantation of a cardioverter defibrillator (ICD) should have the antitachycardic algorithms turned off during the intervention in order not to interfere with the episodes of rapid ventricular pacing.

NONCARDIAC COMPLICATIONS

Vascular Complications

Aortic Dissection

Injury to the aortic wall is a rare complication of TAVI observed in 0.2% of the procedures. It can take different occurrences such as aortic hematoma, and Type A or B aortic dissection. Usually only Type A dissection jeopardizes patient survival.

Aortic hematoma is a frightening complication when it occurs but can be safely managed using a percutaneous technique. This complication relates to manipulation of the 18-F introducer sheath into the ascending aorta either from a femoral approach using an 80 cm long introducer sheath (Case 6) or the subclavian access.

Description of the Technique

After visualization of the aortic wall hematoma on contrast aortography, the extension of the dissection distal to the ascending aorta (to discriminate from Type A dissection) should be evaluated by control angiogram by using a 5-F pigtail catheter positioned higher in the ascending aorta or the TEE. Then the pigtail catheter is carefully re-advanced forward under fluoroscopy guidance and control of the aortic pressure monitoring to the native aortic valve by using rotational maneuvers to avoid re-entry in the false lumen. After control angiogram of the correct position in the true lumen, the valve is crossed using a regular 0.035 straight guidewire through the pigtail catheter then the 0.035 preshaped stiff guidewire (Amplatz stiff) is positioned in the LV. Control aortogram during valve implantation is performed through a pigtail catheter positioned into the noncoronary sinus by using similar technique of progression of the pigtail catheter to avoid the entry into the false lumen.

Type A dissection is a most dramatic complication, and considering the type of patients treated today with TAVI, the decision to operate in those elderly patients with severe comorbid conditions is not to be taken lightly. However, since the extent of the aortic dissection and thus, the complexity of the surgical revision can rarely be judged from the medical images alone, an immediate thoracotomy with surgical revision will be mandatory in the majority of the patients.

Type B dissection tends to be managed medically unless complications develop.

Iliac Ruptures and Retroperitoneal Bleeding

With the decreased size of the introducer sheaths required for CoreValve implantation and careful respect of the basic rules for the femoral approach, it became also a rare complication occurring in less than 2% of the procedures. Whatever the reason for the vessel perforation might be (balloon angioplasty or 18-F introducer advancement in calcified iliac arteries), the most important is the immediate recognition of the complication to stop the internal bleeding before severe hemodynamic consequences ensue. Then depending on the location and severity of the arterial perforation, different options can be discussed. Again, shared experience and judgments of cardiologists and cardiovascular surgeons working together provide a better option for the patient. Without defining strict rules, the following attitudes have prevailed in the following situations.

In case of iliac perforation following peripheral angioplasty balloon dilatation (PTA) of the iliac artery performed before valve implantation to allow the way for the 18F introducer to progress, hemostasis is easily obtained using inflation of the PTA balloon at low pressure at the level of the arterial rupture. A covered stent (size beyond the length of the previous PTA balloon) is then prepared and, except when the control angiogram shows effective sealing of the arterial perforation after prolonged balloon inflation, BP is deeply lowered and the covered stent advanced and expanded at the level of the arterial rupture. Except when the valve prosthesis is already off the glutaraldehyde solution, the valve implantation procedure should be aborted. Otherwise, another access may be discussed (Case 7).

In case of external iliac perforation revealed after withdrawal of the 18-F introducer, hemostasis is obtained using advancement of the 18-F dilator with the guidewire left in place or with the use of a peripheral balloon catheter positioned higher into the common iliac artery from the same or contralateral access side. Then, as previously described, a covered stent is prepared and expanded. In such instances, the stent should insure extensive covering of the external iliac artery from 2 cm above the location of the arterial rupture to the ilio-femoral junction. Preferably a self-expandable covered stent is used and expanded at the same time when the 18-F introducer is slowly retrieved. To conclude, in all difficult femoral accesses, slowly withdrawal of the 18-F introducer under fluoroscopy and repeat control angiograms using contrast injection through the 18-F introducer with a guidewire into the iliac vessel is recommended.

In case of femoral bleeding or retroperitoneal bleeding revealed after the withdrawal of the 18-F introducer at the end of the procedure, hemostasis is generally obtained with manual compression of the femoral access. Correction of the arterial perforation can be obtained using the different options in order of complexity:

Prolonged Manual Compression and Protamine Injection

Prolonged inflation of a peripheral angioplasty balloon at low pressure eventually prolonged by covered stent implantation advanced from the contralateral femoral side in cases of too high puncture (Case 8).

Surgical Revision

Differences in treatment strategies may reflect differences in the expertise of heart teams.

Occlusion of the Femoral Artery Vessel

Severe residual obstruction or complete occlusion of the femoral access on final control angiogram occurs in around 5% of the procedures with femoral access. The correction of this complication can be obtained using prolonged inflation of a peripheral angioplasty balloon at low pressure (Case 9).

Surgical Revision

Peripheral Embolization

In the absence of systematic control angiogram of the peripheral vasculature after TAVI, the rate is unknown. The management is not specific to TAVI.

CONCLUSION

Only increasing knowledge and future efforts to develop measures to decrease the complications rate will ensure the future for a safe and effective procedure for patients—this is the responsibility of the heart team.

21 | Acute and Early Complications of Transcatheter Aortic Valve Implantation with the Balloon-Expandable Edwards System

Jean-Bernard Masson and John G. Webb
St. Paul's Hospital, University of British Columbia, Vancouver, British Columbia, Canada

INTRODUCTION

Transfemoral approach to the aortic valve can be accomplished with antegrade transvenous or retrograde transarterial access. Although transcatheter aortic valve replacement was initially performed through the venous route (1), this approach has been supplanted by the more reproducible transarterial (2), or transapical approaches (3). This chapter will focus on the avoidance and management of complications that may occur during or immediately after a retrograde transarterial procedure using the balloon-expandable Edwards valve (Edwards Lifesciences, Inc., Irvine, California).

Transarterial implantation of the Edwards SAPIEN and CoreValve self-expandable valves shares many similarities and therefore many potential adverse events. However there are some specificities to the Edwards system that need to be acknowledged, namely a shorter valve design, a larger delivery system and obviously, balloon expansion. These features may either be an advantage or a disadvantage with respect to potential complications. Throughout this chapter, challenges specific to the Edwards system are emphasized. Complications related to the transapical access route will not be discussed in this chapter.

Complications range from relatively minor to potentially fatal adverse events. Awareness of potential problems and timely response can sometimes be the difference between successful and unsuccessful outcome. To date, several thousands of Cribier–Edwards and Edwards SAPIEN valve implants have been performed, however only a few single-center and multicenters registries are available, generally with less than 100 patients per publication. Therefore precise evaluation of the incidence of most complications is yet premature and numbers cited in this chapter should be interpreted cautiously.

VASCULAR COMPLICATIONS

Arterial Injury

The current 23- and 26-mm Edwards SAPIEN valves are delivered through 22- and 24-F sheaths respectively, equivalent to 8 and 9 mm in outer diameter. Although delivery systems will likely become smaller in the near future, the large diameter of the current system is a potential source of arterial injury. Careful patient screening with ilio-femoral angiography and computed tomographic angiography (CTA) may be the most effective tool to protect patients from arterial injury. Small ilio-femoral arteries or stenosis, tortuosities, and calcification are risk factors for vascular complications. The combination of circumferential calcification and a small lumen area strongly argues against the transarterial approach.

It is important to ensure puncture of the common femoral artery, particularly if percutaneous arterial closure is planned. Fluoroscopy-assisted needle entry over the femoral head will generally be sufficiently low as to avoid retroperitoneal bleeding and sufficiently high as to avoid injury to the femoral bifurcation. Sonography may be more accurate and may also identify areas of calcification or atheroma that would be best avoided. Angiography or placement of a target catheter from the contralateral leg may also be helpful [Fig. 1(A) and (B)]. Use of a small diameter needle or sheath may allow repeated puncture if needed. Suitability of femoral puncture site for percutaneous closure can be confirmed with injection of contrast through the femoral sheath.

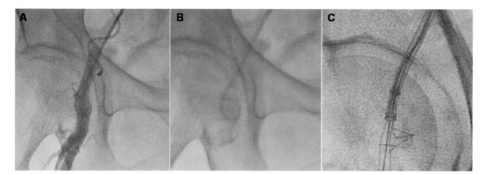

Figure 1 Percutaneous access and closure. (**A**) Placement of a pigtail catheter to select puncture site and (**B**) serve as target for needle insertion. (**C**) Failed attempt at preclosure of the femoral artery. The Prostar XL needles failed to go through the calcified artery.

No percutaneous closure device specifically intended for closure after placement of large diameter sheaths is currently available. However, "preclosure" with either 1 or 2 Prostar XL 10-F devices or 2 or 3 ProGlide devices (Abbott Vascular Inc., Santa Clara, California) are commonly used with success. Extensive femoral calcification or obesity increases the risk of device failure [Fig. 1(C)]. It is prudent to leave a guidewire in place until hemostasis is confirmed. Should this fail a sheath can be reinserted or an occlusion balloon advanced proximal to the bleeding site to allow surgical closure.

Traumatic puncture or sheath insertion may result in arterial injury ranging from minor bleeding to dissection or rupture. Femoral and iliac dissections are often best managed with careful observation but extensive or flow limiting dissection may require stenting or surgical repair. In contrast arterial perforation may result in rapid bleeding and requires immediate control. Unexplained hypotension during or shortly after sheath placement should prompt evaluation for bleeding. However, most often ilio-femoral perforation becomes apparent at the time of sheath removal as evidenced by sudden hypotension. Reinsertion of the sheath, volume expansion, and placement of a dedicated occlusion balloon proximal to the perforation typically provides temporary hemostasis and hemodynamic stability while the bleeding site is appropriately managed (4) (Fig. 2, Video 1). Most cases of vessel perforation can be sealed with a covered stent. In some cases, however, surgical repair may be necessary.

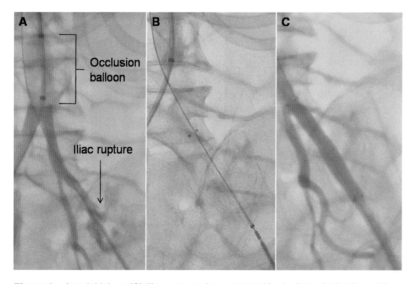

Figure 2 Arterial injury. (**A**) Iliac rupture demonstrated by ipsilateral injection while an occlusion balloon (Coda Occlusion Balloon Catheter, Cook Medical, Bloomington, IN, USA) is inflated in the distal aorta. (**B**) Retrograde deployment of a self-expandable Fluency covered stent (**C**) effectively sealing the bleeding site.

Avulsion of the iliac or femoral artery can occur when the arterial wall becomes adherent to a large, occlusive sheath. This should be suspected when marked resistance to sheath withdrawal is encountered. In such cases, preemptive placement of an occlusion balloon in the distal abdominal aorta can prevent massive bleeding. Angiography during sheath removal can be helpful, providing early detection with contrast injections either through the large sheath itself or with a catheter advanced from the contralateral leg and positioned in the common iliac. The likelihood of vessel adherence may be reduced with periodic rotation of the sheath and early sheath removal.

In the very early TAVI experience, major vascular complications were very common, running 5% to 10% (5). However, the risk of vascular complications continues to fall dramatically largely as a result of screening and careful attention to patient selection.

Aortic Injury

Injury to the aorta may occur due to mechanical trauma during sheath insertion, catheter manipulation, or balloon dilation (6). Aortic dissection, given comorbidities in these patients, is often best managed conservatively. Rarely, however, aortic stenting or surgical management may be necessary. In contrast, perforation may result in hemodynamic collapse. Rapid placement of a compliant occlusion balloon may allow stabilization and controlled management with an endograft or surgery.

Stroke

Atheroembolism from the aortic arch may be the most frequent cause of stroke following transarterial TAVI. Screening for mobile atheroma within the aorta with CTA or TEE may identify patients at higher risk for stroke. Deflection of the steerable catheter tip to avoid resistance and gentle manipulation of the delivery catheter through the aortic arch and across the stenotic valve probably can help reduce the risk of stroke. Hopefully, improvement in catheter technology will bring smaller delivery catheters with nontraumatic tips, which will lessen the risk further. Embolic protection devices to protect the arch vessels from embolization are currently under development.

Other potential causes for stroke include embolization of calcific material from the aortic valve during valvuloplasty or valve deployment, prolonged or marked hypotension particularly in the presence of cerebrovascular disease, thromboembolism from wires or catheters, and, rarely, dissection of an arch vessel (7). Avoidance of unnecessary or overaggressive valve dilation, timely management of hypotension with vasoactive agents, and adequate anticoagulation are strongly recommended.

In the largest series published to date, the stroke rate with transarterial aortic valve implantation using the balloon-expandable Edwards system was 5.3% ($n = 114$) (8). Combined data from REVIVAL II and REVIVE II suggest a similar incidence (6.3%; $n = 161$) of neurological events (unpublished data). A lower stroke rate associated with a transapical access has been suggested by several reports (6,9). Transcatheter valve implantation remains an immature technique that currently uses first- and second-generation devices. While unlikely to be completely eliminated from this procedure, stroke risk is expected to fall as technology matures and operators gain experience.

MALPLACEMENT AND EMBOLIZATION

Malplacement

Optimal results are obtained with full coverage of the aortic leaflets, secure anchoring at and below the level of the leaflets, and avoidance of unnecessary contact with surrounding structures. Proper position prior to inflation is typically guided by fluoroscopic recognition of calcific landmarks, aortography, and echocardiography. Using a fluoroscopic angulation perpendicular to the valve plane will provide more reliable placement whereas a non-coaxial position prior to inflation makes correct positioning more challenging (Fig. 3). During transarterial deployment, the Edwards SAPIEN valve typically moves 1 to 2 mm in the direction of the aorta. Consequently, optimal positioning requires that, prior to balloon inflation, approximately two-thirds of the stent is positioned below the plane of leaflet insertion. At the same time, the prosthesis

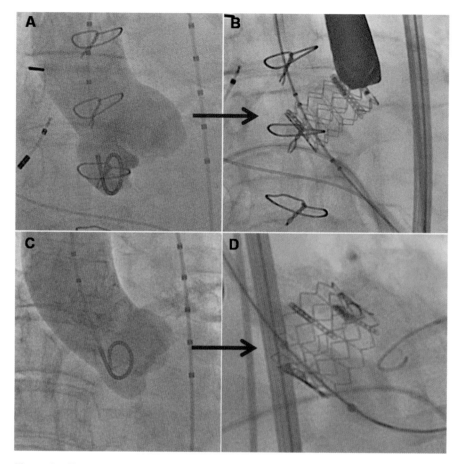

Figure 3 Choosing an angulation perpendicular to the valve plane makes positioning easier. (**A**) The aortic cusps are perfectly aligned on a single plane. (**B**) Deployment in the same angulation as (**A**). (**C**) The aortic cusps are not aligned on a single plane. (**D**) Deployment in the same angulation as (**C**).

needs to be positioned sufficiently high so that the tip of the native valve leaflets will be constrained by the frame. In some cases, anatomical considerations may make it difficult to fully satisfy both requirements. Deployment is generally performed during rapid right ventricular pacing. Reliable capture and loss of pulsatile flow is mandatory to avoid expulsion of the inflated balloon (and valve) toward the aorta. Balloon inflation and deflation must be rapid and pacing must continue until the balloon is fully deflated. Details of valve positioning and deployment are discussed elsewhere.

A prosthesis positioned too low (toward the ventricle) can be associated with residual aortic stenosis if the native leaflets are not held open or problematic paravalvular regurgitation if the sealing cuff is not fully apposed to the left ventricular outflow tract. Placement of a second overlapping prosthesis more completely covering the native leaflets and extending the sealing cuff will generally resolve this problem. A valve positioned even lower into the ventricle may interfere with the mitral valve or left ventricular function and would likely require surgical removal.

A prosthesis positioned too high (toward the aorta) may be also be associated with paravalvular regurgitation due to inadequate apposition of the sealing cuff. If deployed so high that tissue fixation is not achieved embolization may occur.

Embolization
Embolization of the prosthesis to the aorta does not cause hemodynamic compromise so long as the prosthesis is maintained oriented so as not to obstruct flow. Should the valve become

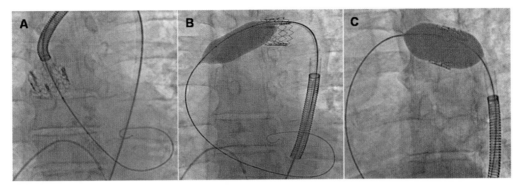

Figure 4 Embolization secondary due premature discontinuation of burst pacing (**A**) Wire position across the embolized valve holds it in correct orientation. (**B**) A semi-inflated balloon is used to pull the valve toward the arch. (**C**) The valve is secured with re-inflation. There was no residual gradient across the valve.

inverted then obstruction to aortic flow could occur (10). The key is to maintain coaxial guidewire position through the device to prevent rotation of the prosthesis. In most cases a semi-inflated valvuloplasty balloon can be used to pull the prosthesis into the aortic arch (Fig. 4, Video 2) or descending aorta (11). When the valve reaches an adequate landing zone where it would not obstruct important side branches, it can be secured with re-inflation.

In most instances, embolization is a consequence of suboptimal initial positioning prior to balloon expansion or technical errors during deployment. If the cause for malposition and device embolization can be identified a second attempt will often prove successful. If the mechanism of embolization cannot be identified and corrected then alternative approaches should be considered.

CARDIAC COMPLICATIONS

Annular Injury
Annular tears may rarely occur due to forceful crossing or dilation of the stenotic aortic valve. Dehiscence of an aortic leaflet may result in acute, severe regurgitation best managed by rapid valve implantation. Rarely rupture of the annulus may result in mediastinal bleeding or septal rupture may result in left to right shunting. Surgical repair, if possible, may be the only option. Severe annular calcification in combination with overly aggressive dilation or device oversizing may be predisposing factors (12).

Mitral Injury
Acute mitral regurgitation may occur due to wire or catheter interference with the mitral apparatus or myocardial ischemia. While interference or laceration of mitral chordae and/or leaflets have been described with the antegrade transvenous and transapical approaches (12), a retrograde approach does not mechanically interfere with the mitral valve function. The Edwards valve is relatively short, measuring ~15 mm in length. Although the valve extends into the outflow tract, contact with the anterior mitral curtain and acute mechanical interference with the mitral valve has not appeared to be a clinical problem. Rarely mitral tears may occur in the presence of severe calcification of the anterior leaflet (Fig. 5) (12).

Tamponade
Cardiac perforation may rarely lead to pericardial effusion or tamponade. Perhaps the most common causes are right heart perforation during placement of a transvenous pacemaker and left ventricular perforation due to guidewire or catheter nosecone trauma (Fig. 6). Guidewires should have a soft J-tip and gentle supportive curve extending well beyond the valve delivery catheter (Fig. 7). Unexplained hypotension should prompt immediate assessment with echocardiography. Generally, hemodynamically important pericardial effusions can be managed with pericardiocentesis.

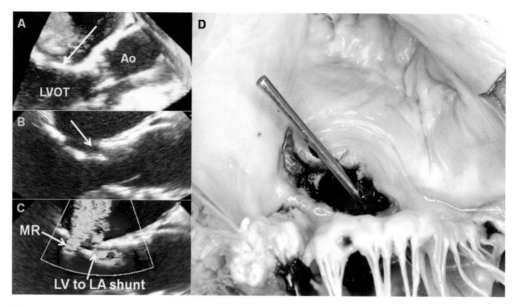

Figure 5 (**A**) Three-dimensional transesophageal echocardiograhic image showing a thick, calcified anterior mitral curtain (*arrow*). (**B**) After valve implantation a tear is created in the anterior mitral curtain (*arrow*), resulting in (**C**) LV to LA shunt in addition to preexisting mitral regurgitation (MR). (**D**) Autopsy-proven tear in anterior mitral leaflet (seen from the left atrium). *Abbreviations*: LVOT, left ventricular outflow tract; Ao, aorta; LV, left ventricular, LA, left atrial.

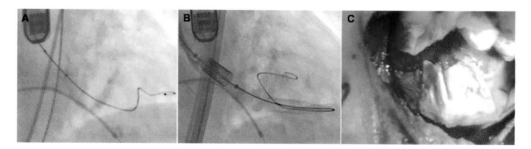

Figure 6 Perforation of the left ventricle. (**A**) An extra-stiff wire is positioned into the left ventricle but is not well elongated. (**B**) As the nosecone is advanced, the relationship between the wire and nose-cone suggest perforation of the ventricle. (**C**) Beating-heart left ventricular patch repair performed under femoro-femoral support.

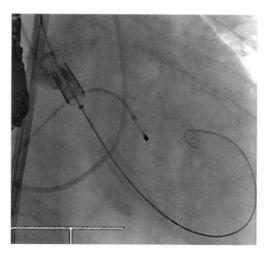

Figure 7 Proper position of the extra-stiff wire, well elongated into the left ventricle.

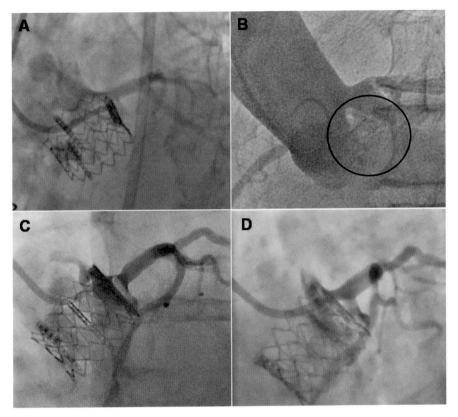

Figure 8 Coronary obstruction. (**A**) The very uncommon situation of a coronary ostium being obstructed by a stent strut. (**B**) Bulky coronary leaflets that warrants further evaluation. (**C**) Left main obstruction by a bulky coronary leaflet. (**D**) Successful stenting of the left main coronary through an open cell of the valved stent.

Coronary Obstruction

Coronary compromise is uncommon with an incidence to date of ~1%. The Edwards SAPIEN valve is designed to be positioned below the coronary ostia and to extend into the aortic root without contacting the ascending aorta at the level of the ostia. Obstruction would not be expected even if the open cells of the valve frame extend over the left coronary ostium. On rare occasions, a very bulky native valve leaflet might be folded up over the left coronary ostium (Fig. 8, Video 3) (2). Presentation is likely to be with ST elevation and hypotension immediately following valve implantation. Although possibly fatal (2,6), successful management with bypass surgery or stenting is possible (9). Examination of a preprocedural echocardiogram and aortogram for an unusually bulky native valve leaflet in close proximity to a coronary ostium may be prudent. CT scanning can identify patients at high risk in whom the distance from the leaflet insertion to the left main ostium is relatively short (<12 mm)(13). Ultimately balloon valvuloplasty in combination with fluoroscopy or angiography may provide the best assessment of the risk of leaflet obstruction of the left main (Fig. 9).

Conduction Abnormalities

Complete heart block or left bundle branch block can occur as the result of pressure-induced injury to the specialized conduction tissues located in the interventricular septum. The Edwards SAPIEN valve is relatively short, a potential advantage with respect to heart block as early data suggest that a prosthesis that contacts a greater length of LVOT and interventricular septum is associated with higher incidence of conduction problems (14). Preexisting right bundle branch block or other infra-nodal conduction delay and aggressive oversizing may be risk factors for complete heart block. Permanent pacemaker implantation, specifically for

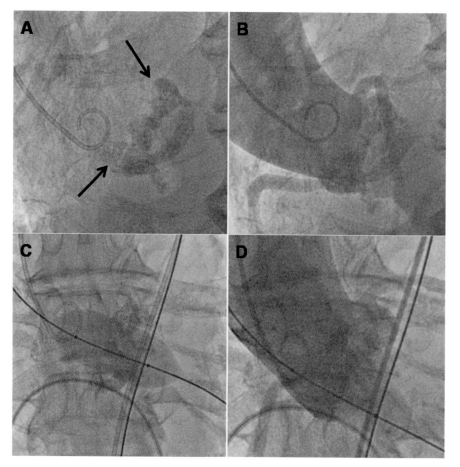

Figure 9 Calcified and bulky coronary leaflets (**A**) in close relationship with the left main coronary ostium (**B**). During balloon valvuloplasty (**C**) a supravalvular aortogram (**D**) shows good opacification of the coronary arteries. The risk of coronary obstruction therefore appears low.

new complete heart block has been reported to be 5.7% in a single-center report of balloon-expandable TAVI (15) which compares favorably with conventional surgical (16) and transcatheter self-expandable experience (14). Heart block almost always occurs immediately after valve implantation. In the some patients, conduction abnormalities can be associated with guidewire position in the left ventricle or balloon aortic valvuloplasty. However, in rare instances block may manifest later; consequently cardiac monitoring is recommended for at least 48 hours (17).

Arrhythmias
Wire and catheter manipulation often causes ventricular ectopy. In the setting of aortic stenosis, frequent or prolonged ectopy can result in hypotension and repositioning the wire may be desirable. Atrial fibrillation may be poorly tolerated and require cardioversion. Ventricular fibrillation can occur, most often triggered by burst pacing. Preemptive placement of defibrillator pads is desirable. If ventricular fibrillation develops during burst pacing at the time of valve implantation, the best course of action may be to deploy the valve first and then proceed with defibrillation.

Cardiogenic Shock
In the setting of severe aortic stenosis, hypotension or tachycardia of any cause can lead to ischemia, myocardial dysfunction and cardiogenic shock. Initial hypotension can be the result

of obvious complications, but the cause can also be more subtle. In patients with cardiomyopathies (left ventricular dysfunction and left ventricular hypertrophy) or coronary disease, arrhythmias or anesthetic agents may be sufficient to significantly lower blood pressure and initiate a downward spiraling effect. Liberal use of vasoactive agents such as phenylephrine and norepinephrine to maintain coronary perfusion is preferred over chronotropic or inotropic agents such as dopamine or epinephrine. Rarely, femoral cardiopulmonary support will be necessary to provide a bridge to myocardial recovery. The need for circulatory support is generally brief with recovery rapidly following successful relief of aortic stenosis. Should chest compressions be required it seems prudent to reassess valve placement and expansion, as stent geometry can be altered. Echocardiographic examination can be very helpful in the diagnosis of hypovolemia, tamponade, aortic or mitral valvular dysfunction.

VALVE FAILURE

Paravalvular Regurgitation

Some degree of paravalvular regurgitation is commonly present after valve implantation. Aortic paravalvular regurgitation is generally mild in severity and without discernable clinical symptoms or hemolysis (18). Early in the transcatheter balloon-expandable experience, problematic paravalvular regurgitation was more frequent but the incidence of severe regurgitation has fallen dramatically with routine oversizing, optimal positioning and incorporation of a lengthened sealing cuff that now extends over two-thirds of the valve length.

Severe paravalvular regurgitation typically presents with a low diastolic pressure immediately after implantation. Rarely, systolic hypotension may develop. Causes of paravalvular regurgitation include positioning errors (too high or too low), undersizing or incomplete expansion. When incomplete expansion is present repeat dilation can be helpful. Postdilation is generally performed with no more than 1 cc of added volume to avoid overstretching the stent and creating noncoaptation of the leaflets. Where paravalvular regurgitation is the result of improper positioning (Fig. 10), the implantation of a second overlapping valve so as to extend the sealing cuff is an effective immediate solution; however this is rarely necessary.

Structural Valve Failure

The potential for injury to prosthetic valve leaflets as a consequence of crimping, catheter delivery and dilation is an obvious concern, but has not been reported. Valves that are designed to adopt an open leaflet position in the absence of a closing pressure gradient may be susceptible to poor leaflet closure should the valve be implanted very low in the left ventricular outflow tract so that an unrestrained native leaflet overhangs a prosthetic leaflet. To date, late structural failure has not been observed.

MISCELLANEOUS COMPLICATIONS

Acute Renal Failure

Improvement in renal function as a result of improved cardiac output is frequently seen within a few days after TAVI. However, acute renal failure may occur as the consequence of atheroembolism, nephrotoxic contrast, and hypotension. Fortunately, severe worsening of renal function is infrequent and the need for temporary dialysis following transarterial TAVI is rare. It is prudent to minimize radiographic contrast in the presence of preexisting renal dysfunction. A potential role for pharmacologic renal protection is controversial and unfortunately routine volume loading may be unwise in patients with aortic stenosis.

SUMMARY

TAVI remains a young procedure with the potential for significant complications. Better understanding of these complications along with their prevention and management will continue to improve outcomes.

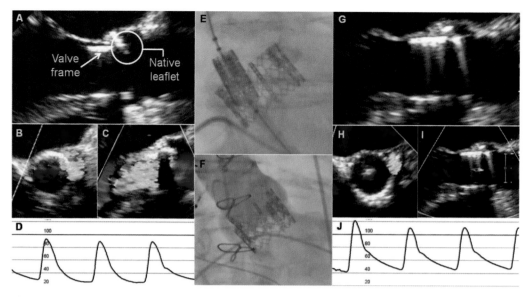

Figure 10 (**A**) Native aortic leaflets are seen to prolapse at the distal edge of a valved stent implanted too low. (**B**) and (**C**) Ensuing severe paravalvular regurgitation. (**D**) Low diastolic pressure associated with severe paravalvular regurgitation. (**E**) Placement of a second, overlapping valve extending the sealing cuff. (**F**) Supravalvular aortogram showing mild residual paravalvular regurgitation. (**G**) The native leaflets are now completely covered by the second prosthesis. (**H**) and (**I**) Mild residual paravalvular regurgitation. (**J**) Normalization of pressure tracing after paravalvular leak resolution.

REFERENCES

1. Cribier A, Eltchaninoff H, Bash A, et al. Percutaneous transcatheter implantation of an aortic valve prosthesis for calcific aortic stenosis: First human case description. Circulation 2002; 106(24):3006–3008.
2. Webb JG, Pasupati S, Humphries K, et al. Percutaneous transarterial aortic valve replacement in selected high-risk patients with aortic stenosis. Circulation 2007; 116(7):755–763.
3. Ye J, Cheung A, Lichtenstein SV, et al. Transapical aortic valve implantation in humans. J Thorac Cardiovasc Surg 2006;131(5):1194–1196.
4. Masson J-B, Al Bugami S, Webb JG. Endovascular balloon occlusion for catheter-induced large artery perforation in the catheterization laboratory. Catheter Cardiovasc Interv 2009; Epub ahead of print.
5. Kodali SK, O'Neill W, Moses JW, et al. Preliminary results from the percutaneous endovascular implantation of valves trial in high risk patients with critical aortic stenosis. Am J Cardiol 2006; 98(abstract suppl):48M.
6. Svensson LG, Dewey T, Kapadia S, et al. United States feasibility study of transcatheter insertion of a stented aortic valve by the left ventricular apex. Ann Thorac Surg 2008; 86(1):46–55.
7. Berry C, Cartier R, Bonan R. Fatal ischemic stroke related to non permissive peripheral artery access for percutaneous aortic valve replacement. Catheter Cardiovasc Interv 2007; 69:56–63.
8. Webb JG, Altwegg L, Boone RH, et al. Transcatheter aortic valve implantation. Impact on clinical and valve-related outcomes. Circulation. 2009; 119(23):3009–3016.
9. Walther T, Falk V, Kempfert J, et al. Transapical minimally invasive aortic valve implantation; the initial 50 patients. Eur J Cardiothorac Surg 2008; 33(6):983–988.
10. Piazza N, de Jaegere P, Serruys PW. The case of the flip-flop valve. EuroIntervention. In press.
11. Al Ali AM, Altwegg L, Horlick EM, et al. Prevention and management of transcatheter balloon-expandable aortic valve malposition. Catheter Cardiovasc Interv 2008; 72(4):573–578.
12. Masson J-B, Kovac J, Schuler G, et al. Transcatheter aortic valve implantation: Review of the nature, management and avoidance of procedural complications. J Am Coll Cardiol Intv 2009; 2(9):811–820.
13. Lu T-L, Huber C, Rizzo E, et al. Ascending aorta measurements as assessed by ECG-gated multi-detector computed tomography: A pilot study to establish normative values for transcatheter therapies. Eur Radiol 2009; 19(3):664–669.
14. Piazza N, Onuma Y, Jesserun E, et al. Early and persistent intraventricular conduction abnormalities and requirements for pacemaking after percutaneous replacement of the aortic valve. JACC Cardiovasc Interv 2008; 1(3):310–316.

15. Sinhal A, Altwegg L, Pasupati S, et al. Atrioventricular block after transcatheter balloon expandable aortic valve implantation. JACC Cardiovasc Interv 2008; 1(3):305–309.

16. Dawkins S, Hobson AR, Kalra PR, et al. Permanent pacemaker implantation after isolated aortic valve replacement: Incidence, indications, and predictors. Ann Thorac Surg 2008; 85(1):108–112.

17. Vahanian A, Alfieri O, Al-Attar N, et al. Transcatheter valve implantation for patients with aortic stenosis: A position statement from the European Association of Cardio-Thoracic Surgery (EACTS) and the European Society of Cardiology (ESC), in collaboration with the European Association of Percutaneous Cardiovascular Interventions (EAPCI). Eur Heart J 2008; 29(11):1463–1470.

18. Murphy CJ, Pasupati S, Webb JG. Hemolysis after transcatheter balloon-expandable aortic valve insertion. Can J Cardiol 2007; 23(Suppl C):260.

22 | Complications of Transapical Aortic Valve Implantation: Tips and Tricks to Avoid Failure

Jian Ye, Anson Cheung, John G. Webb, and Samuel V. Lichtenstein
St. Paul's Hospital, University of British Columbia, Vancouver, British Columbia, Canada

Transcatheter aortic valve implantation (AVI) has been demonstrated to provide relief of aortic stenosis and possibly reduce perioperative risks (1–8). Since the first implant by Cribier (1), transcatheter AVI is ushering in a new era in the surgical treatment of aortic stenosis (2). At present, transcatheter AVI procedures have only been offered to very high-risk patients on a compassionate (no other treatment modality available) basis (3–9) and in the context of randomized clinical trials. Recent clinical experiences have suggested that transcatheter AVI likely mitigates the procedural risks and favorably alters the balance of risks and benefits in the high-risk group of patients. However, transcatheter AVI remains associated with the potential for serious complications despite being less invasive than conventional aortic valve replacement (AVR), and clinical benefits, particularly long-term benefits, remain unproven (4–11).

Currently, approaches for transcatheter AVI include transarterial and transapical. The advantages of the transapical approach compared to the transarterial approach include independence of peripheral vascular and aortic disease, not limited by delivery system sheath sizes, independence of the orientation of the ascending aorta and aortic annulus angle, less instrumentation in the aorta, and better positioning (coaxial alignment) and stabilization (less motion during valve deployment) perhaps because of short, direct distance. Furthermore, the transapical approach is more suitable for transcatheter valve-in-valve implantation (12) and for transcatheter AVI in patients with previous mitral valve implantation. We have been performing transapical AVI since October 2005 when the first successful human case was carried out at our center (13). The significant learning curve for these new technologies has been demonstrated in previous studies. As the technology edges toward widespread availability, we believe it is important for the medical community to disseminate the lessons learned in order to facilitate the learning curves of new implanting centers. To describe critical incidents and complications with transapical AVI, and the accompanying practical lessons on how to avoid such pitfalls from our early experiences would further mitigate perioperative mortality and morbidity. In this chapter, we discuss potential intraoperative and early postoperative complications following transapical transcatheter AVI of a balloon-expandable transcatheter valve. Most of complications are observed in both transarterial and transapical procedures, and unique complications related to transapical AVI are apical bleeding, apical pseudoaneurysm, and wound infection. We summarize pitfalls, and tips to avoid complications and procedural failure.

INTRAOPERATIVE COMPLICATIONS

Apical Laceration and Hemorrhage

Apical bleeding is a unique complication and the Achilles heel of transapical AVI. It occurred mainly in our initial experience with the transapical procedure (7,14). Massive apical bleeding is rare, and may require conversion to sternotomy and could be fatal. The incidence of apical laceration and bleeding is about 5% in our first 70 transapical AVI patients. Risk factors include friable tissue, fatty apex, chronic steroid use, dilated left ventricle with thinned walls, and hypertension during removal of the valve delivery sheath. While patient characteristics are important, the role of good surgical technique cannot be overstated. The most important risk factors are probably the incorrect placement of pursestring sutures or two "U-shape" orthogonal sutures in the apex, and a lack of experience in dealing with apical bleeding in an emergent situation. Achieving good hemostatic control of the LV apex is one of the most critical steps in ensuring the success of the transapical procedure, particularly in the elderly with friable tissue. The consequences following major apical laceration and bleeding include hemorrhagic shock/death, coronary artery injury, impaired left ventricular (LV) function, low cardiac output syndrome, and LV pseudoaneurysm. The following are the important points in avoiding this serious complication.

Selecting an Appropriate Area for Apical Access

In selecting the best position for placement of apical control sutures, several factors should be considered. The most critical point is to avoid an area covered with epicardial fat, which provides no additional strength and obfuscates correct judgment of the depth of suture placement. It is extremely important to take deep bites of myocardium, preferably full-thickness [Fig. 1(A)]. Occasionally, apical fat or large coronary arteries (the left anterior descending artery and diagonal branches) necessitated using a slightly more anterolateral position on the left ventricle; however, the apex is preferable to the free wall for minimizing the risk of lacerating the myocardium (due to greater convexity and reduced wall stress as per LaPlace's law).

Correct Suture Technique

We use 3–0 polypropylene sutures with a large (MH) needle, pledgeted with customized pledgets approximately 1 × 2 cm in size (13,14). Two perpendicular horizontal mattress sutures are snared through tensioning tourniquets. These can be individually tensioned by an assistant when the surgeon is downsizing or removing catheters. The area bounded by the apical sutures should be approximately 1.5 cm in diameter, or larger than the largest delivery sheath (26 Fr)[Fig. 1(A) and (B)]. With two perpendicular horizontal mattress sutures, an approximately

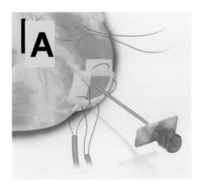
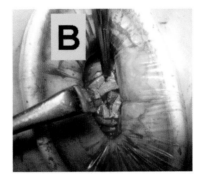
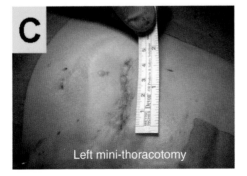

Figure 1 Technique for hemostatic control of the LV apex and left mini-thoracotomy. (**A**) Two perpendicular, pledgeted sutures are placed at the apex to avoid epicardial fat and vessels; A Seldinger needle is passed through the apex at the central point bounded by the sutures. (**B**) Excellent hemostasis following tying two pledgeted sutures. (**C**) Left mini-thoracotomy.

4 to 5 cm skin incision without spread of ribs is usually sufficient [Fig. 1(B) and (C)], which significantly minimizes postoperative pain (7). Other techniques such as using polypropylene pursestring sutures have also been used by other groups (6), however, with this technique a larger skin incision and rib spreading is necessary to allow placement of large pursestring sutures. Both suturing methods give equal satisfactory hemostatic control of apical access site as long as appropriate surgical technique is used [Fig. 1(B)].

Access Point
Once the sutures are placed, it is of utmost importance to then gain access with a needle precisely at the central point within the sutures [Fig. 1(A)]. This reduces the likelihood of extending the enlarging myocardial defect beyond the control sutures as larger sheaths are introduced stepwise. We use a progressive catheter dilation technique and never a scalpel stab wound for fear of biasing a tear along the blade direction.

Control of Hypertension
It is not uncommon to develop significant hypertension following relieve of aortic stenosis after successful deployment of a stented valve. Controlling hypertension is important before removing a large delivery sheath and tying down the sutures, which avoids potential significant tear of the LV wall. This is particularly important in the elderly with friable tissue, dilated cardiomyopathy, and chronic use of steroids. We try to control systolic blood pressure at approximately 100 mm Hg during removal of the delivery sheath. More aggressive control of blood pressure with temporary rapid ventricular pacing has also be advocated and used by some surgeons. However, this may increase risk of myocardial ischemia, infarction or ventricular arrhythmia, particularly in patients with significant coronary artery disease and/or poor LV function. We do not think that rapid ventricular pacing is necessary in the majority of patients.

Caution to Incorporate the Pericardial Edge into the Apical Sutures
In non-reoperative cases, we found it worthwhile to avoid the temptation to incorporate the pericardial edges into pledgeted apical sutures in an attempt to stop bleeding. This unfortunately makes identifying and locating a source of bleeding, as well as repairing the bleeding within the closed pericardium extremely difficult. Missing identification of a bleeding site during the procedure could cause postoperative tamponade and low cardiac output syndrome. Furthermore, in our experience incorporation of the pericardium does not seem to provide any additional strength to the closure since the sutures are already pledgeted. In reoperative cases, the pericardium may be incorporated because there are dense adhesions in the pericardial space and the likelihood of blood tracking unseen is less likely.

Management of Apical Laceration and Bleeding
Transapical AVI should be performed in a cardiac operating room, preferably in a hybrid operating room. Before the procedure is initiated, the following should be prepared as a routine: (i) cardiopulmonary bypass or ECMO system should be primed, (ii) different sizes of catheters for femoral artery and vein cannulation should be immediately available, (iii) one perfusionist is physically in the room, (iv) packed red blood cells are checked and ready for emergent transfusion, (v) surgical instruments for urgent sternotomy are set up, and (vi) two surgeons or one surgeon with an appropriate assistant should be scrubbed. Minor bleeding from the apex can usually be controlled with additional pledgeted sutures. In these elderly patients, the left ventricle is quite friable and easily torn with placement of new sutures, and care is needed to avoid torquing the needles as they are passed through the beating heart. If the apical bleeding cannot be controlled with additional sutures, the following methodologies should be considered: (i) no hesitation in enlarging the thoracotomy to achieve better exposure, (ii) establishment of femoro-femoral cardiopulmonary bypass to unload heart, and (iii) sternotomy if necessary. Although one surgeon with a cardiologist is sufficient to perform the transapical procedure in the majority of cases, it is better to have two surgeons scrubbed at the same time to deal with emergent situations. For the extremely friable tissue, a pericardial patch with BioGlue

is a very useful technique in securing the apical access site following unsatisfactory suture repair of the apex.

Cardiac Arrest

Cardiac arrest during the procedure is rare, but is one of the most devastating complications with this procedure. This can occur anytime during the procedure, but most frequently during initial balloon valvuloplasty and following valve deployment. This is because positioning of a balloon valvuloplasty catheter in the stenotic aortic valve can cause complete obstruction of the aortic valve with significant stress on the already hypertrophic heart and results in myocardial ischemia. In addition, significant acute aortic regurgitation may occur immediately following aortic valvuloplasty. Cardiac arrest following deployment of a transcatheter valve is most likely due to myocardial ischemia, hemorrhage, or newly developed significant valvular abnormalities. Both balloon and valve are deployed during rapid ventricular pacing which increases ischemic stress. Potential causes of cardiac arrest include (*i*) myocardial stress and ischemia, which could be as a result of anesthesia, rapid ventricular pacing, or instrumentation through the stenotic valve; (*ii*) acute hemodynamic compromise due to newly developed rapid atrial fibrillation; (*iii*) rapid ventricular pacing during valvuloplasty or deployment of a transcatheter valve; (*iv*) coronary embolization and potential thrombosis from debris from calcified valve or aorta, or air emboli; (*v*) compromised coronary blood flow due to complete or partial obstruction of a coronary ostium by calcified native valve or valve stent; (*vi*) major hemorrhage due to annulus or aortic rupture; and (*vii*) newly developed severe aortic regurgitation secondary to malposition of a transcatheter valve, or iatrogenic severe mitral regurgitation. Predisposing risk factors for these complications include coronary artery disease, poor LV function, and extreme critical aortic stenosis with bulking calcified leaflets, severe pulmonary hypertension, and significant mitral stenosis. Patients with severe aortic stenosis often have little myocardial flow reserve particularly in the presence of LV hypertrophy or coronary artery disease. We have observed cardiac arrest in 4 out of 70 patients undergoing transapical AVI as a consequence of anesthetic induction, left ostial obstruction, and massive bleeding. Hypotension or tachycardia may initiate a downward spiral of ischemia and myocardial dysfunction leading to shock or cardiac arrest. Our experience has suggested that one should not hesitate to initiate temporary femoro-femoral or sternotomy cardiopulmonary support if there is no sign of improvement with initial resuscitation. Further investigations are then performed to identify causes of the cardiac demise. Sometimes, immediate relieve of aortic stenosis is the only and a good option to stabilize hemodynamics in a downward spiraling clinical condition. If chest compression is required during resuscitation, stent positioning and expansion of the valve must be reevaluated after resuscitation.

Rupture of Aortic Root or Annulus

Rupture of the aortic annulus or aortic root is a rare complication of transcatheter AVI. This complication occurred in one case at our center with an incidence of less than 0.5%. This patient experienced rupture of the porcelain aortic root immediately after deployment of transcatheter valve. Excessive balloon dilation, aggressive valve oversizing, extensive calcification of both mitral and aortic annulus, and significant root calcification appear to be risk factors for this complication. Therefore, it may be particularly important to avoid aggressive overdilation of the aortic annulus and valve oversizing in patients with small heavily calcified aortic annulus and aortic root. The clinical warning signs of this complication include unexplained hypotension following balloon dilation or valve deployment, leading to cardiogenic shock and cardiac arrest due to massive bleeding and/or tamponade. Emergent sternotomy and surgical repair may be the only hope to save the patient.

Heart Block and Arrhythmia

As seen in conventional AVR, heart block also occurs following deployment of a transcatheter valve. This is probably as a result of displacement of calcium that causes permanent pressure on or injury to the atrioventricular conducting system at the noncoronary and right coronary cusp junction. The ventricular end of the valve stent could also be responsible for injury to the conducting systems located in the ventricular septum. The incidence of permanent heart block following transapical AVR is approximately 5% at our center (15). Potential risk factors include aggressive oversizing, small LV outflow tract, subaortic calcification near the membranous septum, preexisting partial atrioventricular (particularly right bundle brunch) block, and deployment of the valve too far below the aortic annulus. It has been suggested that the prosthetic stent extending further below the aortic annulus is associated with increased incidence of conduction abnormalities, particularly left bundle branch block. Heart block usually occurs immediately following valve deployment or during the first 24 to 48 hours after the procedure. Recovery from complete heart block appears less likely in patients undergoing transcatheter AVI, and therefore permanent pacemaker implantation is usually required.

Arrhythmia such as atrial fibrillation or ventricular ectopy may be precipitated by intracardiac instrumentation during the procedure, which is poorly tolerated by the patients with severe aortic stenosis. Fortunately, arrhythmias are uncommon during transapical AVI. Sustained ventricular fibrillation was observed in 1 out of 70 transapical patients (1.4%) as a result of rapid ventricular pacing, which was easily converted with external defibrillation. Therefore, as a routine external defibrillation pads must be applied before the procedure is initiated in each patient.

Myocardial Ischemia or Infarction

Coronary artery disease is present in approximately 70% of our transapical patients. Although prior coronary artery bypass grafting and angioplasty have been performed in the distant past in approximately 30% and 20%, respectively, many patients have residual non-revascularized coronary artery disease. Surprisingly, no perioperative myocardial infarction due to existing coronary artery disease has been observed in the cohort of patients who have undergone transapical AVI (7), which suggests that aggressive interventions for moderate coronary artery disease prior to the transapical procedure may not routinely be necessary. This is an example of the overriding myocardial stress of aortic stenosis and increased afterload versus ischemia from coronary disease. Occasionally, prophylactic preprocedural angioplasty and stenting is performed prior to transcatheter AVI in patients who have a critical coronary artery stenosis with respect to increased risk for ischemia during rapid ventricular pacing. Generally speaking, there is no need to postpone a transcatheter valve procedure following coronary stent deployment because there is no need to stop Plavix prior to transcatheter AVI. In selected patients who have critical stenosis in the left anterior descending artery, combined MIDCAB and transapical AVI through the same skin incision can be an option. However, our early experience suggests that combined MIDCAB and transapical AVI may carry an excessively high risk of operative mortality and morbidity. This option may be more beneficial in younger patients with aortic stenosis and critical stenosis in LAD who are declined for conventional AVR due to a porcelain aorta. Transient myocardial ischemia or infarction may occur as a consequence of repeat or prolonged rapid ventricular pacing, air or particle embolization, or obstruction of a coronary ostium (5,7).

Mitral Valve Apparatus Injury and Worsening of Mitral Regurgitation

Functional mitral regurgitation is common in patients with severe aortic stenosis, and moderate to severe mitral regurgitation is observed in more than 50% of our transapical patients. Our experience has suggested that mitral valve regurgitation is generally well tolerated during transapical procedure, and significantly decreased following AVI in the majority of transapical patients (Fig. 2).

With the transapical approach a guidewire may rarely pass through the mitral chordae before accessing the aortic valve and advancing a balloon catheter and a large delivery sheath over such a wire course may result in temporary distortion of the mitral valve apparatus or laceration of mitral chordae, leading to transient or permanent acute mitral regurgitation (Fig. 3). In another rare situation, mitral regurgitation may result from injury or interference with movement of the anterior mitral leaflet from a valve stent that is inappropriately positioned far below the aortic annulus. To avoid potential injury to mitral chordae, the following points should be kept in mind during the procedure: (i) when a guidewire is advanced into the left atrium, the wire should be completely withdrawn into a delivery sheath before trying to reposition it; (ii) the route from the LV apex to the aortic valve is quite straight, and therefore if the

Mitral regurgitation

p=ns

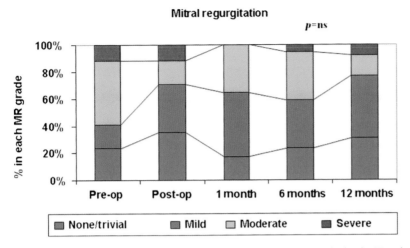

Figure 2 Twelve-month echocardiographic follow-up on mitral regurgitation in 17 patients survived >12 months (matched data). *Abbreviation*: MR, mitral regurgitation.

wire forms an unusual angle before entering the aortic valve, it may suggest that the wire likely passes through and is distorted by the mitral chordae before reaching the aortic valve (Fig. 3); (*iii*) significant worsening of mitral regurgitation during intraventricular instrumentation should also alert the surgeon to this possibility. If there is any concern, rewiring or utilization of a balloon flotation catheter should be considered to avoid passage through mitral chordea.

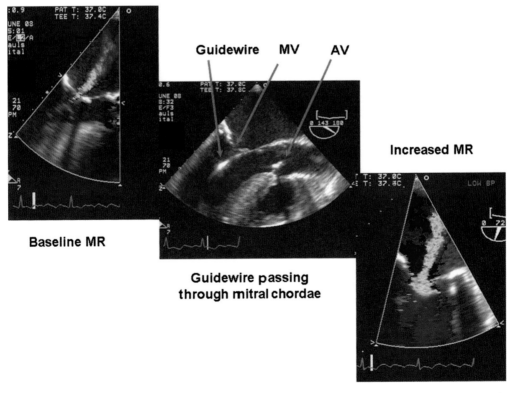

Figure 3 A guidewire passing through the mitral chordae, which results in worsening of mitral regurgitation. *Abbreviations*: MV, mitral valve; AV, aortic valve.

Embolized valve   **Anchoring valve in distal arch**

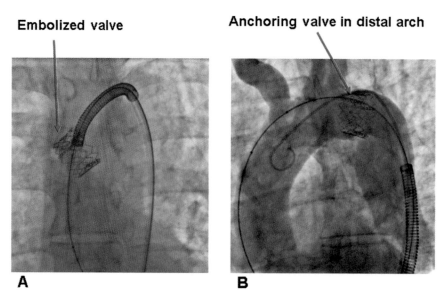

A   **B**

Figure 4 Embolization of transcatheter valve into the ascending aorta immediately following transarterial aortic valve implantation and anchoring of the valve in the distal aortic arch.

Valve Migration and Embolization

Prosthetic embolization occurred mainly in the early experience with transcatheter, particularly transarterial, AVI (3,5) [Fig. 4(A)]. This complication is primarily due to malpositioning of a valve, incorrect measurement of native aortic annulus, incorrect selection of a valve size, or lack of significant valve calcification for prosthetic anchoring. Malpositioning of a valve usually occurs as a result of lack of experience in positioning, poor coaxial alignment, ineffective or failed rapid ventricular pacing to reduce pulsatile blood flow during deployment, or accidentally moving balloon catheter during valve deployment. With increased experience, this complication has decreased significantly. We have not observed valve embolization in our 70 transapical patients. Relative to the transfemoral approach, the transapical approach may carry less risk of this complication because of more accurate positioning, better coaxial alignment, and better catheter stabilization (short straight distance) during valve deployment. The best management of an embolized bioprosthesis is to anchor it to the aorta preferably distal to the origins of arch vessels to avoid compromise of blood flow through the arch vessels (3) [Fig. 4(B)]. This is possible only if the guidewire remains in place to prevent the valve from flipping into a permanently closed position, and therefore the guidewire should not be removed until the end of the procedure. Embolization into the aorta is well tolerated as long as the coaxial wire position is maintained to prevent the valve from flipping over to obstruct antegrade flow. After the embolized valve is anchored in the distal aorta, an additional transcatheter valve can usually be successfully reimplanted into the native aortic valve through either the transfemoral or transapical approach. However, an alternative approach may be advisable when the reason for initial failure cannot be addressed. Delayed migration of a valve was observed in one transapical patient, in whom the valve partially migrated into the LV outflow tract, leading to severe aortic regurgitation (Fig. 5). Retrospective analysis revealed that the possible cause in this patient was a slightly too big aortic annulus (26 mm by TEE, smaller by TTE) and asymmetric calcification (lack of calcification in one cusp). Currently, the largest size of balloon-expandable transcatheter valve is 26 mm. The procedure should be abandoned in patients with borderline sizes of annulus approaching this size, unless the native aortic valve is uniformly and heavily calcified. Embolization of a bioprosthesis into the left ventricle is very rare, but very challenging. Surgical removal is probably the only option, but carries extremely high mortality and morbidity.

Coronary Ostial Obstruction

Coronary ostial obstruction is a fatal complication with transcatheter AVI. Fortunately, this complication is rare (3,5,7). Obstruction to coronary flow by the prosthesis itself appears rare and

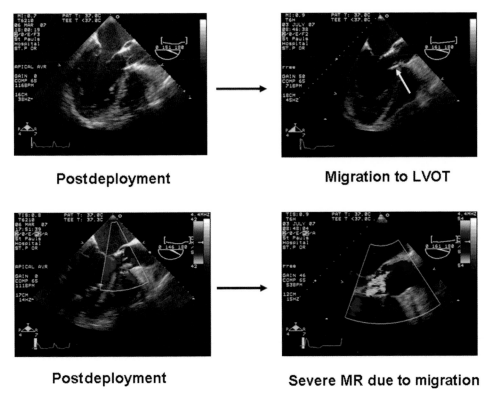

Postdeployment

Migration to LVOT

Postdeployment

Severe MR due to migration

Figure 5 Delayed migration of a transcatheter valve, causing significant aortic regurgitation. Abbreviations: LVOT, left ventricular outflow tract; AR, aortic regurgitation.

the presence of the open cell portion of the valve frame over a coronary ostium is well tolerated. The most common cause of the complication is the displacement of an unusually bulky, calcified native aortic cusp over a coronary ostium [Fig. 6(A)]. This occurred in two of 70 transapical cases at our center, as a result of bulky native valve calcification displaced towards the left main ostium with deployment of valves. Clinical presentations are progressive hypotension, ventricular fibrillation, or cardiac arrest without massive hemorrhage, which does not respond to aggressive resuscitation. Transesophageal echocardiography demonstrates worsening of LV function and new wall motion abnormalities. Immediate establishment of femoro-femoral bypass is critical to promptly stabilize hemodynamics prior to further determination of causes of the event. Aortic and coronary angiography should be then performed to confirm the obstruction of a coronary ostium, and sometimes stenting of the left main is an effective option for managing this complication [Fig. 6(B) and (C)). Coronary bypass surgery is also an option, but at present carries an excessively high risk of operative mortality and morbidity in a patient previously deemed nonoperable.

Preoperative assessment of the bulkiness of the native valve calcification, the distance from the coronary ostia to the annulus, and the ratio of the sinus of Valsalva and annulus diameters may be helpful in predicting the risk of this complication. Presently, no definite criteria exist to exclude patients from transcatheter AVI based on the risk for coronary obstruction. The potential risks for this complication include (*i*) a bulky calcification mass located particularly near the edge of the left coronary cusp, (*ii*) the left main ostium located close to the aortic annulus, particularly the distance between the ostium and the annulus of less than 10 mm, and (*iii*) calcified aortic root with a ratio of the sinus Valsalva and annulus dimensions near 1.0. Echocardiography, aortography, and CT angiography with 3D reconstruction have been used to assess these relationships. Potential procedure-related risks include oversizing of a transcatheter valve and inappropriately positioning a valve too far into the aorta. Intraoperatively, if a bulky calcium load or a heavily calcified cusp is seen to move toward a coronary ostium during

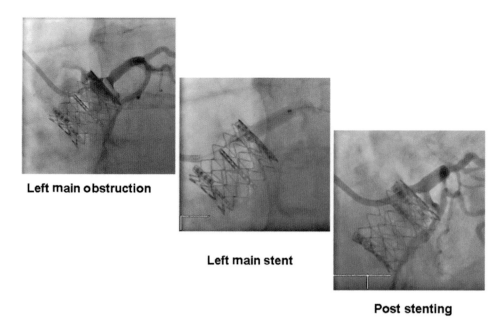

Left main obstruction

Left main stent

Post stenting

Figure 6 Obstruction of the left ostium by the displaced calcified native valve following the deployment of a valve, and stenting of the left main coronary artery.

balloon valvuloplasty, the procedure should be abandoned. Obstruction of the right coronary ostium has not been reported, perhaps because it is usually situated at a greater distance from the aortic annulus.

Paravalvular Leak

Trivial-to-mild paravalvular leaks are common immediately after transcatheter AVI, but remain stable during follow-up (4,5) (Fig. 7). Minimal paravalvular leaks are usually seen at the posterior portion of the annulus where there is relatively less tissue consisting of a thin layer of the fibrotic aorto-mitral curtain. More significant paravalvular leaks are infrequent and most likely result from incomplete deployment or suboptimal positioning of bioprostheses. Incomplete deployment of a valve is easily corrected in the majority of cases by repeat balloon dilation

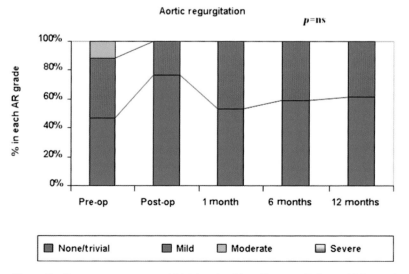

Figure 7 Common occurrence of trivial and mild aortic regurgitation, which remains stable during 12-month follow-up. *Abbreviation*: AR, aortic regurgitation.

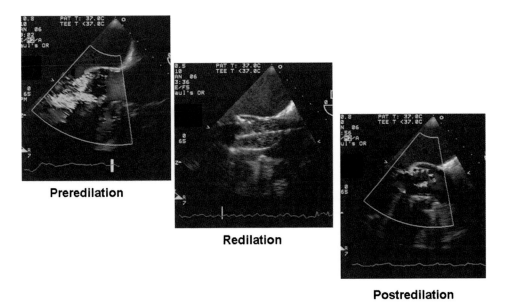

Preredilation

Redilation

Postredilation

Figure 8 Significant improvement in paravalvular aortic regurgitation following redilation.

(Fig. 8). Significant malposition of a valve may require deployment of a second transcatheter bioprosthesis to solve the residual aortic stenosis or significant paravalvular leaks (Fig. 9). Insufficient size of a valve may also cause significant paravalvular leaks, which is difficult to be corrected since excessive overdilation may result in transvalvular leaks. Surgery may be necessary if paravalvular leaks are hemodynamically significant. Clinically important hemolysis has not been observed to date (5,7).

EARLY POSTOPERATIVE COMPLICATIONS

Bleeding Requiring Reexploration of the Chest

As seen in conventional AVR, significant postoperative bleeding requiring surgical reexploration may occur following transapical AVI. Possible sources of bleeding are incomplete hemostasis of the apical access site, injury to epicardial vessels from placement of pacing wires or other

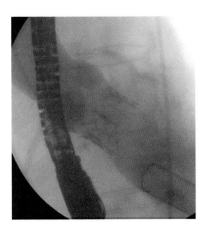

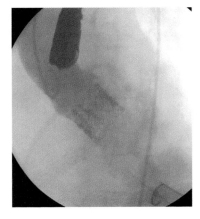

Severe AR after first valve   **Decreased AR following second valve**

Figure 9 Severe aortic regurgitation due to malposition of a valve, which is corrected by implanting another valve inside the first valve. *Abbreviation*: AR, aortic regurgitation

instrumentation, intercostal vessels, or significant coagulopathy. Of 70 transapical patients, three patients had significant postoperative blood loss, which required surgical reexploration. The causes in these three patients were bleeding from the epicardium where pacing wires were placed, intercostal vessels, and a coagulopathy. Careful inspection of the apex, pacing wire sites, and intercostal incision prior to closure of the thoracotomy cannot be overstated, because surgical reexploration significantly increases perioperative mortality and morbidity.

Arrhythmias

Postoperative arrhythmias can be observed following the procedure, such as atrioventricular block, atrial fibrillation, and ventricular arrhythmias. The risks of this complication are similar to those in conventional surgery. Delayed permanent heart block is rare, and hemodynamically significant ventricular arrhythmia has been observed in only one transapical patient. Management of postoperative arrhythmias is similar to those following conventional AVR. Temporary epicardial pacing wires are not routinely left behind in our transapical patients, but this is necessary if new complete or significant heart block occurs immediately during the procedure.

Acute Renal Failure

Since at present the cohort of patients for transapical AVI are the elderly, who usually have many comorbidities, including hypertension, diabetes, and peripheral vascular disease, preoperative chronic renal insufficiency is very common. Furthermore, the kidneys in elderly patients are more sensitive to hypotensive events and renal toxic agents/medications, such as angiographic contrast. Minimizing use of angiographic contrast and avoiding hypotension during the procedure are important in avoiding further deterioration in renal function. We try to eliminate unnecessary aortography to minimize the amount of intravenous contrast used during the procedure in patients with preoperative renal insufficiency. Postoperatively, these patients likely need intravenous fluids, rather than aggressive use of diuretics following the procedure because with critical aortic stenosis and congestive heart failure these patients are usually treated with aggressive diuresis and are hypovolemic preoperatively. Moreover, maintaining high cardiac output and relatively high perfusion pressure is also necessary to prevent deterioration in renal function early after the procedure. Renal artery embolization from debris of the diseased valve or aorta during the procedure can occur, but is less likely to be the cause of postoperative renal dysfunction. In the majority of patients minor deterioration in renal function is common and fortunately transient, and severe renal dysfunction and dialysis requirement is very rare.

Thromboembolic Events and Stroke

It was initially thought that expanding a valve into a calcified native aortic valve would carry a high risk of stroke. However, cumulative experience does not support this concept. Reported incidences of stroke are approximately 4% (5–8). It has been suggested that the incidence of stroke may be lower with transapical approach due to less manipulation in the ascending aorta and aortic arch compared with the transarterial approach, but this remains to be confirmed by a randomized trial or with a large database. Stroke following transcatheter AVI is most likely a result of embolic events, and less frequently as a consequence of ischemic insults due to severe hypotension during the procedure. Common causes of stroke are debris from the calcified native valve, dislodged materials from diseased aortic arch/ascending aorta/carotid arteries, clots on catheters or stented valve, or air. Potential risk factors include history of stroke, atheromatic aortic disease, critical carotid artery stenosis, insufficient heparinization during the procedure, multiple balloon valvuloplasties, extensive instrumentation in the aortic arch and ascending aorta, LV thrombosis, atrial fibrillation, and severe hypotension or hypertension during or following the procedure. Minimized intra-aortic instrumentation with the transapical approach, avoiding repeat valvuloplasty, sufficient heparinization (ACT $\geq$ 300), avoiding prolonged rapid ventricular pacing (repeat pacing should be performed only after recovery from previous pacing) and prolonged blockage of stenotic aortic valve during positioning of a valve, and maintaining good blood pressure are useful ways to potentially reduce the incidence of stroke. LV aneurysm with intramural thrombus may be the only contraindication for transapical approach. A clinically significant embolic event to other organ systems was observed in only one transapical patient who developed ischemic bowel nine days after the transapical AVI, presumed the result of a thromboembolic event. This patient received a second transcatheter valve placed inside the first transcatheter valve that was deployed too low in the ventricular outflow tract. The incidence of late stroke following the procedure has been extremely rare, and there has been no evidence of valve thrombosis with current antiplatelet treatment only, and no evidence to support the use of warfarin after transcatheter AVI unless there are other indications for anticoagulation. Most centers currently recommend one to three months of combination of aspirin and Plavix, followed by daily low dose of aspirin. We prefer three months of combination of aspirin and Plavix.

Left Ventricular Pseudoaneurysms

Apical pseudoaneurysm of the left ventricle is a unique complication following transapical AVI. This complication occurred in 5.7% of our 70 patients who underwent transapical AVI, and was observed mainly in our early experience. The incidence is probably dependent on how aggressively the patients are screened for the complication during follow-up. Our first case of apical pseudoaneurysm was incidentally found during a chest CT scan for other reasons about nine months after transapical AVI (Fig. 10). Following this case, we have aggressively been screening for this complication during follow-up echocardiography. If an apical pseudoaneurysm is suggested, cardiac-gated CT scan of the heart is performed to confirm and characterize the pseudoaneurysm. According to our experience, these apical pseudoaneurysms are generally asymptomatic and possibly less likely to expand significantly because of narrow long necks to the pseudoaneurysms and the usual dense adhesions in the pericardium. We believe that the potential for rupture of these pseudoaneurysms is probably very low. The possible risk factors for the complication include friable cardiac tissue, difficulty achieving apical access hemostasis, unidentified small bleeding into the pericardial space because of incorporation of the pericardium into apical sutures, and requirement of early anticoagulation with intravenous heparin or Coumadin following the procedure. To date, we have identified late LV pseudoaneurysms in four patients (5.7%). Management of these apical pseudoaneurysms can be quite challenging with surgical repair through the same mini-thoracotomy. Conservative treatment with discontinuation of all antiplatelet and anticoagulation medications may be considered in patients at high risk for any surgical procedure. We observed spontaneous thrombosis of a pseudoaneurysm following conservative management in two patients. One patient underwent

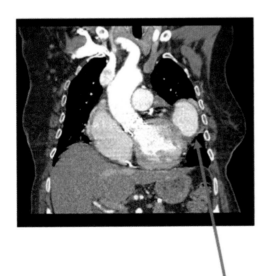
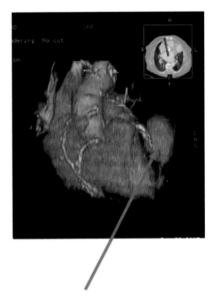

Apical Pseudoaneurysm

Figure 10 Apical pseudoaneurysm of the left ventricle identified by a CT scan.

successful surgical repair without support of cardiopulmonary bypass through the same mini-thoracotomy. With improvement in apical suture techniques and experience, this complication has significantly decreased.

SUMMARY

In this chapter we have tried to systematically review the complications associated with transapical AVI. Since the world experience with this procedure is somewhat limited at present, we have relied in large part on our own recognition and tabulation of complications in our patients. We have no doubt that as transapical AVI becomes more widespread there will be reports of complications not as yet appreciated.

Despite the many complications encountered, it remains a viable procedure in patients for whom there is no other therapeutic modality and high-risk surgical patients. With a better appreciation of these complications and techniques modified to address these, transapical AVI will very likely find a role in even lower risk surgical patients.

REFERENCES

1. Cribier A, Eltchaninoff H, Bash A, et al. Percutaneous transcatheter implantation of an aortic valve prosthesis for calcific aortic stenosis: First human case description. Circulation 2002; 106:3006–3008.
2. Webb JG. Percutaneous aortic valve replacement will become a common treatment for aortic valve disease. JACC Cardiovasc Interv 2008; 1:122–126.
3. Webb JG, Chandavimol M, Thompson CR, et al. Percutaneous aortic valve implantation retrograde from the femoral artery. Circulation 2006; 113:842–850.
4. Ye J, Cheung A, Lichtenstein SV, et al. Six-month outcome of transapical transcatheter aortic valve implantation in the initial seven patients. Eur J Cardiothorac Surg 2007; 31:16–21.
5. Webb JG, Pasupati S, Humphries K, et al. Percutaneous transarterial aortic valve replacement in selected high-risk patients with aortic stenosis. Circulation 2007; 116:755–763.
6. Walther T, Simon P, Dewey T, et al. Transapical minimally invasive aortic valve implantation: Multi-center experience. Circulation 2007; 116(11 suppl):I240–I245.
7. Ye J, Cheung A, Lichtenstein SV, et al. Transapical transcatheter aortic valve implantation: One year outcome in 26 patients. J Thorac Cardiovasc Surg 2009; 137:167–173.
8. Svensson, LG, Dewey T, Kapadia S, et al. United States feasibility study of transcatheter insertion of a stented aortic valve by the left ventricular apex. Ann Thorac Surg 2008; 86:46–55.
9. Webb JG, Lukas A L, Boone RH, et al. Transcatheter aortic valve replacement. Impact on clinical and valve-related outcomes. Circulation. 2009; 119:3009–3016.
10. Al Ali AM, Altwegg LA, Horlick EM, et al. Prevention and managemet of transcatheter balloon-expandabel aortic valve malposition. Catheter Cardiovasc Interv 2008; 72:573–578.
11. Tuzcu ME. Transcatheter aortic valve replacement malposition and embolization: Innovation brings solutions also new challenges. Catheter Cardiovasc Interv 2008; 72:579–580.
12. Ye J, Webb J, Cheung A, et al. Transcatheter transapical aortic valve-in-valve implantation: 16 month follow-up. Ann Thorac Surg. In press.
13. Ye J, Cheung A, Lichtenstein SV, et al. Transapical aortic valve implantation in man. J Thorac Cardiovasc Surg 2006; 131;1194–1196.
14. Lichtenstein SV, Cheung A, Ye J, et al. Transapical transcatheter aortic valve implantation in humans. Initial clinical experience. Circulation 2006; 114:591–596.
15. Sinhal A, Altwegg L, Pasupati S, et al. Atrioventricular block after transcatheter balloon expandable aortic valve implantation. JACC Cardiovasc Interv 2008; 1:305–309.

23 | ICU Care

Axel Linke and Gerhard Schuler

Department of Cardiology, University of Leipzig—Heart Center, Leipzig, Germany

MONITORING ON THE ICU

Immediately after the procedure, patients are typically transferred to an intensive care unit akin to patients undergoing surgical aortic valve replacement. The risk of life-threatening complications can still exist even after a "noncomplicated" transfemoral or transapical aortic valve implantation (TAVI). TAVI is currently performed in patients who are elderly and have major comorbidities—it is axiomatic that these patients can be at high risk for postprocedural complications.

Possible complications may include cardiac (e.g., acute aortic insufficiency associated with prolonged hypotension, acute cardiac failure, ventricular arrhythmias, pericardial tamponade, myocardial infarction (MI), conduction abnormalities), vascular (e.g., overt or covert bleeding related to the access site, vessel perforation or dissection resulting in hypovolemic shock or ischemia), pulmonary (e.g., pulmonary edema from cardiac decompensation, pneumonia, pneumo- or hemothorax, renal failure, infections (e.g., SIRS sepsis), hematological (e.g., thrombocytopenia, disseminated intravascular coagulation), and neurological (e.g., stroke, transient loss of consciousness, seizures, vasovagal) (1–9). Most of the complications manifest within 1 to 3 days of the procedure. Some of the complications become evident soon after the procedure (i.e., immediate) while some can take a few days to become apparent (i.e., delayed).

It is essential, therefore, that clinical and ICU monitoring is performed in a continuous and systematic fashion: neurological (regular assessments of the level of consciousness and for neurological deficits), cardiac (continuous blood pressure and ECG monitoring), pulmonary (arterial oxygen saturation), renal (volume balance, diuresis), infections (body temperature, white blood cell count), etc.

This chapter addresses complications that may occur early after the procedure and strategies to diagnose and treat them.

POTENTIAL COMPLICATIONS AFTER TRANSFEMORAL OR TRANSAPICAL VALVE IMPLANTATION: PREVENTION, RECOGNITION, AND MANAGEMENT IN THE ICU

Cardiac

Conduction Abnormalities

Preimplantation aortic balloon valvuloplasty performed during rapid ventricular pacing is required to facilitate the retrograde or antegrade passage of the aortic prosthesis across the native calcified valve. A temporary pacemaker can protect the patient from the hemodynamic consequences of high-grade AV block, asystole, or bradyarrhythmia that may occur after valvuloplasty alone, after transapical/transfemoral valve implantation, or in the postprocedural period (1,3,4,6,8–12).

According to the literature, the frequency of conduction abnormalities may be somewhat different depending on the type of transcatheter valve implanted (1,3,4,6,8,9). After implantation of the Edwards SAPIEN transcatheter heart valve, approximately 7.5% of patients require permanent pacemaking for complete heart block or bradycardia (3,6). With regard to the CoreValve ReValving system, the risk of conduction abnormalities requiring permanent pacemaking appears to be slightly higher, ranging from 10% to 25% (1,8,9,13). In addition, up to 40% of patients implanted with the CoreValve device may develop a new left bundle branch block. It has been suggested that a deeper implantation within the left ventricular outflow tract

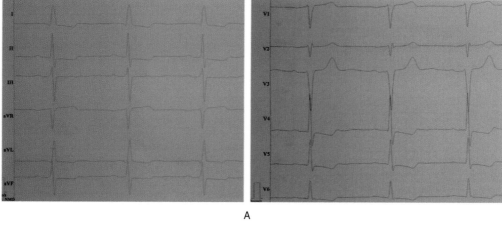

A

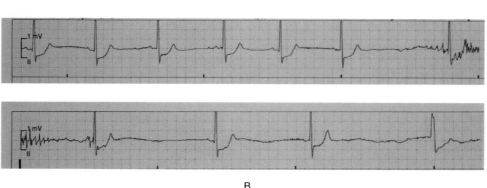

B

Figure 1 (**A**) Baseline ECG recording from a patient prior to transfemoral Edwards SAPIEN valve implantation (50 mm/sec). (**B**) Monitor ECG recording from the same patient after transfemoral Edwards SAPIEN valve implantation (25 mm/sec): Symptomatic bradycardia was evident 7 days after valve implantation. Therefore, a temporary pacemaker was exchanged for a permanent DDD pacemaker. (**C**) Video files: Position of the Edwards SAPIEN valve in the above-mentioned patient in an AP (Video 1) and LAO (Video 2) projection.

may increase this risk (13). Furthermore, patients with a preexisting right-bundle branch block may be at increased risk for complete.

It is important to realize that life-threatening conduction disturbances may develop hours or even days after the index implantation procedure (Figs. 1 and 2). Hence, continuous ECG monitoring in the ICU or the use of telemetry once the patient is on the wards is recommended.

To date, there are no firm recommendations on the duration of the temporary pacemaker period or the duration of in-hospital heart rhythm monitoring. Based on the literature and our own clinical experience, it appears prudent to maintain the temporary pacemaker 48 hours after the procedure (with a backup pacing rate of 30 beats/min) and verify its function every shift in the ICU since the lead might dislodge when the patient moves. Afterwards, further monitoring of the heart rate for 3 days by using a telemetric system is strongly recommend in order to recognize delayed-onset heart block.

Indications for implantation of a permanent pacemaker should follow the recommendations set by guidelines (14). Definite indications for permanent pacemaking include persistent or intermittent second-degree atrioventricular block type II, third-degree (complete) atrioventricular block, asystole, and symptomatic bradycardia. Uncertain indications for permanent pacemaking include the development of new left bundle branch block (with or without first- or second-degree atrioventricular block type I) and asymptomatic bradycardia.

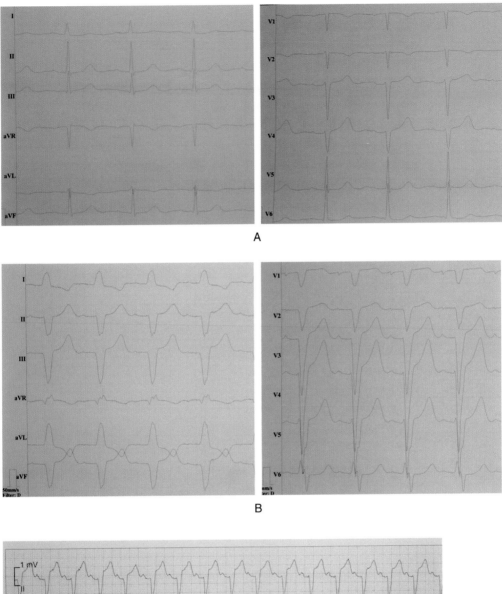

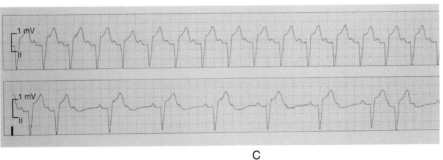

Figure 2 (**A**) Baseline ECG recording from a patient prior to transfemoral CoreValve implantation (50 mm/sec). (**B**) 12-lead ECG recording from the same patient immediately after transfemoral implantation of a CoreValve prosthesis (50 mm/sec). The patient developed a new first-degree AV block and left bundle branch block. (**C**) Monitor ECG obtained one day after implantation of the CoreValve device (25 mm/sec): identification of an asymptomatic, intermittent, second-degree AV block type II led to the implantation of a permanent DDD pacemaker. (**D**) Position of the CoreValve device in the above-mentioned patient in a RAO (Video 3) projection after release of the frame and in a LAO projection shortly before complete deployment (Video 4). High-grade AV block developed in spite of a rather high implantation of the frame.

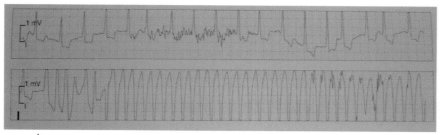

↑Induction of the ventricular tachycardia

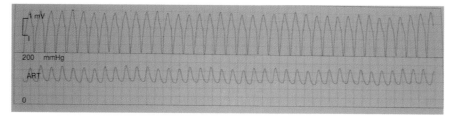

→ Sustained ventricular tachycardia

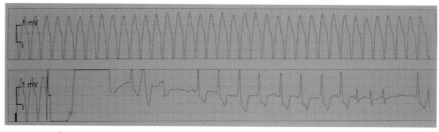

↑Termination by an external shock

Figure 3 ECG recording from a patient who developed ventricular fibrillation shortly after implantation of the CoreValve prosthesis (25 mm/sec)—the patient was successfully resuscitated. The patient had a poor left ventricular function and received an intracardiac defibrillator (ICD).

Ventricular Arrhythmias

The occurrence of significant ventricular arrhythmias or ventricular fibrillation is a rare event (1–3%) and more likely to occur in patients with left ventricular dysfunction and accompanying coronary artery disease (Fig. 3).

A number of preventative or corrective measures can be instituted. In particular, electrolyte abnormalities (e.g., potassium imbalances) should be identified and treated accordingly. In the setting of ventricular arrhythmias, MI should be ruled out.

In patients with impaired left ventricular function, intravenous amiodarone is known to effectively reduce the recurrence of ventricular arrhythmias should they occur (15). In case of torsades-de-pointes, intravenous injection of magnesium remains the therapy of first (16). In these latter patients, it is crucial to verify and discontinue medications that may be associated with long-QT syndromes. An intracardiac defibrillator (ICD) can be contemplated if the arrhythmias become incessant.

Pericardial Effusion

Pericardial effusion and cardiac tamponade are typically observed during the procedure but occasionally become clinically apparent after the procedure while the patient is in the ICU. If there is any reason for concern, an echocardiogram should be promptly performed to rule out

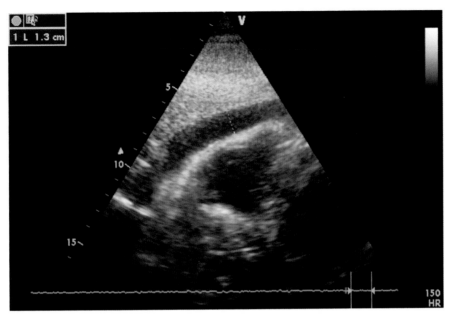

Figure 4 (**A**) Pericardial effusion in a patient after transfemoral implantation of an aortic valve prosthesis. The picture shows 13 mm of effusion in end-diastole from a subphrenical view anterior to the right atrium and ventricle. The effusion became evident 4 hours after the procedure and pericardiocentesis was successfully performed (200 mL venous blood). There was no further evidence of bleeding and the pigtail catheter was removed from the pericardium on the following day. (**B**) Fluoroscopy (LAO projection) during implantation (Video 5). The pacing lead appears suboptimally positioned in the right ventricle and led to the suspicion of a right ventricular perforation.

this potentially life-threatening complication (Fig. 4). The underlying causes include left ventricular perforation by the extra-stiff guidewire, right ventricular perforation by the temporary pacing wire, bleeding from the left ventricular apex access site used for transapical implantation, or aortic root rupture during balloon aortic valvuloplasty.

If the diagnosis is confirmed, immediate actions should consist of the administration of fluids (e.g., colloids, crystalloids, and blood products) pericardiocentesis, or possibly the administration of catecholamines (17). If the bleeding does not stop, definitive repair with direct suturing of the left ventricle by using a thoracotomy can be performed. In certain instances, the pericardial effusion is minor and of no hemodynamic consequence; watchful waiting with continuous monitoring may be an acceptable strategy. Anticoagulants should be stopped temporarily and if required, protamine or Vitamin K can be administered when indicated.

We suggest that if repositioning of the temporary pacing wire is needed, it should be performed under fluoroscopic visualization to avoid right ventricular perforation.

Acute Myocardial Infarction

Acute MI after transfemoral or transapical valve implantation is a rare complication seen in less than 1% of patients (1,3,4,6,8,9). Due to the nature of the procedure, many patients are characterized by negligible elevations in troponin, CK, and CK-MB levels. Potential causes of myocardial ischemia include embolization of calcific debris, displacement of native aortic leaflets or large bulky calcium deposits over coronary artery ostia, or spontaneous plaque rupture. If there is a significant rise in cardiac enzymes, ECG changes or symptoms suggestive of myocardial ischemia, then a coronary angiogram to rule out coronary obstruction should be performed. Neither the Edward SAPIEN nor the CoreValve ReValving system precludes coronary angiography. Treatment of patients with MI should be according to guidelines (18–20).

Low Cardiac Output—Cardiogenic Shock

Cardiogenic shock is defined by sustained hypotension with tissue hypoperfusion despite adequate left ventricular filling pressure. Signs of tissue hypoperfusion include oliguria (<30 mL/h), cool extremities, and altered mentation. Cardiogenic shock can be due to a variety of causes including MI, arrhythmia, cardiomyopathy, or valvular disease. Treatment depends on the underlying cause. In patients with refractory cardiogenic shock, extracorporeal membrane oxygenation or left ventricular assist device may be the only option to regain hemodynamic stability (21) (Fig. 5). Nevertheless, this decision—which is always difficult to make in elderly patients with multiple comorbidities—is best performed by a team approach (interventional cardiologist, cardiac surgeon, and anesthesiologist). In our opinion, this form of aggressive treatment should only be considered for patients who have a reasonable chance of recovery of left ventricular function. Alternatively, cardiac resynchronization in case of asynchrony

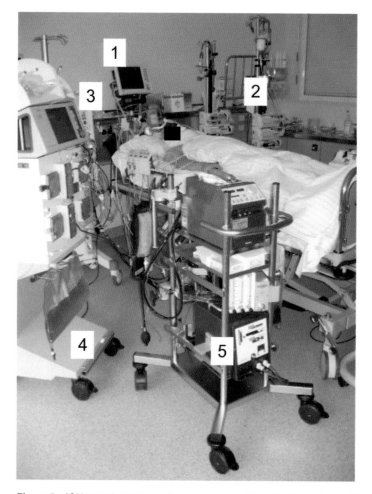

Figure 5 ICU setup in a patient after implantation of the CoreValve device. The patient was diagnosed with severe aortic stenosis and moderately-severe mitral regurgitation (grade 3). Surgery had been refused by two centers. The decision was made to treat the aortic stenosis by TAVI using a CoreValve prosthesis. Although the implantation was straight forward, the patient developed hemodynamic collapse and was connected to the heart-lung machine for reperfusion. He recovered rather quickly and the cannulas were disconnected. The patient was then moved to the ICU. That same night (approximately 8 hours after successful TAVI) the patient became hemodynamically unstable once again and developed cardiogenic shock that was recalcitrant to catecholamines. This figure demonstrates the typical setup in our hospital for a patient with the following needs: (1) constant hemodynamic monitoring (including invasive measurement of pulmonary artery pressures); (2) positive inotropic medication infusion pump; (3) mechanical ventilation; (4) hemodialysis; and (5) extracorporeal membrane oxygenator (ECMO) was implanted via femoral access to achieve hemodynamic stability.

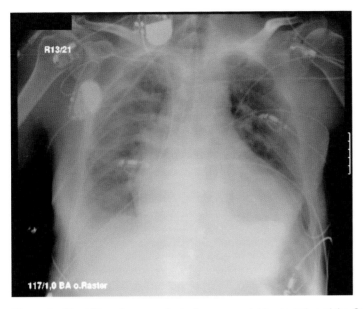

Figure 6   Chest X-ray from a patient after successful implantation of the CoreValve device. The patient was a high risk candidate for conventional surgery due to poor LV function. After CoreValve implantation, the LV function did not recover and it was almost impossible to mobilize the patient due to terminal heart failure. Since the patient had significant left ventricular asynchrony, a temporary coronary sinus pacing lead was introduced through the right jugular vein in an attempt to improve LV function (Videos 6 and 7). LV pacing significantly enhanced left ventricular performance with a subsequent rise in blood pressure by 20 mm Hg. *Abbreviation*: LV, left ventricular.

or implantation of an aortic balloon pump might be taken into account to achieve hemodynamic stabilization (20,21) (Fig. 6). Data, however, proving the effectiveness of these therapies in patients undergoing TAVI are lacking (21). In patients with paravalvular or transvalvular regurgitation, aortic balloon counterpulsion is contraindicated.

Vascular Complications
Vascular complications including access site vessel occlusion, dissection, perforation, and peripheral embolization may occur in up to 12% of patients undergoing transfemoral aortic valve implantation (1,3,6). Risk factors include mismatch between sheath size and access site vessel diameter, circumferential calcification, and severe tortuosity associated with ulcerations and atherosclerosis.

Usually, the complication becomes clinically evident during the procedure. A control peripheral angiogram should be routinely performed at the end of the procedure to recognize any covert bleeding. Dissections and perforations should be treated using self-expanding and covered stents, respectively.

In some cases, small dissections may be considered clinically irrelevant. These small dissections, however, may impair blood flow and induce thrombus formation—peripheral embolization can occur a few hours or days after the procedure. It is essential, therefore, to question patients about symptoms of peripheral ischemia and to regularly examine the extremities for clinical signs of ischemia (pain, paleness, paresthesia, pulselessness, paralysis, prostration). In addition, small perforations in the setting of hypotension may be overlooked during control angiography.

Performing blood gas analysis on a regular basis within the first 8 hours can be helpful in detecting early complications. An increase in blood lactate levels may be an early sign of peripheral ischemia whereas a drop in hemoglobin strongly suggests a bleeding complication.

Peripheral ischemia can be confirmed by Doppler ultrasound interrogation in the ICU, and if the diagnosis is confirmed, a peripheral angiogram should follow to identify the culprit lesion. In the meantime, patients should receive painkillers and the extremity in question should be covered with a warming blanket to avoid further cooling.

In case of access site bleeding, manual compression is often adequate to achieve hemostasis. In some cases, however, the site of bleeding is above the inguinal ligament and manual compression is ineffective. The suspicion of an intra-abdominal or retroperitoneal bleeding should be confirmed by ultrasound in the ICU followed by a CT scan to exactly identify the site of bleeding and to plan further interventions (Fig. 7). Angiography is often necessary and implantation of a covered stent in the perforated vessel usually seals the bleeding.

Renal Failure

Renal failure is considered to be a risk factor and predictor of mortality after conventional valve replacement (22,23). Similar observations are yet to be confirmed in patients undergoing TAVI.

In experienced hands, TAVI can be performed using only 60 mL of contrast medium. Some studies have shown that adequate rehydration before contrast reduces the likelihood of a postinterventional increases in creatinine levels and oliguria/anuria (24). On the other hand, the additional volume challenge in critically ill patients with severe aortic stenosis may lead to cardiac decompensation and pulmonary edema. There is a discrepancy in the literature with regard to acetylcysteine and the prevention of renal failure (24). Given that a recent meta-analysis was able to show a possible benefit, it is our practice to administer 1200 mg of acetylcysteine twice a day with cautious rehydration in patients with preexisiting renal failure. Therapy should be instituted 2 days before TAVI and continued until the third postinterventional day.

Urine output must be monitored and recorded hourly using a urinary catheter. Creatinine levels should be measured every day to detect early changes in renal function (25). Bacterial infections of the urinary tract may exacerbate preexisiting renal dysfunction and if diagnosed, should be treated with antibiotic therapy (26). Urinary catheters should be discontinued at the earliest time feasible to avoid bacterial contamination.

Pulmonary Complications

Approximately one-quarter of patients undergoing TAVI have pulmonary comorbidities (e.g., severe chronic obstructive pulmonary disease, restrictive lung disease) (1,3,4,6,8,9).

Depending on the clinical status of the patient and local hospital practices, TAVI may be performed with local or general anesthesia (1,3,4,6,8,9). If general anesthesia is used, attempts should be made to minimize the total duration of mechanical ventilation and if possible, extubate the patient immediately after the procedure in the hybrid theatre/OR/cath lab (27,28).

In some cases, however, immediate extubation may not be possible. In these patients, weaning should be initiated as soon as possible to avoid complications of long-term mechanical ventilation such as ventilator-associated pneumonia (VAP) and deconditioning of the diaphragm and other respiratory muscles. (27,28) Another disadvantage of general anesthesia is the delayed recognition of procedure-related neurological complications. In cases where there is an altered level of consciousness, the question is whether it is due to the anesthesia itself or whether a stroke or intracranial bleed has occurred. In most cases, a CT scan with contrast must be performed to rule out the latter possibility. Furthermore, general anesthesia may impair the early mobilization of patients after TAVI.

Auscultation of the lungs should be performed at least twice daily to detect clinical signs of pneumonia or pulmonary edema. If either is suspected, the diagnosis should be confirmed by chest X-ray and appropriate treatment instituted (29) (Fig. 8). Moreover, one has to keep in mind that early mobilization is the key to avoid hypostatic pneumonia (29).

Neurological Complications

Transient Ischemia Attack, Prolonged Reversible Ischemic Neurological Deficits, and Stroke

The incidence of neurological complications was high during the early experience of TAVI (3,6,8,9) (Fig. 9). This raised the question of whether this method is really applicable to a broader patient population since neurological defects are usually associated with life-long disabilities. More recently, however, it has become evident that the stroke rate has declined considerably. The exact reasons for this are unknown, but the development of smaller sized delivery catheters, steerable catheters, and the growing experience are thought to play a role (1,3,4,6,8,9).

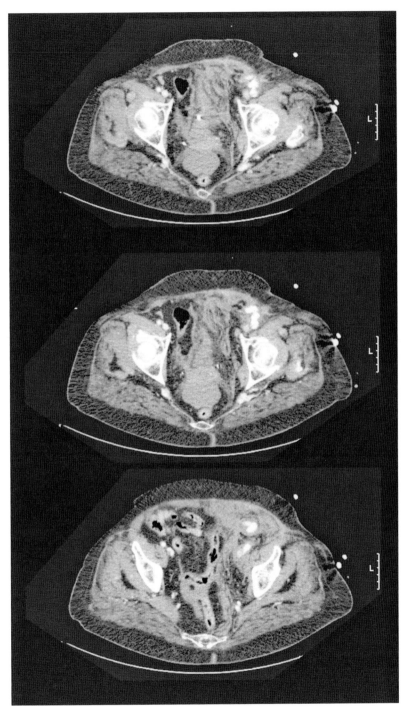

Figure 7 Case example—A patient who underwent successful TAVI developed sudden hemodynamic instability approximately 4 hours after the procedure. This was associated with a drop in hemoglobin from 6.0 to 4.0 mmol/L within 30 minutes of the event. Echocardiography was normal and there was no evidence of pericardial effusion. Ultrasound of the abdomen showed a massive retroperitoneal bleeding. (**A**) CT scan of the abdomen confirmed the retroperitoneal bleeding originating from the iliac artery. (**B**) Angiography of the left femoral access site after transfemoral implantation of the aortic valve prosthesis. Massive bleeding from the left iliac artery (Video 8) was sealed by deployment of a covered stent (Videos 9 and 10). Proximal to this lesion, the vessel appeared to be dissected (Video 11) and another stent was placed (Video 12, still frame). The final angiogram confirmed a successful result with no evidence of residual bleeding (Video 13).

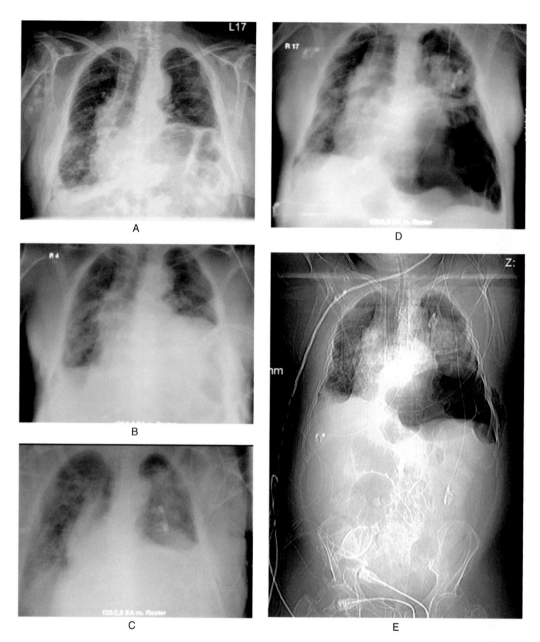

Figure 8 Chest X-rays and CT scans of the thorax from a patient after implantation of the CoreValve device. (**A**) A chest X-ray obtained three days after the procedure demonstrated a partially resected left lung as a result of cancer years before the procedure. In addition, the patient had severe chronic obstructive pulmonary disease. There was no evidence of pulmonary congestion or pneumonia and the patient was spontaneously breathing and doing fine. (**B**) The procedure was performed under general anesthesia using the subclavian approach (due to peripheral arterial occlusive disease). The patient was extubated 2 hours after the procedure, recovered quickly and was transferred to the normal ward on postprocedure day 3. Unfortunately, the patient developed hospital-acquired pneumonia 6 days after the procedure requiring antibiotic therapy. (**C**) Progressive bilateral infiltrations resulted in a further deterioration of pulmonary status and the patient needed mechanical ventilation. (**D**) The patient developed sudden hypotension and the chest X-ray confirmed a pneumothorax that was already suspected on physical examination (**E**) The topogram of the CT scan confirmed the diagnosis of the pneumothorax. (**F**) CT scan of the chest demonstrates the left pneumothorax, bilateral pneumonic infiltrates and pulmonary congestion.

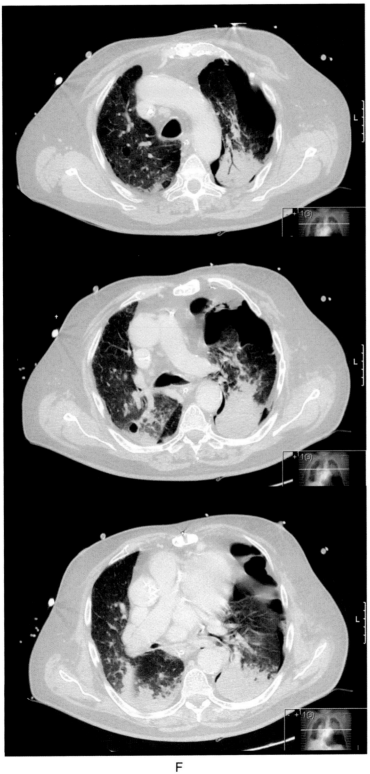

F

Figure 8 (*Continued*)

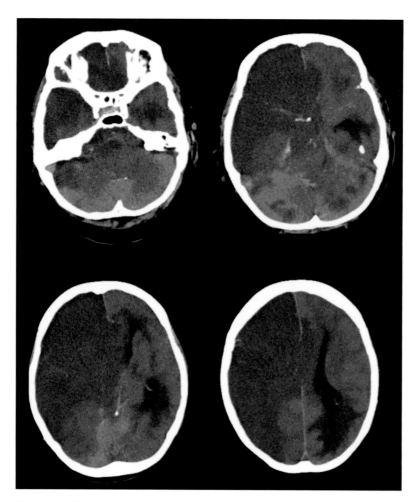

Figure 9 CT scan of the brain after percutaneous aortic balloon valvuloplasty was performed as a bail-out procedure during cardiopulmonary resuscitation in a patient with severe aortic stenosis. After the procedure, the patient was hemodynamically stable, catecholamines were discontinued and the patient started to breath spontaneously on the respirator. On hospital day 3, however, the patient was not triggering the ventilator and became respirator-dependent. The suspicion of a large stroke was confirmed on CT scan of the brain.

The majority of neurological complications are recognized immediately during the procedure—that is, if the patients are not under general anesthesia. Interestingly, some patients experience a stroke several hours or days after the intervention (1). The reasons for these delayed events are not clear. Fortunately for some, the deficits are transient and disappear over a period of hours or days.

A complete neurological exam should be performed at least once per day while in the ICU. When a neurological complication is suspected, a brain CT scan with contrast should be performed to rule out a bleed or a perfusion defect. In the setting of large strokes (e.g., complete occlusion of the medial cerebral artery), direct angiography to evaluate the perfusion defect and, if possible, intervention by angioplasty should be considered (30). Alternatively, local thrombolysis might be administered (31). In most cases, however, it is unclear whether embolized calcific debris or thrombotic material is the cause of the perfusion defect. Calcified material might be thrombolysis naive and the decision to infuse thrombolytic drugs carries the risk of bleeding (31). On the other hand, if thrombotic material were responsible for the occlusion, local thrombolysis might be the only therapy to prevent life-long disability and even death. Since no recommendations exist for this cohort of patients, a consensus should be reached by the team of physicians (interventional cardiologist, cardiac surgeon, and anesthesiologist) taking care of the patient.

In case of neurological complications, early physiotherapy (two to three times a day) is absolutely essential to improve function (30,31). In addition, physiotherapy should not be restricted to the postinterventional in-hospital period and all attempts should be made to continue it in a rehabilitation unit or outpatient clinic until independence of the patient is largely re-established.

Symptomatic Transitory Psychotic Syndrome
A reduction in consciousness is often seen after interventions and operation. The symptoms are usually mild and transient in nature. The likelihood of developing delirium significantly increases with age and is modulated by many cofactors, for example, individual predisposition, alcohol or drug abuse, postoperative pain, stress due to the intervention, sleeplessness, side effects of medication, changes in the electrolyte balance, infections, fever, and dehydration (32). Treatment of the underlying reasons and mobilization of the patient often leads to the complete disappearance of the symptoms within a couple of hours. In case of severe disorientation and aggressive behavior, a combination of neuroleptic drugs and benzodiazepines may be indicated (32).

Hematological Complications
Severe and prolonged thrombocytopenia identified within days of the procedure was a concern during the early experience, especially after CoreValve implantation (8). This was primarily attributed to the use of the heart-lung machine (8). Theoretical considerations led to the advice of preprocedural administration of a clopidogrel loading dose of 300 mg in an attempt to block platelet activation and consumption (1,8,9). Once this practice was instituted, postprocedural thrombocytopenia, if it occurred, was only mild and transient (8).

Within the first week of TAVI, platelet counts should be measured daily. Platelet infusions should be administered if (1) platelet counts $< 10 \times 10^9$; (2) platelet counts $< 10–20 \times 10^9$; (3) platelet counts $< 50 \times 10^9$ associated with active bleeding, disseminated intravascular coagulation, or coagulopathy; (4) platelet counts $< 50 \times 10^9$ and need for extracorporeal membrane oxygenation; and (5) active bleeding in association with qualitative platelet defects (33).

Of note, clopidogrel or ticlopidine can be associated, albeit rarely, with thrombotic thrombocytopenic purpura (TTP). This condition is characterized by intravascular coagulation, thrombocytopenia, and bleeding (typically in the brain) (34). Platelet administration is contraindicated except in situations of life-threatening bleeding. Plasma apheresis and the administration of fresh frozen plasma are the only known therapies known to improve survival (34).

General Inflammatory Response and Infections
Periprocedural antibiotics should be administered according to local practice guidelines. Despite this practice, some patients are characterized by an increase in inflammatory markers (e.g., leucocytes, blood sedimentation rate) in the setting of elevated body temperature. In these case, further diagnostic tests are necessary to identify a potential focus of infection, e.g., urinalysis (rule out urinary tract infection), chest X-ray (to detect pneumonia), and blood cultures. Vascular access lines and urinary catheters should be changed or discontinued when they cannot be ruled out as a source of infection. If judged necessary, broad spectrum antibiotics should be instituted according to guidelines (26,29,35).

If severe septic shock develops, catecholamines might be required to achieve hemodynamic stabilization. Hematological parameters should be monitored for evidence of disseminated intravascular coagulation. (Fig. 10).

NUTRITION
Patients recovering quickly after percutaneous aortic valve implantation should receive a balanced diet. Some patients, however, might be mechanically ventilated for prolonged period of time that may negatively impact on their alimentation (36). According to current recommendations, enteral feeding should be initiated as soon as the gastrointestinal tract is functioning. One disadvantage of enteral feeding is the possibility of underfeeding associated with inadequate

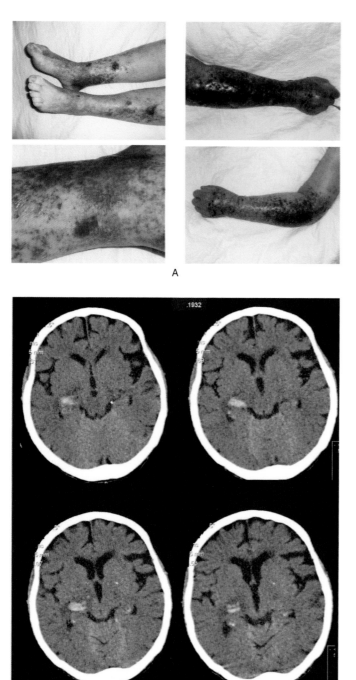

Figure 10 (**A**) Skin lesions in a patient 14 days after TAVI suggestive of disseminated intravascular coagulation (left upper panel: both feet, right upper panel: right arm, left lower panel: higher magnification form the left foot, right lower panel: right left arm). The patient was characterized by a massive drop in platelets and 6 out of 6 blood cultures revealed the presence of staphylococci. (**B**) The patient went into a state of coma. The brain CT scan demonstrated diffuse bleeding into the thalamus. (**C**) In addition, a perfusion defect of the lower left leg was recognized by physical examination (paleness of the left foot [(**A**), left upper panel], pulselessness of the popliteal artery) and this was confirmed by angiography. The popliteal artery was almost completely occluded (Video 14) and successfully revascularized by stent implantation (Video 15). However, diffuse microthrombi were evident in the peripheral circulation of both legs in accordance with the results from the physical examination (Video 16).

energy and protein intake—coupled with an increased risk of morbidity, for example, higher rates of infection, delayed wound healing, prolonged mechanical ventilation, and delayed recovery (36). A recent meta-analyses of ICU studies provided ample evidence that parenteral nutrition is not related to excessive mortality, but in the contrary, may even contribute to improved survival. Therefore, supplemental parenteral nutrition combined with enteral nutrition should be strongly considered to cover the energy and protein targets when enteral nutrition alone does not achieve the caloric goal (36).

REFERENCES

1. Piazza N, Grube E, Gerckens U, et al. Procedural and 30-day outcomes following transcatheter aortic valve implantation using the third generation (18 Fr) corevalve revalving system: Results from the multicentre, expanded evaluation registry 1-year following CE mark approval. EuroIntervention 2008; 4(2):242–249.
2. Walther T, Simon P, Dewey T, et al. Transapical minimally invasive aortic valve implantation: Multicenter experience. Circulation 2007; 116(11 suppl):I240–I245.
3. Webb JG, Pasupati S, Humphries K, et al. Percutaneous transarterial aortic valve replacement in selected high-risk patients with aortic stenosis. Circulation 2007; 116(7):755–763.
4. Cribier A, Eltchaninoff H, Tron C, et al. Treatment of calcific aortic stenosis with the percutaneous heart valve: Mid-term follow-up from the initial feasibility studies: The French experience. J Am Coll Cardiol 2006; 47(6):1214–1223.
5. Walther T, Falk V, Kempfert J, et al. Transapical minimally invasive aortic valve implantation; the initial 50 patients. Eur J Cardiothorac Surg 2008; 33(6):983–988.
6. Webb JG, Chandavimol M, Thompson CR, et al. Percutaneous aortic valve implantation retrograde from the femoral artery. Circulation 2006; 113(6):842–850.
7. Lichtenstein SV, Cheung A, Ye J, et al. Transapical transcatheter aortic valve implantation in humans: Initial clinical experience. Circulation 2006; 114(6):591–596.
8. Grube E, Laborde JC, Gerckens U, et al. Percutaneous implantation of the CoreValve self-expanding valve prosthesis in high-risk patients with aortic valve disease: The Siegburg first-in-man study. Circulation 2006; 114(15):1616–1624.
9. Grube E, Schuler G, Buellesfeld L, et al. Percutaneous aortic valve replacement for severe aortic stenosis in high-risk patients using the second- and current third-generation self-expanding CoreValve prosthesis: Device success and 30-day clinical outcome. J Am Coll Cardiol 2007; 50(1):69–76.
10. Klein A, Lee K, Gera A, et al. Long-term mortality, cause of death, and temporal trends in complications after percutaneous aortic balloon valvuloplasty for calcific aortic stenosis. J Interv Cardiol 2006; 19(3):269–275.
11. Percutaneous balloon aortic valvuloplasty. Acute and 30-day follow-up results in 674 patients from the NHLBI Balloon Valvuloplasty Registry. Circulation 1991; 84(6):2383–2397.
12. Hara H, Pedersen WR, Ladich E, et al. Percutaneous balloon aortic valvuloplasty revisited: Time for a renaissance? Circulation 2007; 115(12):e334–e338.
13. Piazza N, Onuma Y, Jesserun E, et al. Early and persistent intraventricular conduction abnormalities and requirements for pacemaking after percutaneous replacement of the aortic valve. JACC Cardiovasc Interv 2009; 1:310–316.
14. Epstein AE, Dimarco JP, Ellenbogen KA, et al. ACC/AHA/HRS 2008 Guidelines for Device-Based Therapy of Cardiac Rhythm Abnormalities: A report of the American College of Cardiology/American Heart Association Task Force on Practice Guidelines (Writing Committee to Revise the ACC/AHA/NASPE 2002 Guideline Update for Implantation of Cardiac Pacemakers and Antiarrhythmia Devices): Developed in collaboration with the American Association for Thoracic Surgery and Society of Thoracic Surgeons. Circulation 2008; 117(21):e350–e408.
15. Vassallo P, Trohman RG. Prescribing amiodarone: An evidence-based review of clinical indications. JAMA 2007; 298(11):1312–1322.
16. Gupta A, Lawrence AT, Krishnan K, et al. Current concepts in the mechanisms and management of drug-induced QT prolongation and torsade de pointes. Am Heart J 2007; 153(6):891–899.
17. Spahn DR, Cerny V, Coats TJ, et al. Management of bleeding following major trauma: A European guideline. Crit Care 2007; 11(1):R17.
18. Bassand JP, Hamm CW, Ardissino D, et al. Guidelines for the diagnosis and treatment of non-ST-segment elevation acute coronary syndromes. Eur Heart J 2007; 28(13):1598–1660.
19. Van de WF, Bax J, Betriu A, et al. Management of acute myocardial infarction in patients presenting with persistent ST-segment elevation: The Task Force on the Management of ST-Segment Elevation Acute Myocardial Infarction of the European Society of Cardiology. Eur Heart J 2008; 29(23):2909–2945.

20. Sjauw KD, Engstrom AE, Vis MM, et al. A systematic review and meta-analysis of intra-aortic balloon pump therapy in ST-elevation myocardial infarction: Should we change the guidelines? Eur Heart J 2009; 30(4):459–468.
21. Westaby S. Destination therapy: Time for real progress. Nat Clin Pract Cardiovasc Med 2008; 5(8): 477–483.
22. Alexander KP, Anstrom KJ, Muhlbaier LH, et al. Outcomes of cardiac surgery in patients > or = 80 years: Results from the National Cardiovascular Network. J Am Coll Cardiol 2000; 35(3):731–738.
23. Urso S, Sadaba R, Greco E, et al. One-hundred aortic valve replacements in octogenarians: Outcomes and risk factors for early mortality. J Heart Valve Dis 2007; 16(2):139–144.
24. Kelly AM, Dwamena B, Cronin P, et al. Meta-analysis: Effectiveness of drugs for preventing contrast-induced nephropathy. Ann Intern Med 2008; 148(4):284–294.
25. McCullough PA. Contrast-induced acute kidney injury. J Am Coll Cardiol 2008; 51(15):1419–1428.
26. Guay DR. Contemporary management of uncomplicated urinary tract infections. Drugs 2008; 68(9):1169–1205.
27. Fassl J, Walther T, Groesdonk HV, et al. Anesthesia management for transapical transcatheter aortic valve implantation: A case series. J Cardiothorac Vasc Anesth 2009; 23(3):286–291.
28. Ender J, Borger MA, Scholz M, et al. Cardiac surgery fast-track treatment in a postanesthetic care unit: Six-month results of the Leipzig fast-track concept. Anesthesiology 2008; 109(1):61–66.
29. Rotstein C, Evans G, Born A, et al. Clinical practice guidelines for hospital-acquired pneumonia and ventilator-associated pneumonia in adults. Can J Infect Dis Med Microbiol 2008; 19(1):19–53.
30. Ringleb PA, Bousser MG, Ford G, et al. Guidelines for management of ischaemic stroke and transient ischaemic attack 2008. Cerebrovasc Dis 2008; 25(5):457–507.
31. Albers GW, Amarenco P, Easton JD, et al. Antithrombotic and thrombolytic therapy for ischemic stroke: American College of Chest Physicians Evidence-Based Clinical Practice Guidelines (8th edition). Chest 2008; 133(6 suppl):630S–669S.
32. Pun BT, Ely EW. The importance of diagnosing and managing ICU delirium. Chest 2007; 132(2): 624–636.
33. Dellinger RP, Levy MM, Carlet JM, et al. Surviving Sepsis Campaign: International guidelines for management of severe sepsis and septic shock: 2008. Crit Care Med 2008; 36(1):296–327.
34. Bennett CL, Kim B, Zakarija A, et al. Two mechanistic pathways for thienopyridine-associated thrombotic thrombocytopenic purpura: A report from the SERF-TTP Research Group and the RADAR Project. J Am Coll Cardiol 2007; 50(12):1138–1143.
35. Pepin J. Vancomycin for the treatment of Clostridium difficile Infection: For whom is this expensive bullet really magic? Clin Infect Dis 2008; 46(10):1493–1498.
36. Heidegger CP, Darmon P, Pichard C. Enteral vs. parenteral nutrition for the critically ill patient: A combined support should be preferred. Curr Opin Crit Care 2008; 14(4):408–414.

24 | Postdischarge and Follow-Up Care

Dominique Himbert, Gregory Ducrocq, and Alec Vahanian
Department of Cardiology, Bichat Claude Bernard Hospital, APHP, Paris, France

INTRODUCTION

The evaluation of patients at discharge and during follow-up after transcatheter aortic valve implantation (TAVI) is overall similar to that of patients after surgical aortic valve replacement using a bioprosthesis. However, there are some specificities due to the following reasons:

In comparison to the current knowledge on surgically implanted bioprostheses, our knowledge of TAVI relies on limited data reported mostly in oral communications and by a few articles in peer-reviewed journals, and is temporarily limited since the long-term results of TAVI are largely unknown. After two to three years, conclusions regarding the incidence of complications and the frequency and mode of valve dysfunction are yet to be made (1–8).

Patients treated by TAVI are usually more ill than those included in surgical series, in particular, because of their age and the presence of comorbidities, which should be taken into account for follow-up (6–9).

Finally, as can be expected at the present time, there are no precise guidelines on the postoperative management of patients after TAVI, in contrast to what is available for patients with surgically implanted bioprostheses (10,11).

Evaluation Before Hospital Discharge

Clinical Evaluation

Clinical evaluation is the key for the evaluation of cardiac and extracardiac status.

This evaluation includes clinical assessment, chest X-ray, ECG, transthoracic echocardiography, and blood testing. This reference assessment is of utmost importance for interpreting subsequent changes in murmurs and prosthetic sounds, as well as changes in ventricular function and transprosthetic gradients as assessed by Doppler echocardiography.

The status of vascular access in the case of the transfemoral approach or the thoracic scar in the case of the transapical approach should be carefully examined.

The exact incidence, timing, and predictors of atrioventricular block have yet to be identified precisely. The occurrence of AV block may be delayed after several days and justify further evaluation in patients at risk, such as those with previous bundle branch block with new conduction defects which appeared during or after implantation (12,13). In case of doubt it seems reasonable to perform Holter monitoring and electrophysiological studies before discharge to indicate pacemaker implantation.

Details on *Echocardiographic evaluation* are provided in chapter 25.

Medical Treatment

In patients with a surgically implanted bioprosthesis, even if it is not evidence based, the current guidelines recommend anticoagulation during the first three months (10,11). There is also no evidence to support the long-term use of antiplatelet agents in patients with a bioprosthesis who have no indication other than the presence of the bioprosthesis itself.

After TAVI, both manufacturers currently recommend a combination of aspirin and clopidogrel for three up to six months and then to take aspirin alone indefinitely, even if there is only limited evidence to support this strategy (Edwards Lifesciences Inc., Irvine, CA, USA, and Medtronic Int. Trading, Tolochenaz, Switzerland). In practice, when there is a high bleeding risk it is advisable to stop one antiplatelet agent as soon as possible.

Vitamin K blockers should be continued in patients in whom they are indicated, or those with atrial fibrillation, or a history of embolism. In such cases it is necessary to shorten as much as possible the use of antiplatelet therapy. During this period, weekly monitoring of INR is advised and any over-anticoagulation should be avoided.

Other medications should be continued such as medication for the treatment of heart failure, antiarrhythmic agents as well as the agents necessary for the treatment of extra-cardiac diseases.

Education

Before discharge, it is useful to improve patient education on endocarditis prophylaxis according to the recent guidelines (11) and, if needed, on anticoagulant therapy, as well as emphasizing that new symptoms should be reported as soon as they occur.

Rehabilitation

It is not routinely recommended after TAVI. It could be important in patients presenting pleural effusion after transapical approach. Patients are discharged either at home or in a general hospital, or finally in a rehabilitation clinic depending of their cardiac or more importantly their extra-cardiac status.

Follow-Up

General Comments

Taking into account the limitations mentioned before on the limited knowledge of long-term outcome, the following recommendations can be proposed.

All patients who have TAVI require lifelong follow-up by a cardiologist to detect early deterioration in prosthetic or ventricular function, or the further progression of disease in a heart valve. In the early phase of the technique it seems advisable that the team that performed TAVI has a leading role in the follow-up, keeping precise records of each individual patient and including them in registries. This should be done in close collaboration with the other physicians, such as the GP, and other specialists, such as geriatricians, if needed, according to the specifics of the extra-cardiac condition of the patient. It is of utmost importance that all these physicians are informed about the procedure.

Similar to the recommendations for surgically implanted bioprostheses, a complete baseline assessment should be performed, ideally one month after TAVI. This will include clinical assessment, which is the cornerstone of follow-up, chest X-ray, ECG, transthoracic echocardiography, and blood testing to detect silent bleeding in patients under anticoagulant therapy, or suffering from pathological hemolysis. In addition, it will probably be useful to assess quality of life and make a global assessment of the extracardiac condition by using scores such as the Lee or Charlson score (14,15). This visit is also useful to improve patient education.

Thereafter, clinical assessment could be performed at 3, 6, and 12 months after implantation and then twice a year. Functional deterioration or change in auscultation during late follow-up raise the question of valve dysfunction and require prompt echocardiographic examination.

There is no consensus regarding the usefulness of systematic echocardiographic follow-up, however it seems reasonable at this early stage in the technique to recommend that echocardiographic examination is performed during these visits. Transprosthetic gradients during follow-up are best interpreted in comparison to the baseline values in the same patient, rather than in comparison to theoretical values for a given prosthesis, which lack reliability. Transesophageal echocardiography (TEE) should be considered only if transthoracic echocardiography is of poor quality in all cases of suspected prosthetic dysfunction or endocarditis.

The clinical performance of valvular substitutes is judged according to the "Guidelines for Reporting Mortality and Morbidity After Cardiac Valve Intervention" (16).

Management of Complications

The specific complications associated with cardiac valve prostheses are structural valve degeneration (SVD), nonstructural dysfunction, delayed displacement, thromboembolism and thrombosis, and prosthetic valve endocarditis.

Structural Deterioration

SVD occurs in all bioprostheses if they remain in place long enough. Bioprosthesis failure occurs via several mechanisms: regurgitation via leaflet tears, stenosis due to leaflet calcification, or perforations unrelated to calcification.

Mid-term clinical outcome at up to five years (though only two years in most studies) is reported in a limited number of patients and is encouraging since serial echocardiographic studies have consistently shown good prosthetic valve function with no structural deterioration of valve tissue.

Structural deterioration may be detected in several circumstances: new heart failure, changes in auscultatory findings with detection of a diastolic murmur or changes in the characteristics of the systolic murmur that becomes louder, or finally changes in echocardiographic parameters. Auscultatory and echocardiographic findings should be carefully compared with previous examinations in the same patient.

The management of this complication after TAVI is difficult to define due to several reasons:

The long-term durability of these new bioprostheses as well as their mode of degeneration remain largely unknown, which does not allow us to give precise recommendations as regards the timing of reintervention.

The extra-cardiac condition and especially the multiple comorbidities of the patients currently treated by TAVI should be taken into account when deciding on the indication and the type of intervention used.

The feasibility of subsequent surgical aortic valve intervention is largely unknown (17). Preliminary case reports have shown that valve-in-valve implantation is feasible especially in the case of acute failure of TAVI, and this leads us to expect that if these initial findings are confirmed it will be the preferred option in case of SVD (18).

Finally, percutaneous balloon dilatation should be avoided in the treatment of stenotic left-sided bioprostheses because of the risk of embolism and cusp rupture leading to massive regurgitation (19).

The decision to reintervene should take into account the risk of reoperation, which increases with age, high functional class, LV dysfunction, comorbidities, and, above all, the emergency situation.

Reintervention will be advised in symptomatic patients with significant prosthetic dysfunction (significant increase in transprosthetic gradient or severe regurgitation) if their life expectancy is acceptable. Reintervention should be considered early, since its risk rapidly increases in patients in NYHA class III or IV.

Asymptomatic patients with any significant prosthetic dysfunction should be carefully followed up at shorter time intervals but it does not seem advisable to recommend reintervention at this stage on the basis of the current knowledge on TAVI.

Valve Prosthesis–Patient Mismatch

Data on valve prosthesis–patient mismatch after TAVI is very limited and suggests that it will be unlikely.

Nonstructural Dysfunction

Paraprosthetic regurgitation has been reported in 6% of patients after surgical aortic valve replacement. Even mild paraprosthetic regurgitation may cause hemolysis (10).

In the field of TAVI, long-term consequences of paravalvular leaks (PVL) have not been reported. However, it is to be anticipated that mild to moderate regurgitation will not have significant clinical consequences in this population. Conversely, severe aortic regurgitation may lead to heart failure.

Blood tests for hemolysis should be part of routine follow-up. Haptoglobin measurement is too sensitive, and lactate dehydrogenase, although nonspecific, is better related to the severity of hemolysis. The diagnosis of hemolytic anemia often requires TEE to detect a paravalvular leak. Even in surgical literature only limited data is available regarding therapeutic options. In the field of TAVI there is very limited data suggesting that in the acute setting balloon dilatation within the stented valve may decrease the magnitude of paravalvular regurgitation, but the risk-to-benefit ratio of such an approach is unknown since the technique may induce acute intravalvular leakage. There is no data on the performance of this technique at a later stage. Thus surgery seems to be the only option if reintervention is needed for paravalvular leakage causing hemolysis. In the guidelines on valve disease there is a consensus to recommend reoperation if PVL is related to endocarditis, or if PVL causes hemolysis needing repeated blood transfusions or leading to severe symptoms. In patients with severe hemolytic anemia and PVL where surgery is contraindicated, or in those unwilling to undergo reoperation, medical therapy includes iron supplementation, β-blockers, and erythropoietin if hemolysis is severe.

Transcatheter closure of paravalvular regurgitations is feasible but complex, and concerns exist regarding its efficacy. Little information is available since most evaluations of transcatheter closure of paravalvular regurgitations are case reports. A small series showed improvement of symptoms but no efficacy on hemolysis in most patients. This explains why transcatheter intervention is not considered as an alternative to surgery in guidelines (10,20) but it may be an interesting approach to be explored after TAVI.

Delayed Displacement
Although the vast majority of percutaneously implanted prothesis migrations occurred during, or just after the procedure, one case of delayed dislocation occurring 3 weeks after implantation has been published (21).

Endocarditis
Infective endocarditis prophylaxis is of particular importance in patients with a heart valve prosthesis, who are considered at high risk for endocarditis in all guidelines (11). This also applies after TAVI even if only 2 cases have yet been reported (1,22) due to the limited duration of follow-up. The current trend is to encourage good dental hygiene but limit antibiotic prophylaxis to dental procedures that involve the manipulation of either the gingival tissue, the periapical region of teeth, perforation of the oral mucosa, or interventions on the upper respiratory track. Surgery will be the only option if reintervention is needed in the case of hemodynamic compromise or persistent sepsis or recurrent embolism. However, the high surgical risk or even the absolute contraindication for surgery in many patients will probably often lead to medical treatment alone, which could be successful in the case of nonvirulent microorganisms. These anticipated problems with surgical intervention should lead to a reinforcement of the measures for prophylaxis of endocarditis and the avoidance of unnecessary procedures at high risk of endocarditis in this population.

Prosthetic Thrombosis
Occlusive prosthetic thrombosis is characterized by impaired motion of the mobile part of the prosthesis. It is rare after surgical implantation of an aortic bioprosthesis and its incidence after TAVI is unknown. Only one case has been reported to date. If it occurs it is likely that the principles used for the other bioprosthesis implanted surgically may be used.

This high-risk complication justifies a particular awareness and should lead to prompt performance of transthoracic echocardiography, and most often TEE. Occlusive prosthetic thrombosis is usually treated by redo surgery, which carries a relatively higher risk, particularly when patients are in poor hemodynamic condition. Thrombolysis is an alternative but it is associated with high mortality rates due to failure or embolic events. According to recent guidelines, thrombolysis is mainly considered if surgery is contraindicated, which may well be the case in patients currently treated by TAVI. On the other hand, a careful search for contraindication for thrombolysis should be done in this elderly population.

Thromboembolism after valve surgery is multifactorial both in its etiology and its origin. Although many thromboembolic events will have originated from thrombus, a vegetation on a prosthesis or as the result of the abnormal flow conditions created by a degenerated prosthesis, many others will have arisen from other sources as the result of other pathogenic mechanisms and be a part of the background incidence of stroke and transient ischemic attack in the general population.

Thorough investigation of each episode of thromboembolism is therefore essential (including cardiac and noncardiac imaging when appropriate) to allow for appropriate management.

Nonocclusive prosthetic thrombosis may be diagnosed on TEE after an embolic event. First-line treatment is oral anticoagulation, or the addition of antiplatelet drugs in patients who are already on vitamin K blockers, under close echocardiographic monitoring. Surgery can be considered in large nonocclusive prosthetic thrombosis (≥ 10 mm), in particular, if it is complicated by an embolic event or if it persists despite intensification of anticoagulant therapy. Here again the decision to operate will be very rare in the TAVI population because of an unfavorable risk-to-benefit ratio.

The prevention of further thromboembolic events involves the treatment or reversal of remediable risk factors such as atrial fibrillation, hypertension, hypercholesterolemia, diabetes, smoking, chronic infection, and prothrombotic blood test abnormalities.

For patients on oral anticoagulation, the optimization of anticoagulation control is necessary, if possible, with patient self-management, on the basis that better control is more effective than simply increasing the target INR. This should be discussed with the neurologist in case of recent stroke.

Heart Failure
Heart failure after valve surgery or TAVI should lead to a search for the following:

- Prosthesis-related complications: structural dysfunction, paravalvular leakage, or rarely, valve thrombosis.
- LV dysfunction: Systolic LV dysfunction may be due to (*i*) persistent pre-TAVI LV dysfunction, which is unlikely in isolated aortic stenosis but may occur in case of ischemic disease, especially after myocardial infarction leading to large myocardial scars and (*ii*) myocardial infarction occurring during or after TAVI.
- In the elderly population heart failure may be also due to diastolic LV dysfunction related to severe LV hypertrophy.
- Persistence or progression of another valve disease. This concerns especially the patients with severe organic mitral regurgitation in whom TAVI has been performed because the degree of regurgitation has been underestimated. However, one case of mitral valve injury occurring late after TAVI has been described (23).
- Nonvalvular related causes such as coronary disease, hypertension or sustained arrhythmias should also be considered.

The management of patients with persistent LV dysfunction should follow the guidelines on the management of chronic heart failure (24).

CONCLUSIONS
Currently, the limited knowledge of long-term follow-up after TAVI limits the possibility of issuing firm recommendations as regards the management of these patients during follow-up. The main principles for follow-up of patients after TAVI can be summarized as follows:

Follow-up should be done by a cardiologist and a team of physicians working together. A comprehensive assessment of the cardiac and extracardiac condition is necessary before discharge. Education of the patient is crucial. Sequential follow-up visits including clinical examination and in most cases echocardiography is recommended at this stage of our knowledge.

To make further progress, all patients receiving TAVI should be included in registries led by scientific societies and managed at national and international levels. This will allow us to better assess the durability and long term outcomes of TAVI and provide us with evidence-based guidance.

REFERENCES
1. Webb JG, Altwegg L, Boone RH, et al. Transcatheter aortic valve implantation: Impact on clinical and valve-related outcomes. Circulation 2009; 119:3009–3016.
2. Grube E, Buellesfeld L, Mueller R, et al. Progress and current status of percutaneous aortic valve replacement: Results of three device generations of the CoreValve revalving system. Circ Cardiovasc Interv 2008; 4(2):242–249.

3. Piazza N, Grube E, Gerckens U, et al. Procedural and 30-day outcomes following transcatheter aortic valve implantation using the third-generation (18Fr) CoreValve ReValving System—Results from the multicentre, expanded evaluation registry 1-year following CE mark approval. EuroIntervention 2008; 4(2):242–249.
4. Walther T, Simon P, Dewey T, et al. Transapical minimally invasive aortic valve implantation: Multi-center experience. Circulation 2007; 116: I240–I245.
5. Svensson LG, Dewey D, Kapadia S, et al. United states feasibility study of transcatheter insertion of a stented aortic valve by the left ventricular apex. Ann Thorac Surg 2008; 86(1):46–55.
6. Eltchaninoff H, Zajarias A, Tronc C, et al. Transcatheter aortic valve implantation: Technical aspects, results and indications. Arch Cardiovasc Dis 2008; 101:126–133.
7. Vahanian A, Alfieri O, Al-Attar N, et al. Transcatheter valve implantation for patients with aortic stenosis: A position statement from the European Association of Cardio-Thoracic Surgery (EACTS) and the European Society of Cardiology (ESC), in collaboration with the European Association of Percutaneous Cardiovascular Interventions (EAPCI). Eur Heart J 2008; 29:1463–1470.
8. Rosengart TK, Feldman T, Borger MA, et al; American Heart Association Council on Cardiovascular Surgery and Anesthesia; American Heart Association Council on Clinical Cardiology; Functional Genomics and Translational Biology Interdisciplinary Working Group; Quality of Care and Outcomes Research Interdisciplinary Working Group. Circulation 2008; 117:1750–1767.
9. Iung B, Baron G, Butchart EG, et al. A prospective survey of patients with valvular heart disease in Europe: The Euro Heart Survey on valvular disease. Eur Heart J 2003; 24:1231–1243.
10. Vahanian A, Baumgartner H, Bax J, et al. Guidelines on the management of valvular heart disease. The Task Force on the management of valvular heart disease of the European Society of Cardiology. Eur Heart J 2007; 28:230–268.
11. A Report of the American College of Cardiology/American Heart Association Task Force on Practice Guidelines. (Writing committee to revise the 1998 guidelines for the management of patients with valvular heart disease). Focused update incorporated into the ACC/AHA 2006 guidelines for the management of patients with valvular heart disease. Circulation 2008; 118(15):e523–e661.
12. Piazza N, Onuma Y, Jesserun E, et al. Early and persistent intraventricular conduction abnormalities and requirements for pacemaking after percutaneous replacement of the aortic valve. Am J Cardiol 2008; 1:310–316.
13. Sinhal A, Altwegg L, Pasupati S, et al. Atrioventricular block after transcatheter balloon expandable aortic valve implantation. JACC Cardiovasc Interv 2008; 1:305–309.
14. Charlson ME, Pompei P, Ales KL, et al. A new method of classifying prognostic comorbidity in longitudinal studies: Development and validation. J Chronic Dis 1987; 40(5):373–383.
15. Lee SJ, Lindquist K, Segal MR, et al. Development and validation of a prognostic index for 4-year mortality in older adults. JAMA 2006; 295:801–808.
16. Akins CW, Miller C, Turina MI, et al. Guidelines for reporting mortality and morbidity after cardiac valve interventions. J Thorac Cardiovasc Surg 2008; 135:732–738.
17. Litzler P, Cribier A, Zajarias, et al. Surgical aortic valve replacement after percutaneous aortic valve implantation: What have we learned? J Thorac Cardiovasc Surg 2008; 136:697–701.
18. Walther T, Kempfert J, Borger MA, et al. Human minimally invasive off-pump valve-in-a-valve implan-tation. Ann Thorac Surg 2008; 85(3):1072–1073.
19. Vahanian A, Palacios IF. Percutaneous approaches to valvular disease. Circulation 2004; 109(13):1572–1579.
20. Shapira Y, Hirsch R, Komowski R, et al. Percutaneous closure of perivalvular leaks with Amplatzer occluders: Feasibility, safety, and short term results. J Heart Valve Dis 2007;16(3):305–313.
21. Maroto LC, Rodriguez JE, Cobiella J, Silva J. Delayed dislocation of a transapically implanted aortic bioprosthesis. EJTCS 2009; (in press).
22. Comoglio C, Boffini M, El Quarra S, et al. Aortic valve replacement and mitral valve repair as treatment of complications after percutaneous CoreValve implantation. J Thorac Cardiovasc Surg 2009; (in press).
23. Wong DR, Boone RH, Thompson CR, et al. Mitral valve injury late after transcatheter aortic valve implantation. J Thorac Cardiovasc Surg 2009; 137:1547–1549.
24. Dickstein K, Cohen-Solal A, Filippatos G, et al. Guidelines for the diagnosis and treatment of chronic heart failure: The task force for the diagnosis and treatment of CHF of the European Society of Cardiology. Eur Heart J 2008; 29:2388–2442.

25 | Tips and Tricks for Imaging Percutaneously Implanted Aortic Valve Prostheses

Carl Schultz, Nicolo Piazza, Robert Jan van Geuns, P. de Feyter, Patrick W. Serruys, and Peter de Jaegere

Department of Interventional Cardiology, Erasmus University Medical Center, Thoraxcenter, Rotterdam, The Netherlands

INTRODUCTION

An understanding of the anatomy of the aortic valvar complex is a prerequisite for the correct interpretation of postimplant images that can be obtained by echocardiography, fluoroscopy, multislice computed tomography (MSCT), and MRI (1).

During surgical aortic valve replacement, densely calcified native leaflets are removed to make space for the prosthesis. In contrast, calcifications remain in situ during transcatheter aortic valve implantation (TAVI). The dense annular calcification and the dense metal struts of the prosthesis cause signal loss, which can affect all imaging modalities to a variable degree. The loss of signal, in addition to limitations imposed by echocardiographic windows, can severely restrict the ability of echocardiography to evaluate the three-dimensional (3D) geometry and position of the implanted prosthesis. This evaluation may be better achieved by 3D MSCT or using multiple views on cine-angiography. On the other hand, echocardiography remains the most frequently used modality for assessment of flow and prosthesis integrity. The particular set of difficulties and limitations that can affect imaging of the implanted prosthesis are shown in Table 1. Table 2 indicates the relative strengths and weaknesses of each imaging modality.

We briefly describe the indications for imaging post-TAVI and then explain the utility of echocardiography, fluoroscopy, MSCT, and MRI in more detail.

INDICATIONS

Clinical indications for postprocedural imaging include (*i*) evaluation of procedural success (i.e., valve position and valve function), (*ii*) assessment and management of procedural complications, (*iii*) evaluation of persistent or recurrent symptoms, and (*iv*) surveillance of device integrity.

Evaluation of Valve Position and Function

The optimal function of the prosthesis relies on correct sizing, correct positioning of the prosthesis, and adequate expansion and adequate apposition of the prosthesis to the surrounding tissue (2,3). The residual gradient and degree of aortic regurgitation are the most important parameters to be assessed. Additional information such as the position of the prosthesis within the aortic root (i.e., depth of implantation), angulation and geometry of the prosthesis, as well as displacement of the calcified leaflets relative to the coronary tree is required. A combination of imaging modalities is ideally needed. If significant regurgitation or a residual gradient is detected, the cause needs to be identified and managed correctly (e.g., prosthesis implanted too deep, underexpanded or malapposed prosthesis).

Serial investigations of valve integrity and function will eventually provide important data on long-term durability. Furthermore, deformation of the valve prosthesis after implantation with respect to its nominal dimensions can potentially impact the long-term durability of the valve (4,5). This concept is further discussed in a subsequent section.

Assessment of Procedural-Related Complications

During TAVI, complications such as device embolization or the need for a valve-in-valve may require postprocedural imaging to assess the safety and efficacy of these practices. In both situations, we have appreciated that the frame of the prosthesis may become severely deformed with potential clinical consequences (3,6) (Figs. 1 and 2). For instance, it is important to establish

Table 1 Factors Complicating Imaging of Implanted PAVR Prostheses

Patient related

- Frail patients, limited mobility, difficult to position, poor echo windows, claustrophobia
- Heavy calcification of the aortic root and ascending aorta causing signal loss (annular calcification is removed during surgical AVR but not PAVR)
- High incidence of arrhythmia including atrial fibrillation and frequent ventricular ectopy can reduce image quality in gated acquisitions (MSCT and MRI)
- Renal impairment: risk of contrast nephropathy (MSCT, cine-angiography) or gadolinium toxicity (CMRI)

Prosthesis related

- Multiple dense metal struts in addition to native calcification causing signal loss (ECHO>MRI>MSCT)
- Complex 3D morphology of the aortic root and PAVR prostheses (especially CoreValve), axial views can be difficult to obtain with 2D imaging modalities

whether the embolized valve may impinge on the carotid arteries or whether the prosthesis that is too low may affect left ventricular or mitral valve function.

Investigation of Persistent or Recurrent Symptoms

TAVI is highly effective in reducing the transaortic gradient and alleviating patient symptoms, but not all patients will symptomatically improve and some may deteriorate after an initial improvement (7). The lack of improvement of symptoms may be caused by cardiac factors or noncardiac comorbidities. Cardiac factors may include valvular hemodynamic perturbations (central or paraprosthetic aortic regurgitation, residual stenosis, incorrect sizing, mitral regurgitation, left ventricular impairment, coronary embolism or jailing, cardiac arrhythmia, or heart failure). Management will depend on the underlying cause of the symptoms.

Surveillance of Device Integrity

Long-term data on device is integrity is not yet available. To date, there have been no stent or frame fractures reported with either the Edwards SAPIEN or CoreValve ReValving system (CRS), respectively. This topic is further discussed later.

IMAGING MODALITIES

Echocardiography

Doppler echocardiography is the gold standard imaging modality for the serial assessment of valve function and left ventricular performance (8,9). In patients with suspected prosthetic valve dysfunction, echocardiography can provide information on valve structure, hemodynamics, and left ventricular function and evaluate for conditions such as prosthetic valve thrombosis or endocarditis. An echocardiographer who is skilled at assessing prosthetic valves is in a position to significantly impact patient care.

This section discusses aspects relating to (*i*) estimations of transaortic prosthetic valve gradients, (*ii*) effective aortic valve orifice areas, and (*iii*) the approach to the patient with suspected prosthetic valve dysfunction. Many of the principles discussed here are extrapolated from what is known about the evaluation of native aortic valves and surgically implanted prosthetic aortic valves.

Assessment of Prosthetic Valve Function

Following implantation, transthoracic echocardiography should be performed at least once before hospital discharge so as to provide baseline values for future comparison. Until further experience accumulates and "norm" is established, it may be prudent to perform serial transthoracic echocardiograms at each follow-up visit (e.g., 3 months, 6 months, 12 months, and twice a year thereafter).

Table 2 Strengths and Weaknesses of Each Imaging Modality for Postprocedural Imaging of PAVR

	TTE	TOE	Cine-angiography (noncontrast)	MSCT	CMRI
Availability	+++[a]	+++	+++	+++	++
Ease of use	+++	++	+++	++	++
Tolerance by patients	+++	++	+++	+++	+
Quality of images in the presence of signal loss due to:					
Calcium	++	++	+++	++(+)	+++
Metal struts	+	++	+++	+++	+
Assess of flow:					
Stenosis	+++	++(+) (Origin of paravalvular jets can be difficult to locate)	−	−	++
Regurtitation	++ (+)	+++	−	+	++
Ability to assess axial geometry	+	++	+	+++	+
Additional information	LV and mitral valve function	LV and mitral valve function		LV and mitral valve function, coronary anatomy, peripheral vasculature	LV and mitral valve function, peripheral vasculature
Safety in renal impairment	+++	+++	+++	++ (Risk of contrast nephropathy). Avoid if GFR < 30	++ (Risk of gadolinium toxicity). Avoid if GFR < 30

[a] +++, very good; ++, moderate; +, poor; −, absent/none.
Abbreviation: LV, left ventricular.

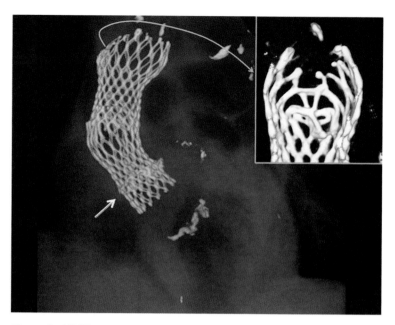

Figure 1 MSCT images of a sequential valve implantation. The first prosthesis was implanted correctly but was displaced following withdrawal of a pigtail catheter from the left ventricle. The MSCT images subsequently demonstrated that the tip of the pigtail catheter had inadvertently passed through the struts of the CRS during passage to the left ventricle. This resulted in entanglement with the frame on withdrawal (*inset*). A second CRS was implanted with clinically success result.

Transaortic Prosthetic Valve Gradients

The simplified Bernoulli equation relates blood flow velocity through a narrowed orifice to the pressure gradient between two chambers such that $\Delta P = 4V^2$ (where ΔP is the pressure gradient (mm Hg) and V is the velocity (m/sec) through the narrow orifice). The maximal instantaneous (peak) pressure gradient is obtained by estimating the maximal (peak) velocity across the valve orifice by using continuous wave Doppler. The mean gradient can be estimated by sketching out the envelope of the jet velocity profile obtained by continuous wave Doppler. Various acoustic windows (apical, suprasternal, right parasternal) should be evaluated to detect the highest velocity signal.

False low gradients can be associated with left ventricular dysfunction or due to improper alignment of the Doppler beam to the jet velocity. High gradients can be associated with prosthetic valve obstruction/stenosis, prosthetic valve regurgitation, or high output states such as anemia, tachycardia, or sepsis. Prosthetic valve obstruction/stenosis can be due to patient–prosthesis mismatch, valve thrombosis, endocarditis, incomplete valve expansion due to dense calcifications, and prolapse of native valve leaflet or calcific nodules into the prosthetic valve impeding normal leaflet excursion. A more complete discussion on prosthetic valve regurgitation can be found below.

Discrepancies in estimated pressure gradients can occur between cardiac catheterization and Doppler echocardiography. These observations should be confirmed by at least two experienced echocardiographers. There can be several potential explanations for the discrepancies—nonsimultaneous pressure recordings, interrogation of the mitral regurgitation jet instead of the aortic stenosis jet, high jet velocities within the left ventricular outflow tract or supravalvular regions, or the pressure recovery phenomenon.

The pressure recovery phenomenon implies that valve gradients estimated by Doppler echocardiography are "overestimated" when compared to those at cardiac catheterization (10–12). These differences can range from 1 to 53 mm Hg (mean 20 mm Hg) (13). As blood flow passes through the prosthesis or narrowed orifice, jet velocity increases and pressure decreases based on Bernoulli's principle (the law of conservation of energy). The maximum velocity and peak pressure drop occur at the level of the vena contracta, located a short distance distal to the

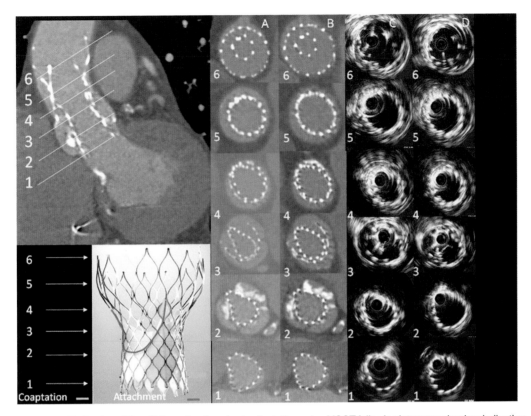

Figure 2 Evaluation of CoreValve valve–in-valve implantation using MSCT following intraprocedural embolization of the CRS implanted first. MSCT and intravascular ultrasound images are shown of the CRS implanted first that embolized (higher and outside) and the second CRS (lower and inside the first). Axial images are shown at levels of interest (1–6) of the functionally important second CRS both before (**A** and **C**) and after (**B** and **D**) balloon valvuloplasty. *Source*: From Ref. 3. Levels of the second CRS are 1 = Ventricular end, 2 = nadir of CRS leaflets, 3 = central coaptation of CRS leaflets, 4 = commissures, 5 = nominally the widest point of second CRS (central coaptation of first CRS), 6 = apex of outflow.

location of maximal anatomic constriction. Distal to the vena contracta, blood flow decelerates and pressure increases (i.e., "pressure recovery"). It then follows that the transaortic pressure gradient estimated with a fluid-filled catheter positioned in the ascending aorta represents the pressure difference between the left ventricle and the region distal to the vena contracta. On the other hand, the transaortic pressure gradient estimated by Doppler echocardiography represents the pressure difference between the left ventricle and the vena contracta. Neither modality is inherently wrong. An appreciation of these "natural" discrepancies is essential in the proper management of patients.

Following TAVI, peak and mean transaortic valve gradients decrease significantly (15–20 mm Hg and 5–15 mm Hg, respectively) (14–17). These results are comparable to those reported for surgical aortic valve replacement (18).

Continuity Equation for Calculation of Aortic Valve Area

Calculation of the effective aortic orifice area is based on the continuity principle where $EOA = CSA_{LVOT} \times VTI_{LVOT}/VTI_{Transprosthesis}$ (EOA, effective orifice area; CSA, cross-sectional area; LVOT, left ventricular outflow tract; and VTI_{LVOT}, velocity time integral obtained by pulse wave Doppler; $VTI_{Transprosthesis}$, velocity time integral obtained by continuous wave Doppler). Potential sources of variability include accurate measurements of the left ventricular outflow tract, eccentric jets leading to underestimation of jet velocities or settings of altered volume status or heart rate. Transesophageal echocardiography can provide more reliable estimates of the diameter of the left ventricular outflow tract than transthoracic echocardiography.

After successful TAVI, there is an important and sustain increase in effective aortic orifice area to approximately 1.5 to 2.0 cm^2 (15,16). The effective orifice area may vary depending on valve type and valve size.

Paravalvular Aortic Regurgitation

Following TAVI, mild paravalvular aortic regurgitation can be observed in 50% to 70% of patients and appears to be well tolerated clinically (14,15,19,17). Anecdotal experience dictates that this percentage decreases over time but confirmatory evidence is lacking.

Specific guidelines on how to quantify and classify the severity of paravalvular regurgitation in the context of TAVI are lacking. Semiquantitative indices suggesting more severe degrees of aortic regurgitation include longer duration of the regurgitant signal, eccentricity of the jet (Coandă effect), extension of the jet signal deep into left ventricular cavity, and a mosaic jet suggesting high velocities and turbulent flow.

Briefly listed, the potential causes of paravalvular aortic regurgitation include undersized prosthetic valve, aggressive preimplant balloon dilatation, valve implantation too high or too low, inadequate frame or stent expansion, dense calcifications causing deformity of prosthesis, and prolapse of native valve leaflet or calcific nodules into prosthetic valve impeding normal leaflet excursion.

Mild degrees of aortic regurgitation can be recorded in 6% to 73% of patients after surgical aortic valve replacement (20–22). In most instances, this is known as "closing regurgitation" that fortuitously prevents stasis and thrombus formation by a "washing mechanism." This effect is more prominent with mechanical than bioprosthetic valves.

Mitral Valve Function

Current evidence would suggest that the severity of mitral regurgitation does not change appreciably after TAVI (15,19). There are some patients, however, who seem to improve or worsen in this respect. Details of the frequency, pathophysiological mechanisms, and prognostic implications of these findings require further study.

The following case example illustrates a patient who presented three months after implantation of the CRS with fever and positive blood cultures for corynebacterium. Transesophageal echocardiography showed severe mitral regurgitation due to a perforated aneurysm of the anterior mitral valve leaflet at the level of the ventricular edge of the metal frame. The patient underwent surgical aortic valve replacement with a 23-mm Carpentier-Edwards bioprosthetic valve and pericardial patch repair of the anterior mitral valve leaflet. A vegetative lesion was observed on the transcatheter aortic valve cusp (Figs. 3 and 4 and Videos 1, 2, 3). (Figures

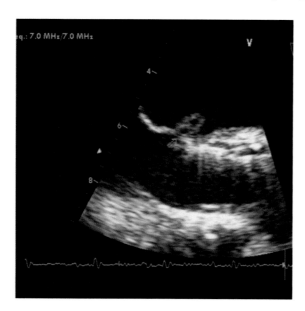

Figure 3 Transesophageal echocardiogram (105°) long-axis view of the left ventricular outflow tract (zoom in). The inflow portion of the CoreValve prosthesis is impinging upon the anterior mitral valve leaflet. An aneurysm of the anterior mitral valve leaflet can be observed at the hinge point between the ventricular edge of the metallic frame and anterior mitral valve leaflet. (Courtesy of Sebastiano Marra, MD, Maurizio D'Amico, MD, Mauro Rinaldi, MD, Fabrizio Sansone, MD, Chiara Comoglio MD, Paolo Scaciattella from the University of Turin, San Giovanni Battista Hospital, Turin, Italy).

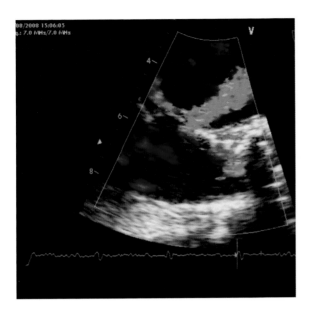

Figure 4 Transesophageal echocardiogram (105°) long-axis view of the left ventricular outflow tract (zoom in) with color Doppler of the mitral valve. Moderate to severe mitral regurgitation is secondary to a perforation of the anterior mitral valve leaflet. (Courtesy of Sebastiano Marra, MD, Maurizio D'Amico, MD, Mauro Rinaldi, MD, Fabrizio Sansone, MD, Chiara Comoglio MD, Paolo Scaciattella from the University of Turin, San Giovanni Battista Hospital, Turin, Italy).

and videos for this case provided courtesy of Sebastiano Marra, MD, Maurizio D'Amico, MD, Mauro Rinaldi, MD, Fabrizio Sansone, MD, Chiara Comoglio MD, Paolo Scaciattella from the University of Turin, San Giovanni Battista Hospital, Turin, Italy). Video 1 also demonstrates the inflow portion of the prosthesis impinging upon the anterior mitral valve leaflet. Contrast aortography and echocardiography confirmed the relatively deep placement of the prosthesis within the left ventricular outflow tract [Fig. 5(A) and 5(b)]. The patient underwent successful antibiotic and surgical therapy.

The second case example represents a patient who presented eight months after implantation of the CRS with spontaneous rupture of the chordae tendineae attached to the anterior mitral valve leaflet. Transesophageal echocardiography revealed (*i*) the inflow portion of the prosthesis to be impinging upon the anterior mitral valve leaflet and (*ii*) severe mitral regurgitation due to a flail anterior mitral valve leaflet (Video 4). The relationship, if any, between the depth of implantation and the development of the patients' clinical syndrome is not clear.

Left Ventricular Function

Patients with severe aortic stenosis invariably have diastolic dysfunction with or without systolic dysfunction. According to published literature, it is reasonable to assume that left ventricular systolic performance is preserved following TAVI (23,24). In a study by Bauer et al., echocardiography performed within 24 hours after TAVI demonstrated acute improvements in global and regional left ventricular systolic function by using strain and strain rate imaging techniques (24). De Jaegere et al. showed that in approximately two-thirds of patients diastolic function is unchanged whereas it improves or worsens in the remaining minority of patients (19).

The clinical outcomes of patients with left ventricular dysfunction with or without contractile reserve undergoing TAVI should be the focus of future studies.

Suspected Prosthetic Valve Dysfunction

Patients with prosthetic valve dysfunction associated with obstruction or regurgitation most commonly present with dyspnea. Other symptoms related to bacteremia, thromboembolism, or hemolytic anemias are possible as well.

Several questions need to be addressed concerning the patient with suspected prosthetic valve dysfunction: (*i*) Is the valve well seated? (*ii*) Is the valve opening and closing properly? (*iii*) Is there any expected or unexpected valve regurgitation? (*iv*) Is there evidence for prosthetic valve stenosis? (*v*) Is there an unexpected mass (e.g., endocarditis, thrombus, or pannus) on the valve structure or leaflets? (*vi*) Is there involvement of other cardiac structures (e.g., perivalvular abscess, fistulous tracts, etc.)?

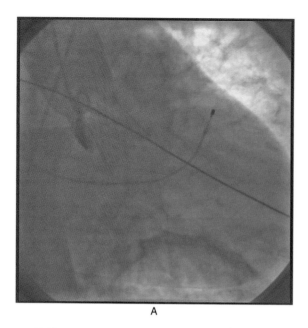

A

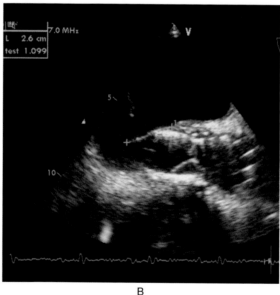

B

Figure 5 Deep implantation of the CoreValve prosthesis (in this case ~12 mm below the aortic valve annulus) shown by (**A** Contrast aortography and (**B** transesophageal echocardiography (105°). (Courtesy of Sebastiano Marra, MD, Maurizio D'Amico, MD, Mauro Rinaldi, MD, Fabrizio Sansone, MD, Chiara Comoglio MD, Paolo Scaciattella from the University of Turin, San Giovanni Battista Hospital, Turin, Italy).

There should be an extremely low threshold to perform transesophageal echocardiography after screening transthoracic echocardiography. Doppler-derived parameters such as pressure-half time and the ratio of $TVI_{LVOT}/TVI_{Transprothesis}$ can be useful to differentiate between valve regurgitation and obstruction. If the cardiac output, two-dimensional (2D) and color flow exam, and gradients are all within normal limits, then it is safe to assume that the effective orifice area will be within acceptable range. If any of these three aforementioned conditions are not satisfied, then the effective orifice area should be calculated using the continuity equation.

In the absence of symptoms and a normal transesophageal echocardiogram, close follow-up is recommended.

Fluoroscopy

The frame of the CRS is composed of Nitinol whereas the Edwards SAPIEN prosthetic valve is composed of stainless steel. In the fields of peripheral vascular and coronary intervention, stent fractures (Nitinol or stainless steel based) have been reported; in vivo pulsatile fatigue effects are thought to play an important role (25). There are no published reports on the in vivo durability or fractures of the CRS or Edwards SAPIEN prosthetic valve. The implications of such fractures would require further study.

Comparing ECG-gated fluoroscopic sequences obtained immediately after implantation with those obtained at follow-up can be useful to assess the integrity of the frame of the prosthesis. It is essential that similar gantry positions obtained during the implantation procedure and two further orthogonal views are used for comparison. Importantly, a rotational cine is essential—otherwise it may be possible to miss a fracture depending on the location and orientation of the fracture. A fracture may be recognized as an interruption or discontinuation of a strut of the frame and/or missing part of the frame.

Serial fluoroscopic assessments for valve integrity are currently being performed in the context of research protocols.

Multislice Computed Tomography

In contrast to transthoracic echocardiography, a cardiac MSCT data set allows visualization beyond both calcification and metal struts and provides images of a 3D virtual heart that can be viewed from any plane thereby allowing true axial orientation for accurate measurement of valve geometry (Video 5).

Frame Geometry and Apposition

MSCT can clearly demonstrate both the struts of the CoreValve prosthesis and the tissue it is apposed to (2,3). As a result, it should be regarded as the method of choice for the evaluation of patient anatomy and geometry of the implanted CoreValve prosthesis. With respect to the latter point, MSCT can provide insights into the undersymmetrical or asymmetrical expansion or malapposition of the CoreValve frame (Fig. 6). A recent MSCT study showed that incomplete apposition of the CoreValve prosthesis was common (3). In addition, asymmetrical and incomplete expansion was frequently seen at the lower levels of the leaflets, although this was minimal over the leaflet coaptation segment that is considered important for valve function (Fig. 7). The long-term implications of these observations are not known.

In approximately 30% of patients, the coaptation of the CRS leaflets can be seen on functional MSCT (Video 6). Native aortic valve leaflet calcification can be assessed in detail including volume, density, distribution, and shift in position following prosthesis implantation. The proximity and apposition of the frame and displaced calcium relative to the coronary ostia can also be clearly seen (Video 6).

Frame Fractures

The struts of transcatheter valves can be clearly visualized by MSCT—this allows deformation of the frame to be detected and quantified (3). However, the significant blooming effect caused by the radio-dense struts would tend to obscure subtle frame fractures. The blooming effect may be reduced by using an edge preserving reconstruction kernel (e.g., b46f) at the expense of some loss in signal to noise ratio (26). In addition, however, the detection of possible frame fractures is restricted by the resolution of MSCT (0.5 mm × 0.5 mm × 0.5 mm) relative to the thickness of struts (~0.4 mm). As a result, only significant displacement of struts may be reliably detected using MSCT whereas point fractures are likely to be missed. Currently, frame fractures have not been reported.

Frame–Mitral Valve Interaction and Left Ventricular Function

In addition to geometry, dynamic functional data throughout the cardiac cycle may be obtained using a retrospective scan technique with limited dose modulation and image reconstruction throughout the cardiac cycle. This allows evaluation of left ventricular function including evaluation of regional wall motion abnormalities and evaluation of movement of the mitral valve

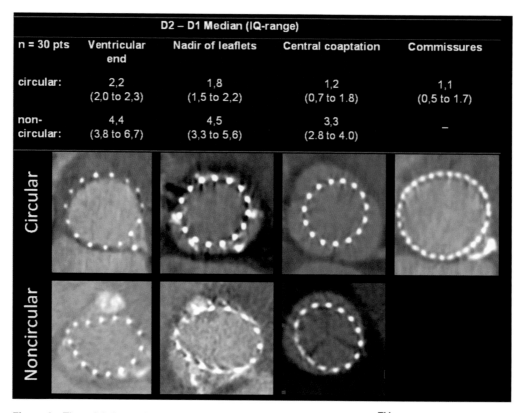

D2 – D1 Median (IQ-range)			
n = 30 pts	Ventricular end	Nadir of leaflets	Central coaptation	Commissures
circular:	2,2 (2,0 to 2,3)	1,8 (1,5 to 2,2)	1,2 (0,7 to 1.8)	1,1 (0,5 to 1.7)
non-circular:	4,4 (3,8 to 6,7)	4,5 (3,3 to 5,6)	3,3 (2.8 to 4.0)	–

Figure 6 The axial shape, dimensions, and apposition of the frame of the CRS[TM] can be assessed at various levels of interest. D2: largest diameter; D1: smallest diameter. *Source*: From Ref. 2.

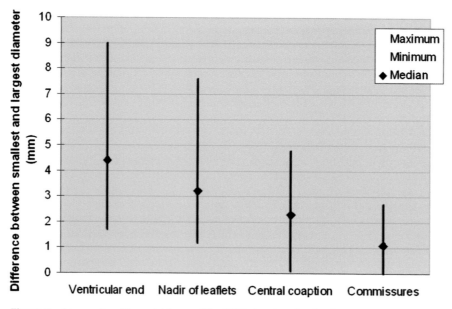

Figure 7 Asymmetry of the axial frame of the CRS at various levels. *Source*: From Ref. 2.

leaflets (27,28). The interaction of the anterior mitral valve leaflet with the inflow of the prosthesis can also be seen (Video 7).

Vascular Complications

In addition to evaluation of the aortic root and prosthesis, the rest of the aorta and large vascular access routes (subclavian, axillary, and femoral) can be assessed in the same MSCT scan provided that this information is requested before the scan is performed. In this way, vascular access related complications such as dissection or retroperitoneal bleeding can be evaluated simultaneously. Furthermore, one can also appreciate the proximity of the displaced calcified native aortic valve leaflets relative to the coronary ostia. Dense and widely distributed coronary calcification is present in a large proportion of these patients, which can limit visualization of the lumen of the coronary tree.

Limitations

A limitation of MSCT technique is that flow cannot be measured. Although the retrospective scanning technique requires high-radiation doses, there is unlikely to be any significant stochastic increase in risk of malignancy in the long-term in the elderly comorbid patient populations receiving PAVR. Considering that radiographic contrast is required and that patients currently treated with TAVI have a high prevalence of impaired renal function (5–25%) (17), it is important to cautiously hydrate patients and administer acetylcysteine. In patients with severe renal impairment (glomerular filtration rate <30 mL/min), MSCT with contrast is generally contraindicated.

Indications

There is currently no literature to support routine use of MSCT post-PAVR. However, in selected cases it may prove very useful, as discussed later.

Case 1: Failure to Improve After Valve-in-Valve PAVR

A man aged 81 years with severe (transaortic peak gradient of 109 mm Hg) symptomatic (NYHA 3) aortic stenosis and a logistic EuroScore of 21.6 was accepted for PAVR, following evaluation by a multidisciplinary team (3). During the procedure, a CoreValve prosthesis with 29 mm inflow was in an acceptable position but was found to be asymmetrically underexpanded at the level of the native aortic leaflets. Postdilatation during rapid ventricular pacing resulted in embolization of the CRS due to premature discontinuation of the pacing. Following implantation of a second CRS the aortic regurgitation was reduced to grade 1. He was discharged with a transvalvular gradient of 10 mm Hg on transthoracic echocardiography (TTE), but at follow-up seven weeks later he was found to be highly symptomatic (NYHA 4) with a functional gradient on TTE. A MSCT demonstrated the geometry of both the CRS's implanted first and second (Fig. 2). Severe underexpansion was noted of the CRS implanted second at the level of coaptation of the CRS leaflets. In view of the high level of symptoms a further procedure was performed with postdilatation of the CRS frame at the level of the restriction. This resulted in an improvement of the CRS geometry and an increase in the cross-sectional area of the CRS leaflet coaptation by 23%, which was accompanied by a reduction in the transvalvular gradient and improvement of the patient symptoms following the procedure.

Case 2: Unexplained Valve Embolization

A woman aged 83 years with severe aortic stenosis (transaortic peak gradient of 77 mm Hg), debilitating symptoms (syncope, NYHA 3), and multiple comorbidities (renal impairment, chronic obstructive pulmonary disease, coronary disease, and left ventricular impairment) was accepted for PAVR. A 26-mm inflow CRS was successfully implanted in an optimal position in the left ventricular outflow tract. After removal of a pigtail catheter from the left ventricular cavity without fluoroscopy, the CRS embolized into the ascending aorta. A second CRS was implanted in the LVOT and the patient left the hospital eight days later (6). At follow-up in out-patients a MSCT showed the second prosthesis positioned correctly in the LVOT and well expanded. The second CRS was positioned in the ascending aorta just below the right carotid artery. The curved tip of the catheter entangled in the outflow of the second CRS frame

Table 3 Timetable for Routine Imaging post-PAVR

	Time after implant		
Modality	**Before leaving the interventional suite**	**Predischarge**	**Annually**
TTE	Gradient, AR, LV fx	Gradient, AR, LV fx, MV fx	Gradient, AR, LV fx, MV fx
TOE	AR, LV fx, MV fx		
X-ray fluoroscopy (noninvasive, noncontrast)	Position of frame in LVOT		Strut fracture
MSCT		Position of frame in LVOT, apposition, frame geometry	

TTE, transthoracic echocardiography; TOE, transesophageal echocardiography; MSCT, multislice computed tomography; AR, aortic regurgitation; LV, left ventricle; fx, function; MV, mitral valve; LVOT, left ventricular outflow tract.

indicating that the catheter had crossed through the struts of the frame into the central lumen of the prosthesis (Fig. 1). During blind withdrawal the pigtail portion had become entangled during removal resulting in the first CRS prosthesis being pulled out of position.

Cardiac MRI
Cardiac MRI is not an absolute contraindication after TAVI. At the moment, however, there is little experience with this imaging modality.

WHEN TO DO WHAT
Table 3 provides a schedule for when different modalities are most likely to be useful. Table 2 indicates the relative strengths and weaknesses of each imaging modality that may guide the selection of the optimal modality(s) to answer specific clinical questions.

CONCLUSIONS
PAVR is still a novel field and there is much to be gained from multimodality imaging postimplantation procedure. Transthoracic echocardiography is the most commonly used modality for determining valve hemodynamics and the presence of regurgitation, whereas transesophageal echocardiography is usually the best modality to accurately locate the origin of paravalvular regurgitation. MSCT can provide a 3D data set that allows evaluation of prosthesis geometry and apposition. Frame fractures may be best detected using X-ray cine/fluoroscopy.

REFERENCES
1. Piazza N, de Jaegere P, Schultz C, et al. Anatomy of the aortic valvar complex and its implications for transcatheter implantation of the aortic valve. Circ Cardiovasc Intervent 2008; 1:74–81.
2. Schultz C, Weustink A, Piazza N, et al. Geometry and degree of apposition of the CoreValve Revalving System with multislice computed tomography after implantation in patients with aortic stenosis. J Am Coll Cardiol 2009; 54(10):911–918.
3. Schultz C, Piazza N, Weustink A, et al. Valve in valve percutaneous aortic prosthesis for acute regurgitation is not a benign procedure: An analysis of Corevalve® geometry using MSCT and IVUS. EuroIntervention. In press.
4. Zegdi R, Ciobotaru V, Noghin M, et al. Is it reasonable to treat all calcified stenotic aortic valves with a valved stent? Results from a human anatomic study in adults. J Am Coll Cardiol 2008; 51(5):579–584.
5. Thubrikar M, Piepgrass W, Shaner T, et al. The design of the normal aortic valve. Am J Physiol 1981; 241:H795–H801.
6. Otten A, Piazza N, Schultz C, et al. Implantation of two self-expanding aortic bioprosthetic valves during the same procedure. Sequential valve implantation. EuroIntervention 2008; 4(4):on-line version.
7. Piazza N, Schultz C, de Jaegere PP, et al. Implantation of two self-expanding aortic bioprosthetic valves during the same procedure-Insights into valve-in-valve implantation ("Russian doll concept"). Catheter Cardiovasc Interv 2009; 73(4):530–539.

8. Bonow RO, Carabello BA, Chatterjee K, et al. 2008 Focused update incorporated into the ACC/AHA 2006 guidelines for the management of patients with valvular heart disease: A report of the American College of Cardiology/American Heart Association Task Force on Practice Guidelines (Writing Committee to Revise the 1998 Guidelines for the Management of Patients With Valvular Heart Disease): Endorsed by the Society of Cardiovascular Anesthesiologists, Society for Cardiovascular Angiography and Interventions, and Society of Thoracic Surgeons. Circulation 2008; 118(15):e523–e661.

9. Vahanian A, Baumgartner H, Bax J, et al. Guidelines on the management of valvular heart disease: The Task Force on the Management of Valvular Heart Disease of the European Society of Cardiology. Eur Heart J 2007; 28(2):230–268.

10. Garcia D, Dumesnil JG, Durand LG, et al. Discrepancies between catheter and Doppler estimates of valve effective orifice area can be predicted from the pressure recovery phenomenon: Practical implications with regard to quantification of aortic stenosis severity. J Am Coll Cardiol 2003; 41(3):435–442.

11. Baumgartner H, Stefenelli T, Niederberger J, et al. "Overestimation" of catheter gradients by Doppler ultrasound in patients with aortic stenosis: A predictable manifestation of pressure recovery. J Am Coll Cardiol 1999; 33(6):1655–1661.

12. Niederberger J, Schima H, Maurer G, et al. Importance of pressure recovery for the assessment of aortic stenosis by Doppler ultrasound. Role of aortic size, aortic valve area, and direction of the stenotic jet in vitro. Circulation 1996; 94(8):1934–1940.

13. Krafchek J, Robertson JH, Radford M, et al. A reconsideration of Doppler assessed gradients in suspected aortic stenosis. Am Heart J 1985; 110(4):765–773.

14. Grube E, Buellesfeld L, Mueller R, et al. Progress and Current Status of Percutaneous Aortic Valve Replacement: Results of Three Device Generations of the CoreValve Revalving System. Circ Cardiovasc Intervent 2008; 1(3):167–175.

15. Webb JG, Pasupati S, Humphries K, et al. Percutaneous transarterial aortic valve replacement in selected high-risk patients with aortic stenosis. Circulation 2007; 116(7):755–763.

16. De Jaegere P, Piazza N, Galema T, et al. Early echocardiographic evaluation following percutaneous implantation with the self-expanding CoreValve ReValving System aortic valve bioprosthesis. EuroIntervention 2008; Published ahead of e-print.

17. Piazza N, Grube E, Gerckens U, . Procedural and 30-day outcomes following transcatheter aortic valve implantation using the third generation (18 Fr) CoreValve ReValving System—Results from the multicenter, Expanded Evaluation Registry 1-year following CE mark approval. EuroIntervention 2008; 4(2):242–249.

18. Jamieson WR, Munro AI, Miyagishima RT, et al. Carpentier-Edwards standard porcine bioprosthesis: Clinical performance to seventeen years. Ann Thorac Surg 1995; 60(4):999–1006; discussion 1007.

19. De Jaegere PP, Piazza N, Galema TW, et al. Early echocardiographic evaluation following percutaneous implantation with the self-expanding CoreValve Revalving System aortic valve bioprosthesis. EuroIntervention 2008; 4(3):351–357.

20. O'Rourke DJ, Palac RT, Malenka DJ, et al. Outcome of mild periprosthetic regurgitation detected by intraoperative transesophageal echocardiography. J Am Coll Cardiol 2001; 38(1):163–166.

21. Rallidis LS, Moyssakis IE, Ikonomidis I, Nihoyannopoulos P. Natural history of early aortic paraprosthetic regurgitation: A five-year follow-up. Am Heart J 1999; 138(2 Pt 1):351–357.

22. Ionescu A, Fraser AG, Butchart EG. Prevalence and clinical significance of incidental paraprosthetic valvar regurgitation: A prospective study using transoesophageal echocardiography. Heart 2003; 89(11):1316–1321.

23. Meliga E, Piazza N, de Jaegere P, et al. Pressure-volume loops in patients with aortic stenosis undergoing percutaneous aortic valve implantation. EuroIntervention. In press.

24. Bauer F, Eltchaninoff H, Tron C, et al. Acute improvement in global and regional left ventricular systolic function after percutaneous heart valve implantation in patients with symptomatic aortic stenosis. Circulation 2004; 110(11):1473–1476.

25. Pelton A, Schroedera V, Mitchell M, et al. Fatigue and durability of Nitinol stents. J Mech Behav Biomed Mater 2008; 1(2):153–164.

26. Seifarth H, Raupach R, Schaller S, et al. Assessment of coronary artery stents using 16-slice MDCT angiography: Evaluation of a dedicated reconstruction kernel and a noise reduction filter. Eur Radiol 2005; 15(4):721–726.

27. Guo YK, Yang ZG, Ning G, et al. Sixty-four-slice multidetector computed tomography for preoperative evaluation of left ventricular function and mass in patients with mitral regurgitation: Comparison with magnetic resonance imaging and echocardiography. Eur Radiol 2009; 19(9):2107–2116.

28. Willmann JK, Kobza R, Roos JE, et al. ECG-gated multi-detector row CT for assessment of mitral valve disease: Initial experience. Eur Radiol 2002; 12(11):2662–2669.

Appendix 1
Second-Generation Transcatheter Aortic Valve Implant System

Reginald Low
University of California, Davis, Sacramento, California, U.S.A.

INTRODUCTION

The standard of care for the treatment of symptomatic severe aortic valve stenosis has been surgical aortic valve replacement (AVR). The surgical risk may be prohibitive for both the patient and surgeon and hence, a significant number of patients have gone untreated. Percutaneous transcatheter aortic valve implants (TAVI) and techniques have been developed and these provide alternative therapy for such high-risk patients. The experiences of first-generation percutaneous aortic valves have been reported for the Edwards–Cribier and CoreValve systems (1–4), and have shown this procedure to be truly revolutionary.

The present generation implants have demonstrated good hemodynamic performance with low gradients and good valve areas along with positive intermediate term durability. Displacement of the native valve, securement with no embolization, no interference of the coronary ostia, and freedom from thrombus formation are strengths of the available systems. However, there continue to be limitations with these systems such as with positioning, repositioning and retrieval, and handling issues that require rigorous training. Extensive efforts are now directed at second-generation devices to improve on the prosthesis, delivery systems and implantation techniques.

To better understand the goals of second-generation devices, a review of desirable features of a percutaneous transcatheter aortic valve system is useful (Table 1). These properties can be classified into functional features and deliverability attributes. Functional features include a large effective orifice area (EOA), low gradients, and excellent durability since the benchmark is the standard surgical valve. In addition, these implants should have good apposition (sealing) to the annulus so as to minimize paravalvular leak and the prosthesis must be secure so there is no risk for valve embolization. The prosthesis must not extend too high into the aorta to avoid coronary ostial obstruction. Various size options or prosthesis design must be available to treat the many different aortic annular dimensions. Finally, safety is paramount and the implant should have low risk for thrombus formation and clot embolization.

The ideal features for deliverability include low delivery profile, flexibility, and trackability of the delivery system along with repositioning and retrieval abilities. Importantly, the positioning of the implant must be precise, which can be difficult in a beating heart that is ejecting blood. Repositioning and retrieval of the valve would be necessary.

The innovative and technical prowess of biomedical device companies will surely result in significantly improved next-generation devices. As new concepts of valve design are developed, safety and efficacy are paramount. Each component of the implant will be carefully designed and optimized to not only meet the necessary requirements, but to also meet or exceed the desirable features of a percutaneous transcatheter valve. For example, leaflet technology will not only include bovine and porcine pericardial tissue but may also include plasticized metal fabricated with nanotechnology. Support frames will be both metallic and nonmetallic. Fixation, sealing, and securement may become mechanical and active, which may help expand the use of TAVI to aortic insufficiency. Implant designs are using materials to have the tissue become incorporated with the prosthetic to increase longevity and stability. Moreover, fixation will continue to use radial strength or new techniques that provide axial strength or a combination of the two. For example, manufactures have designed the prosthesis to capture and secure the native leaflet

Table 1 Overview of Emerging Transcatheter Aortic Valve Devices

	Leaflet material	Support structure	Profile (F)	Repositionable	Retrievable	Functional assessment ability	Rapid pacing requirement
Direct flow	Bovine pericardium	Dacron	18	Yes	Yes	Yes	No
Heart Leaflet Technology	Porcine pericardium	Nitinol	16 or 17	Yes	Yes	Yes	No
Sadra Medical	Bovine pericardium	Nitinol	21	Yes	Yes	Yes	No
JenaValve Technology	Porcine aortic root	Nitinol	32 or 16	Yes	With limitations	Yes	No

anatomy for axial fixation, and another system expands and clips on to the stenotic valve like a paperclip.

A major departure from the current generation transcatheter valve procedure is the focused attention on the ability to perform early evaluation of the hemodynamic and functional assessment before final device implantation. Measuring hemodynamics (gradient and valve area), paravalvular leakage, stability or disruptions of mitral valve function is directly tied into a delivery system that is allows for repositioning. Ideally, this delivery system will offer finer control, but at the same time the procedure itself must not be complicated and the efficiency of the procedure must be maintained. Reducing lengthy steps with intuitive design can decrease the overall operation time. In addition, measuring functional capacity before final placement reduces the overall time by reducing the overall complication rate. Slimmer profiles and more flexible delivery systems delivered with a retrograde approach, percutaneously via the femoral artery may increase the overall patient base. Valve material selection or prosthesis loading techniques for stent-based frames permit the catheter to be more flexible to track the anatomy more effectively. Complications from the procedure such as vascular injury, stroke, and inability to deliver the device to the aortic annulus should be reduced with improved profile and flexibility.

Despite the great enthusiasm for next-generation percutaneous TAVI systems, there are significant obstacles that must be addressed. Improvements in some properties must not come at the expense of function, safety, and durability. These challenges include compromises in design to achieve smaller, more flexible implantation systems. As the delivery system profile decreases, the loading of the valve may become more aggressive, possibly reducing the overall longevity or durability of the prosthesis. Moreover, the materials used to decrease size may also have an adverse effect, such as thinner porcine tissue, or narrower or less robust stent frames. Clinical challenges include understanding acute functional and hemodynamic measurements with long-term outcomes. Additional clinical challenges consist of knowing when to reposition or remove the device entirely. For example, will a mild but acceptable gradient be deemed too high, knowing the device is infinitely positionable? What gradient or paravalvular leakage warrants repositioning versus retrieval? Other clinical concerns will be patient selection, and determining when this procedure should be performed on younger more active patients. Additional concerns include economic challenges for research and development, lack of a good animal model for testing, and development and regulatory barriers. Clinical trial design and expense are additional challenges especially as the field evolves and devices are approved for clinical use.

The ability to percutaneously implant an aortic valve prosthesis for symptomatic aortic stenosis in high surgical risk patients is truly impressive. As new-generation devices are developed to optimize the function, durability, and deliverability of the implanted valve while minimizing complications and enhancing recovery, the standard surgical aortic valve replacement will be challenged.

REFERENCES

1. Cribier A, Eltchaninoff H, Tron C, et al. Treatment of calcific aortic stenosis with the percutaneous heart valve: mid term follow-up from the initial feasibility studies: the French experience. J Am Coll Cardiol 2006; 47(6):1214–1223.

2. Webb JG, Chandavimol M, Thompson CR, et al. Percutaneous aortic valve implantation retrograde from the femoral artery. Circulation 2006; 113(6):842–850.
3. Cribier A, Eltchaninoff H, Bash A, Borenstein N, et al. Percutaneous transcatheter implantation of an aortic valve prosthesis for calcific aortic stenosis: First human case description. Circulation 2002; 106(24):3006–3008.
4. Grube E, Laborde JC, Gerckens U, et al. Percutaneous implantation of the CoreValve self-expanding valve prosthesis in high-risk patients with aortic valve disease; the Siegburg first-in-man study. Circulation 2006; 114(15):1616–1624.

Appendix 2
Direct Flow Medical

Reginald Low

University of California, Davis, Sacramento, California, U.S.A.

The Direct Flow Medical (DFM) percutaneous aortic valve is designed to have the performance (function, durability, and safety) of a surgical valve while incorporating the desirable attributes for transcatheter delivery (low profile, flexibility, and trackability). It offers excellent securement, sealing, precise positioning, repositioning, and, if necessary, retrieval. Assessment of function and placement with hemodynamic measurements may be completed before final deployment.

The bovine pericardial leaflets include anticalcification treatment and are attached to an inflatable polyester fabric cuff that conforms to the aortic valve annulus and tissue to form a tight seal to minimize paravalvular leak. The slightly tapered implant is designed as an hourglass shape, with independently inflatable ventricular and aortic rings, which encircle and capture the native valve annulus ensuring positive axial anchoring of the device [Fig. 1(A)]. Inflation of the cuff with a saline and contrast solution renders the valve immediately functional and permits fluoroscopic visualization. Before final deployment, the saline and contrast mixture is exchanged under pressure, maintaining cuff shape and position, with a solidifying inflation media (IM) that hardens to form the permanent support structure. The IM is a biocompatible, two component liquid containing a water soluble epoxy and a radiopacifier. After the exchange, the IM gels in minutes and achieves 95% of its final hardness in hours (1).

The prosthesis is attached to three position-fill lumens (PFLs), used to position and align the prosthesis precisely, and loaded into the 18-F delivery system [Fig. 1(B)]. The delivery system works over a 0.035 in. guidewire, and an atraumatic nosecone tip allows smooth transition from the guidewire to the housing sheath. In addition, the delivery system includes an accessory recovery sheath that allows a smooth and straightforward retrieval of the DFM valve through an 18-F introducer sheath.

Arterial access is achieved percutaneously or by cut-down with an 18-F sheath followed by standard balloon aortic valvuloplasty to prepare the stenotic aortic valve. The delivery system is tracked over the guidewire into the left ventricle and the outer sheath is retracted to expose the prosthetic implant. Inflation of the ventricular ring makes the prosthesis immediately functional and ready for positioning, all without rapid pacing or cardiac support. Positioning is achieved by independently manipulating the PFLs to place the ventricular ring evenly against the aortic annulus. The aortic ring is then inflated to secure the valve and permit functional assessment. The implant can be repositioned easily until optimal conditions are achieved. If a different size implant is required, the device is deflated and retrieved. Once final device function is confirmed, the IM is introduced into the pressurized implant and then the delivery system is detached and the procedure is completed.

STUDY PHASE

DFM has performed over 100 preclinical animal studies and cadaver studies. Initial clinical experience included a series of nine temporary implants performed in South America in October 2006, at a single center. Two patients had open surgical implants and seven had percutaneous implants. Overall, excellent hemodynamic valve function and few adverse events were observed. In addition, two transfemoral recoveries of the DFM valve were performed; the first ever reported percutaneous recoveries (2).

A European feasibility trial was also conducted on the 22-F system between October 2007 and August 2008. This was a prospective, nonrandomized clinical evaluation at two centers to determine clinical feasibility and safety of treating patients at high risk for cardiac surgery with a EuroScore $\geq$ 20%, age $\geq$ 70 years, and severe symptomatic aortic valve stenosis. A total of

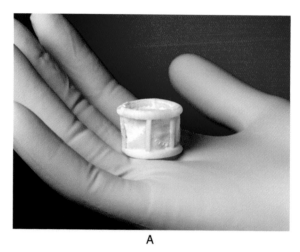

A

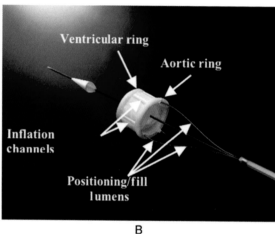

Ventricular ring

Aortic ring

Inflation channels

Positioning/fill lumens

B

Figure 1 (**A**) Direct Flow transcatheter bio-prosthetic valve constructed of inflatable polyester fabric cuffs to which a bovine pericardial tissue valve is attached. (**B**) The Direct Flow valve is attached to the delivery system by three catheter lumens that are used to position the valve and fill the supporting ventricular and aortic rings.

31 patients were enrolled in the trial. The study showed the valve is immediately competent, repositionable, retrievable, and resulted in excellent hemodynamics (3). The new 18-F system is scheduled to be in clinical trials by mid-2009.

REFERENCES

1. Bolling S, Rogers J, Babaliaros V, et al. Percutaneous aortic valve implantation utilising a novel tissue valve—Preclinical experience. Eurointervention 2008; 4:148–153.
2. Low RI, Bolling SF, Yeo KK, et al. A Direct Flow Medical percutaneous aortic valve: Proof of concept. EuroIntervention 2008; 4:256–261.
3. Schofer J, Schluter M, Treede H, et al. Retrograde transarterial implantation of a nonmetallic aortic valve prosthesis in high-surgical-risk patients with severe aortic stenosis. A First-in-Man Feasibility and Safety Study. Circ Cardiovasc Interv 2008; 1:126–133.

Appendix 3
Heart Leaflet Technologies, Inc., Transcatheter Aortic Valve

Spencer H. Kubo, John Gainor, William Mirsch, Richard Schroeder, Jonas Runquist, and Robert F. Wilson

Heart Leaflet Technologies, Inc., Maple Grove, Minnesota, U.S.A.

The Heart Leaflet Technologies (HLT) transcatheter aortic valve is a replacement heart valve that is delivered via a conventional interventional procedure. The device is designed to address critical aortic stenosis in patients who are at high risk for surgical valve replacement. The HLT valve is a tricuspid porcine pericardial valve attached to a self-expanding and self-inverting superelastic Nitinol structure that supports the valve within the native annulus. Three sizes are being developed including 21, 23, and 25 mm. The HLT valve is delivered through a 16- or 17-F delivery system, using a positioning device (the Backstop) that facilitates reliable positioning of the valve and enables deployment without rapid pacing. Importantly, the HLT valve can be repositioned and fully retrieved during the implant procedure.

DEVICE DESCRIPTION
The HLT valve (Fig. 1) is composed of four primary elements: (*i*) a glutaraldehyde cross-linked tricuspid porcine pericardial tissue valve, (*ii*) a superelastic Nitinol wireform that supports the valve structure, (*iii*) a superelastic Nitinol mesh, which supports the prosthetic valve and keeps the valve fixed within the native valve annulus, and (*iv*) a braided polyester liner integrated within the support structure to prevent regurgitant flow around the valve.

DELIVERY SYSTEM
There are six components of the HLT valve delivery system (Fig. 2) including (*i*) the 16 to 17 F delivery catheter that delivers the valve from the femoral artery through the aortic annulus, (*ii*) the dilator, which is designed to provide a smooth transition from the delivery catheter tip to the guidewire (0.035 in.) and aids in initial crossing the native aortic valve, (*iii*) the funnel catheter, designed to protect the tissue portion of the aortic valve prosthesis during loading and delivery, (*iv*) the valve retention cables that provide three attachment points to the HLT valve that are released once the proper anatomical position is achieved, (*v*) the loader catheter, which in conjunction with the funnel catheter and the valve retention cables provides a means for loading and advancing the valve into the delivery catheter, and (*vi*) a Backstop, a tool positioned against the ventricular aspect of the aortic annulus to ensure proper valve placement. The Backstop is also used as a dilation tool to help expand and seat the valve prosthesis following delivery. The Backstop uses a unique "flow-through" configuration that does not restrict blood flow and therefore eliminates the need for rapid ventricular pacing when expanded.

IMPLANT PROCEDURE
The HLT valve implant procedure includes many elements common to other percutaneous valve technologies. The device is delivered via the femoral artery and access can be obtained using a conventional percutaneous puncture. Valve sizing is performed with transesophageal echo (TEE) measurements at the time of implantation, with critical measurements being obtained from the midesophageal long-axis view during systole. Catheter guidance, valve positioning, and delivery are achieved utilizing standard fluoroscopic imaging techniques and planes.

There are several specific procedural steps related to the HLT valve. After standard aortic valvuloplasty, the HLT delivery catheter, and dilator are advanced across the native aortic valve

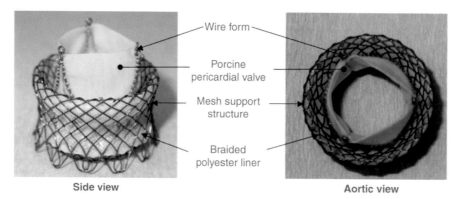

Figure 1 HLT valve prosthesis.

over a guidewire into the left ventricle. The catheter is biased toward the septum. The dilator and guidewire are then removed. The loader catheter, containing the loaded HLT valve and Backstop, is then mounted to the proximal hub of the delivery catheter and the HLT valve is advanced through the delivery catheter across the native aortic valve. The Backstop is deployed against the ventricular aspect of the aortic annulus. The HLT valve is then pushed out of the catheter against the Backstop. When sufficient cuff has been deployed, the cuff inverts on itself, further increasing radial force. The valve is then pushed out of the catheter. Correct valve position and function are verified by TEE and fluoroscopic imaging. The valve can be dilated utilizing the Backstop to ensure that the support structure is round and well seated in the aortic annulus. The valve can be retrieved and the procedure re-started if the desired results are not achieved. If the results are satisfactory, the valve retention cables are released and the procedure completed.

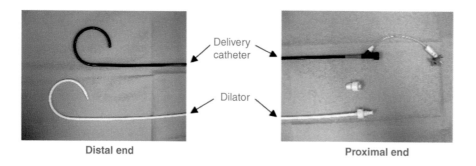

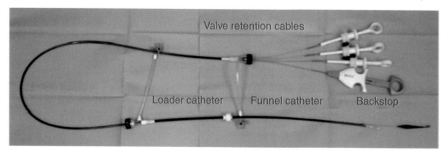

Figure 2 HLT delivery system.

POTENTIAL ADVANTAGES

There are three potential advantages of the HLT valve: (*i*) The delivery system is 16 or 17 F, depending on the valve size. This should expand the potential patient population to include patients with smaller peripheral arteries and eliminate the need for surgical cut-down. (*ii*) The valve can be either repositioned or retrieved in cases of incorrect placement. (*iii*) Since the devices are flow-through, there is no need for rapid ventricular pacing.

CURRENT STATUS

Studies in a chronic animal model suggest that the cuff structure is appropriately fibrosed into the native aortic valve annulus and that valve function over time is normal. Estimated orifice area for the 25 mm valve is 1.8 cm^2. Accelerated wear testing is in progress. We plan "first-in-man" implants in the third quarter of 2009.

Appendix 4
Sadra Medical Lotus Valve System

Ken Martin, Amr Salaheih, Jill Amstutz, and Leah Lepak
Sadra Medical, Inc., Los Gatos, California, U.S.A.

The Lotus valve system is designed to be the first fully repositionable technology for transcatheter aortic valve replacement. In addition to its repositioning and self-centering features that are designed to facilitate optimal positioning of the valve, the device provides physicians with more control over the procedure because of its proprietary delivery system, early leaflet function during deployment, and the ability to be resheathed and retrieved prior to final release.

The Lotus valve system consists of the Lotus valve, a bovine tissue trileaflet bioprosthetic aortic valve, and the Lotus delivery catheter, a delivery system for guidance and placement of the Lotus valve. The device is introduced percutaneously via the femoral artery by using conventional catheterization techniques.

LOTUS VALVE

The valve implant is made of bovine pericardium, which was selected for its long history of durability in bioprosthetic valves (Fig. 1). A Nitinol self-expanding structure holds the valve securely in position, while adapting to the variations in annular geometry among patients. The implant is positioned below the coronary ostia, minimizing the chance of coronary occlusion and enabling straightforward access in subsequent procedures if required. Adaptive seal technology on the outer diameter of the structure is designed to minimize or eliminate perivalvular leakage. The valve is deployed in a beating heart with no dependence on rapid pacing and begins to function early in the release process, providing stabilized hemodynamic functionality immediately.

LOTUS DELIVERY CATHETER

The Lotus valve system provides fine operator control over valve unsheathing, seating, and deployment to aid in precision placement and to help the operator to avoid coronary obstruction and minimize interference with the mitral valve. The delivery system enables a gradual, phased deployment that is both predictable and controllable. It enables positioning of the implant by using small increments to optimize placement in patients. This is of particular importance in patients that present anatomical challenges, such as a restrictive "landing zone." Prior to releasing the Lotus valve in its final position, the valve may be recaptured into the sheath of the delivery system for repositioning and redeployment or removal, as determined necessary by the physician.

The delivery catheter is introduced using transcatheter techniques. The first clinical units had a 21-F shaft, and in the future the shaft profile will be reduced to enable a percutaneous procedure. By using fluoroscopy, the system is advanced over the aortic arch and across the aortic valve. The physician turns the handle on the delivery system to control expansion of the valve. As the valve expands, an assessment of the positioning relative to the mitral valve and coronary ostia can be made. At any point during valve expansion, the physician can make slight or larger adjustments in the valve positioning. The valve can be fully expanded and the flow dynamics assessed prior to releasing the valve. If the physician believes that the implant needs to be repositioned or needs to be removed and exchanged for a different size implant, the physician may withdraw the valve partially or completely back into the sheath and move the valve as needed. Once the final implant position is determined and established, the physician deploys the release mechanism detaching the delivery system from the implant and removes the delivery system from the patient.

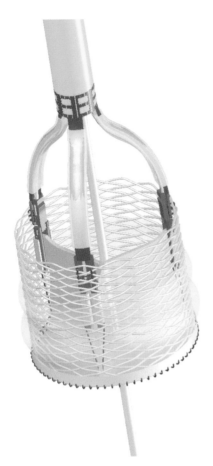

Figure 1 Diagrammatic representation of the Lotus valve attached to the catheter delivery system.

The intuitive, user-friendly delivery system was engineered to make the transcatheter aortic valve implantation (TAVI) procedure more routine, simplifying the steps while providing the physician with precision control and the ability to reposition or remove the device as needed.

First clinical use of the Lotus valve system took place in July 2007. Professor Eberhard Grube and Dr. Ralf Müller performed the procedure in the cath lab at Helios Klinikum Siegburg. They have since treated several more patients. Early clinical work has confirmed the value of accurate placement, repositionability, and retrievability of the valve.

Caution: This device is for investigational use only. It is not available for sale or commercial distribution. It is not approved for sale or use in the United States.

Appendix 5
The JenaValve Technology

Hans Figulla

Division of Cardiology, University Hospital of Jena, Jena, Germany

In 1995, Figulla and Ferrari applied for a German patent (DE 195 46 692 C 2) describing a self-expanding aortic stent valve. When we initiated the development, the purpose of our invention was to replace native aortic valve via a minimally invasive procedure with a prosthesis, a self-expanding stent with a biological valve. To achieve sufficient fixation of the prosthesis that is exposed to enormous mechanical forces, high friction on the aortic wall was achieved by extending the stent in its length to the ascending aorta. The first animal experiments were successfully performed; however, the disadvantages of the extended stent (6–10 cm in length) were obvious.

- First, the crossing of the aortic arch became difficult.
- Second, the ascending aorta was exposed to radial forces and its "Windkessel" function was disturbed which increases afterload of the beating heart and impaired flexible interface between the beating heart and the ascending aorta resulting in the transfer of mechanical forces to the stent struts.
- Third, a transapical route became impossible due to the length of the prosthesis.

Thus, the next steps in the design were to shorten the self-expanding stent to overcome the above-mentioned disadvantages. However, by shortening the stent, the radial forces needed to be increased to achieve enough friction in the surrounding tissue for reliable fixation of the prosthesis. At that time high-radial forces on the aortic wall were considered potentially dangerous due to aneurysm generation caused by remodeling of the tissue. It was decided that the stent should have some active form of fixation. In the first models, hooks were applied to the self-expanding stent to assist the fixation. However, these hooks penetrated the aortic wall. In the following years, stent deployment was developed in two steps: first, so-called "feeler" elements that can be protruded behind the cusps of the naïve valve were used, and second, the prosthesis needed to be deployed by pressing the diseased leaflets against the aortic wall. Such a device had the potential to clip the diseased valve leaflets between the two parts of the stent like a paper clip. That enables the device to transfer the mechanical forces directed toward the left ventricle during the diastolic closing of the valve to the cusps of the diseased native valves. In addition, the protrusion of the "feeler" elements allows deployment of the stent at the exact orthotopic position for the new valve that avoids mispositioning.

The mechanical features of the prosthesis and the delivery system were challenging to develop. Moreover, engineering required the possibility of device repositioning. In addition, the JenaValve device has to fulfill the durability requirements of 400 million cycles without any fracture.

A transapical device has been developed and a transfemoral device is in developing stage. The transapical device will be available first, as we decided to attach a well-known biological porcine valve to our stent. This biological valve has been marketed in the surgical community since many years. Once the procedure has been proven with long-term results, it is expected that the treatment will be available for a larger patient group, not only high-risk patients.

The transfemoral JenaValve device is being developed in parallel, with a pericardial bovine valve, which has been tested in animal trials.

In its final version, the characteristics of the JenaValve device will be:

- unique, smooth and precise positioning, making deployment easy,
- the possibility of repositioning,
- catheter deployment via the transapical route with a porcine biological valve, and
- catheter deployment via the transfemoral route with a pericardial bovine valve.

Neither JenaValve devices will interfere with the "Windkessel" function nor the flexible interface between the heart and aorta, and will not rely on calcification for stability and may also be deployed in aortic insufficiency cases.

Therefore the JenaValve devices will have superior versatility according to the route of application, kind of biological valves used and aortic valve function treatment.

JenaValve is a trademark of JenaValve Technology GmbH. The JenaValve products are protected by pending and granted patent, design, and utility model rights.

Index